T0314097

SOCIAL DETERMINANTS OF HEALTH IN EUROPE

Direct and Indirect Consequences of War

Edited by
Adrian Bonner

With a foreword by
Cornelius Katona

First published in Great Britain in 2025 by

Policy Press, an imprint of
Bristol University Press
University of Bristol
1–9 Old Park Hill
Bristol
BS2 8BB
UK
t: +44 (0)117 374 6645
e: bup-info@bristol.ac.uk

Details of international sales and distribution partners are available at policy.bristoluniversitypress.co.uk

British Library Cataloguing in Publication Data
A catalogue record for this book is available from the British Library

ISBN 978-1-4473-7327-8 hardcover
ISBN 978-1-4473-7328-5 paperback
ISBN 978-1-4473-7329-2 ePub
ISBN 978-1-4473-7330-8 ePdf

Cover design: Andrew Corbett
Bristol University Press and Policy Press use environmentally responsible print partners.
Printed and bound in Great Britain by CPI Group (UK) Ltd, Croydon, CR0 4YY

FSC
www.fsc.org
MIX
Paper | Supporting responsible forestry
FSC® C013604

This book is dedicated to the people in Ukraine and those who have been displaced to other parts of Europe and beyond.

The UNHRC continues to document their situation at https://data.unhcr.org/en/situations/ukraine

Contents

Contents

List of figures and tables

Figures

Tables

List of case studies

Notes on contributors

Fern Barber has an MA in philosophy from Durham University and leads the Policy, Partnerships, Insights & Scrutiny Team at the London Borough of Sutton. She began her career in education policy research, focusing on safeguarding in schools, before transitioning into local government and working on a number of service improvement programmes in Children's Services Departments. In her current role, she works closely with voluntary and community sector organisations to coordinate partnership responses to emerging issues including migrant and refugee resettlement support and the cost of living crisis.

Anne Barrington spent 40+ years in Ireland's Department of Foreign Affairs and the Department of the Taoiseach (Prime Minister's Office). She retired as Ambassador to Japan in 2018 and served as a Special Envoy of the Government for Ireland's Security Council Campaign 2019–2020. Anne was Joint Secretary in the North-South Ministerial Council, Ambassador to Tanzania, Kenya and Burundi and in Ireland's Embassy in Washington, DC, Consulate General of Ireland and Ireland's Permanent Mission to the UN, both in New York. When in Dublin, Anne's positions included Director General Europe Division and Director of the National Forum on Europe. Anne currently chairs an affordable housing cooperative, O Cualann, and the Shared Island/ESRI research body.

Nick Baum has enjoyed a multifaceted career spanning media, advertising and social impact. Graduating from the University of Portsmouth with a BA honours degree in geography in 1995, he embarked on a 25-year journey in the media and advertising industry. His rapid progression culminated in his appointment as Managing Director of VCCP Media, a prominent global agency based in London. In 2022, driven by a passion for social change and community wellbeing, Nick made a significant transition to the charity sector. This transition was deeply rooted in his prior volunteer work for Volunteer Centre Sutton. Currently, he spearheads the charity's community projects, overseeing dedicated volunteers committed to supporting a wide array of community initiatives. These projects encompass areas such as healthcare, youth development and the integration of migrant groups, all guided by a singular vision of building a more inclusive and integrated society. Nick's transition reflects a profound commitment to harnessing his professional acumen for the greater good and making a meaningful impact on the community.

Joanne Beale is an engineer by training, at the University of Cambridge, with 15 years' experience in the international development sector, most of it as a water, sanitation and hygiene (WASH) specialist but with a growing interest in more holistic community development, particularly through a faith-based lens. Joanne has worked for several secular and faith-based organisations in an employment and freelance capacity, including many years with WaterAid which saw her offering technical support to a large number of country programmes. She also spent three years living and working in rural Mozambique for the Anglican church where she designed and managed a highly effective WASH programme. She currently works as the International Community Development Lead at The Salvation Army's International Headquarters where she is focused on building partnerships, capacity and strategy across a range of technical areas.

Adrian Bonner's current research focuses on the impact of economic austerity policies on health, social care and housing strategies, reflected in the publications *Social Determinants of Health: An Interdisciplinary Approach to Social Inequality and Wellbeing* (Policy Press, 2018) and *Local Authorities and Social Determinants of Health* (Policy Press, 2020). A key theme emerging from these books is the recognition of the need for relationships at an individual level, and partnerships between the public and third sectors in addressing the range of complex issues (*wicked issues*) related to the social determinants of health.

Adrian's early research was concerned with neurobiological aspects of alcohol, as reflected in publications and teaching activities in the 1990s at the Universities of Surrey and Kent. At this time, he became Chairman of the Congress of the European Society for Biomedical Research into Alcohol. *Social Exclusion and the Way Out: An Individual and Community Response to Human Social Dysfunction* (2006) provided the basis for research into *The Seeds of Exclusion* (2008), a major report that continues to influence Salvation Army strategic planning. These activities were undertaken while he was a Reader in the Centre for Health Service Studies, University of Kent, and was Director of the Addictive Behaviour Group, which facilitated the development of undergraduate and postgraduate teaching and research activities.

From 2010 to 2012, he was seconded from the University of Kent to become the Director of the Institute of Alcohol Studies. This involved participating in the UK government's Responsibility Deal and membership of the European Alcohol Health Forum, an advisory group supporting the work of the European Commission. These insights into UK and European policy development have influenced his current activities, which include interdisciplinary international research into health inequalities. The previous book in this series, *COVID-19 and Social Determinants of Health: Wicked Issues and Relationalism*, published in 2023, highlighted the need to consider the global factors which exacerbate inequalities.

Currently, Adrian is working with leaders of The Salvation Army and partner universities in order to understand the *structural* and *intermediate* determinants of health at this time of war in Europe. Extending this collaborative network to consider the global determinants of climate justice is providing data and grounded insights to be published in the fifth book of this Policy Press series, *Global Determinants of Health in an Unstable World: Drivers of Climate Justice*.

He is an honorary professor in the Faculty of Social Sciences, University of Stirling, and a Commissioner on the Caring Communities Review, Essex County Council.

Gillian Bonner is a graduate in social science from the University of Leicester and has a PGCE from the University of Southampton. She has taught in both primary and secondary schools in the London Boroughs of Redbridge, Havering and Merton. Gillian first volunteered to work with refugees in Leicester at the time of the arrival of thousands of Ugandan Asians following their expulsion by Idi Amin. More recently she has had first-hand experience of the Home Office Community Sponsorship Scheme for Syrians and is currently involved in supporting the Homes for Ukraine Scheme by leading a support programme within the London Borough of Sutton in connection with The Salvation Army.

Richard Bradbury has worked for The Salvation Army since 2005 in an overseas setting in Bangladesh, Kenya and Zambia. His roles overseas have involved running The Salvation Army's Chikankata Hospital and being responsible for the projects and emergency work of The Salvation Army in Kenya. Richard, a Salvation Army Captain, was appointed to International Headquarters in 2021, where he currently serves as International Development Officer. Richard has a background in criminal justice work and initially worked in the Edinburgh High Court of Justiciary followed by a spell working at the social work and psychology units in Barlinnie Prison in Glasgow. Immediately prior to working for The Salvation Army, Richard was Regional Manager for the East of England in the National Probation Service and Government Adviser in the Home Office. Richard is the co-author of a number of research journals and newspapers articles and is a contributor to the book, *Sense and Sensibility in Health Care* (BMJ Publications).

Marija Branković is Research Associate at the Institute for Philosophy and Social Theory and Associate Professor at the Faculty of Media and Communications in Belgrade, Serbia. She researches the psychology of intergroup relations, social identities and their psychological foundations, especially in the post-conflict societies of the Balkans. She is currently engaged in a Reason4Health project supported by the Science Fund of the Republic of Serbia, focusing on the psychological determinants of questionable health behaviours. She serves as Social Psychology Ambassador of the European Association of Social Psychology to promote the benefits of social psychology and contribute to the further international integration of the region of South and East Europe. She is devoted to a socially engaged science and the effort to apply scientific insight to create a society for the benefit of humans, other animals and the environment.

Michael Burton has spent over 30 years as a journalist and editor covering the public sector. After training on local newspapers he was for 20 years editor of *The Municipal Journal (MJ)*, the market-leading weekly title for UK local government and then editorial director of *MJ* and its events business where, among other duties, he arranged conference agendas with senior civil servants and public and private sector senior executives. He also a board director of *MJ*'s parent publishing and events company, the Hemming Group, and is the author of two books, *The Politics of Public Sector Reform from Thatcher to the Coalition* (Palgrave Macmillan, 2013) and *The Politics of Austerity: A Recent History* (Palgrave Macmillan, 2016).

Agnieszka Cieciura-Miszczak is currently working for The Salvation Army, Republic of Ireland. Agnieszka has over 15 years of experience working with the homeless population. Since 2019 she has been Service Manager of two family hubs in Dublin. Agnieszka holds an MA in psychology, HDip in psychotherapy studies and a degree in addiction studies.

Elaine Douglas is Associate Professor of Ageing and Public Health at the University of Stirling. Her research interests include the social and economic determinants of health, life course and global ageing research, including Healthy Ageing in Scotland. Elaine also works as the Social, Behavioural and Design Research Programme Manager with the UK Research and Innovation Healthy Ageing Challenge. Elaine has a PhD in public health from University College London.

Yrjö Engeström is Professor Emeritus of Education at the University of Helsinki, Finland and Professor Emeritus of Communication at the University of California, San Diego, USA. He is Director of the Center for Research on Activity, Development and Learning. He is the founder of the theory of expansive learning and the Change Laboratory approach, and a foremost international expert in their development and applications.

Damaris Frick is Director of The Salvation Army International Emergency Services. Her involvement in the humanitarian field commenced in January

2006 with a deployment to northern Pakistan for the earthquake relief programme. For several years she held mainly field based or field supporting positions managing disaster relief operations in locations including Myanmar, Indonesia, Eastern DRC, Haiti, Pakistan, Uganda, the Philippines and Vanuatu. She now oversees the management of relief and recovery operations of The Salvation Army worldwide and provides technical and strategic support to Salvation Army leadership and humanitarian personnel worldwide. Her team has been instrumental in shaping the global support to the COVID-19 crisis and now also the locally led but internationally supported response to the war in Europe. Since 2009 she has also been involved in facilitating disaster preparedness and response workshops, training and conferences. Damaris holds an MA (diploma) in social work (Freiburg, Germany) and an MA in development and emergency practice (Oxford Brookes).

Helen Froud was commissioned at the Royal Military Academy, Sandhurst, and she served in overseas logistics and policy roles before moving into local government, where she was deputy Chief Executive of the Western Isles Council and Director of Corporate Services at Worcestershire County Council. She also worked in consulting for KPMG. Helen holds an MBA from Henley Management College and a master's degree in theology from the University of Aberdeen. She has also been a Non-Executive Director of the UK's Health Protection Agency, for the National Records of Scotland, and was a Trustee of One-Parent Families, Scotland. She currently sits on OFCOM's Advisory Committee for Older and Disabled People and their Communications Consumer Panel. Currently Helen is the Assistant Director – Research for The Salvation Army.

Raelton Gibbs is a Salvation Army officer, currently appointed to International Headquarters, serving in the Europe zone, resourcing and supporting the work of The Salvation Army. Previously he had responsibility for The Salvation Army's work in Yorkshire South with Humber Division, in the United Kingdom and Ireland Territory as the Divisional Commander. He has also served for many years in the field of homelessness and also had the opportunity of taking up appointments in overseas work, both in emergency response and in Singapore, Malaysia and Myanmar. Raelton also has a professional doctorate in social work.

Ben Gilbert holds a master's degree in international development and education and has 20 years' experience of teaching and international development spanning South Asia, the Middle East and the UK. He serves as Head of the International Projects Office for The Salvation Army UK. He specialises in supporting Salvation Army territories seeking to development effective community engagement through a church-based approach.

Peter Hain has led a colourful life. The child of South African parents jailed, banned and forced into exile during the freedom struggle, from 1969 to 1970 Peter Hain led anti-apartheid campaigns to stop all-white South African sports tours. He was MP for Neath from 1991 to 2015 and a Privy Councillor, and he served in the UK government for 12 years, seven of these in the Cabinet.

He negotiated the 2007 settlement to end the conflict in Northern Ireland and was a foreign minister with successive responsibilities for Africa, the Middle East and Europe. He has chaired the United Nations Security Council and negotiated international treaties. He was also Secretary of State for Work and Pensions, Secretary of State for Wales, Leader of the House of Commons and Energy Minister. His concise readable biography, *Mandela His Essential Life*, was published in 2018, his memoirs *Outside In* in 2012, and his co-authored *Pitch Battles: Protest, Prejudice and Play* in May 2020. He has written or edited 27 books, and has also appeared regularly on television and radio and written for most UK newspapers. Peter is married with two sons and seven grandchildren, he has degrees from Queen Mary University London and Sussex University.

Therese Trygg Hannevik holds a bachelor's degree in child protection and child welfare from Norwegian University of Science and Technology. After completing her education, she worked for two years at centres for refugees and asylum seekers, first as a Volunteer Coordinator, where she organised and led volunteers who contributed to the residents' daily well-being and integration into society. She then transitioned to the role of Child Welfare Specialist, where she ensured that the rights and needs of the children at the centre were met, and tailored activities and measures for them. Therese has since moved on to other projects in the Salvation Army, and is currently working at the headquarters in Norway, at the youth and children's department.

Rebecca Harrocks is Action Researcher at The Salvation Army Territorial Headquarters in London. She has an MA in theology and religious studies from the University of Nottingham, and a doctorate in theology from King's College London. Her PhD thesis looked at belonging, inclusion and boundary markers within the Jewish communities of ancient Alexandria and Egypt, through the lenses of sex, gender, marriage and procreation. She occasionally lectures in ancient history and biblical studies. Rebecca spent seven years working with single-parent families and coordinating a peer-support group for solo parents, experiencing some of the many legal, social, emotional, mental and physical health challenges encountered by others in this cohort. She is passionate about the support of families in all their diversity, not only through policy and the traditional roles of statutory services, but particularly via proactive and inclusive efforts of churches, other places of worship, and faith-based organisations.

Catherine Hagan Hennessy is Professor of Ageing at the University of Stirling. With a background in public health and anthropology, her research interests are in older people's health, well-being and social inclusion. From 1991-2001, Catherine worked in public health gerontology at the US Centers for Disease Control and Prevention. Subsequently at the University of Sheffield, she was Deputy Director of the Economic and Social Research Council's 'Growing Older Programme on Extending Quality Life' and the UK National Collaboration on Ageing Research. From 2005-2015 she was Professor of Public Health and Ageing at Plymouth University. Catherine holds a doctorate in public health from the University of California at Berkeley.

Cedric Hills, Commissioner, is Secretary for Europe, The Salvation Army. Commissioned as a Salvation Army officer in 1986, his international humanitarian experience began in 1996. Whilst managing a welfare centre for NATO troops serving in Sarejevo, he was tasked to establish an emergency feeding and winterisation programme for families impacted by the Bosnian war in the small village of Sipovo. Witnessing at first-hand the impact of war and conflict had a profound impact upon him. Further emergency management deployments to conflict zones included the Republic of Georgia, Afghanistan, Albania, Kosovo and Iraq. In his current role, he has oversight of TSA activities in the 34 countries of The Salvation Army's Europe Zone, including the UK, Russia, Germany, the Netherlands, Finland, Switzerland, France, Norway, Sweden, Austria, Iceland, Greece, and Spain. He holds a BA in theology and ministry.

Cornelius Katona was trained in general and old age psychiatry at Cambridge and St George's Medical Schools. After teaching psychiatry in elderly care at University College he was appointed Foundation Professor of the Elderly, then Dean of the Royal College of Psychiatrists. His expertise in assessing psychiatric patients has led to him assessing and reporting on the mental health of asylum seekers and refugees. He is an honorary professor at University College and Medical Director of the Helen Bamber Foundation (a leading charity supporting traumatised asylum seekers and refugees).

Petra Kjellen Brooke has an MA and PhD in Diaconal Studies from VID Specialised University in Oslo. Her PhD explored Salvation Army church-based social work and the role of faith in social outreach. It further investigated organisational perspectives relating to building competance and knowledge amongst staff and volunteers using a social learning theoretical approach. Petra is a trained nurse but has worked for The Salvation Army social services for the past 12 years, covering issues such as anti human trafficking, leadership development and competance building. Petra is a member of The Salvation Army international theological council, an advisory body for the General of The Salvation Army. She is interested in topics relating to migration, immigration, refugees and local community development. She is also passionate about how faith-based perspectives affect organisational development and priorities.

Johnny Kleman, Commissioner, was formerly Secretary for Europe Zone, International Salvation Army. He has been The Salvation Army (TSA)'s national leader in a number of countries, last of which was Sweden. He currently has oversight and is responsible for the governance of TSA activities in the TSA Europe Zone, which includes the UK, Russia, Germany, the Netherlands, Finland, Switzerland, France, Norway, Sweden, Austria, Iceland, Greece, Spain and others. He is mentor and teacher at the TSA's training college in Sweden.

Milica Ninković is a PhD candidate and research assistant at the University of Belgrade, Department of Psychology and Laboratory for Research of Individual Differences. Her research interests follow two research lines: intergroup relations, focusing on social identities and interventions that reduce intergroup bias in post-conflict societies; and socio-psychological determinants of health behaviours. She is engaged in the Reason4Health project, funded by the Science Fund of the Republic of Serbia, focusing on psychological antecedents of questionable health behaviours. She cooperates with non-governmental and civil society organisations that apply scientific psychological knowledge with the aim of societal improvement through evidence-based interventions.

Andrii Parkhoma studied at the Ukrainian Gestalt Institute, completing two stages of the programme. He specialises in 'crisis and trauma' and is currently furthering his education in the specialisation of 'Group Psychotherapy in the Gestalt Method'. He is employed by the London Borough of Sutton to support people displaced from Ukraine. He previously worked at a rehabilitation centre focused on addiction prevention, which he founded, and is the centre's director. Currently, he works with Ukrainian refugees and maintains a private online practice with Ukrainians.

Martin Pělucha is Professor of Economic Policy at the Prague University of Economics and Business and also works as an independent expert at IREAS in the Czech Republic. Martin is an expert in the field of evaluation of regional and rural development policy. During his career he was and currently is a coordinator of several research projects related to the field of programme evaluation and methodology of the evaluation (addressed to the Ministry of Regional Development, the Ministry of Agriculture in the Czech Republic, the Ministry of the Environment of the Czech Republic). Martin is a national ambassador of the Regional Studies Association in the Czech Republic, and is also a member of the Czech Evaluation Society and European Evaluation Society.

Amy Quinn-Graham is a PhD student in theology and religious studies at the University of Leeds and a member of the Centre for Religion and Public Life. Her research focuses on responses to domestic violence and abuse in the contexts and structures of The Salvation Army. Amy is also an Action Researcher for The Salvation Army and has a background in gender and international development, with a keen interest in the role of faith-based organisations. Her previous work with the Institute of Development Studies utilised participatory research methods to support women from religious minorities in Pakistan, Iraq and Nigeria to identify the key issues affecting their lives at the intersection of their gender and religious minority status.

Kaia Rønsdal is Associate Professor in the field of leadership, ethics, spiritual and existential counselling/chaplaincy in plural contexts at the Faculty of Theology, University of Oslo, Norway. Her research interests are in the lived practices and human encounters in civil society, addressing issues such as marginality, migration, borders and peripheries, from perspectives including spatial theory, urbanity, phenomenology and theological ethics. Her research also includes methodological explorations within these perspectives and fields. She is involved with several projects allowing for further explorations on the concept of hospitality in the context of migration. She is the co-editor of *Contemporary Christian-Cultural Values: Migration Encounters in the Nordic Region* (Routledge, 2021).

Annalisa Sannino is Professor of Education and Culture and lead of the Engagement for Sustainability and Equitable Transformations Group. RESET Change Laboratory runs projects into the eradication of youth homelessness in Finland. Sannino is Distinguished Research Fellow, Faculty of Education, Monash University, Melbourne, Australia, Visiting Professor, Faculty of Education, Rhodes University, South Africa and Visiting Professor, Work-integrated Learning, University West, Sweden.

Svitlana Semaniv is a psychologist with a wide range of lecturing experience across public and private healthcare services. She worked at a Regional Clinical Oncology Centre in Ukraine, until the invasion of Ukraine, after which she was displaced to the UK. Currently she is employed by the London Borough of Sutton to support Ukrainians affected by the war, in the UK and Ukraine. She has a diploma from Ivano-Frankivsk Medical

College, Ukraine, graduated from Vasyl Stefanyk Precarpathian National University, and has a Family Consultant Certificate from the National Academy of Educational Sciences of Ukraine and a Certificate of a Basic Consultant in Positive Psychotherapy from the World Association of Positive and Transcultural Psychotherapy.

Alexander Shemetev currently holds a candidate of sciences degree in economics (the equivalent of a PhD, awarded for completing a three- to five-year research programme), and also is a PhD student in the Regional Development study programme at the Prague University of Economics and Business from February 2020. He has a US degree in applied economics from CERGE-EI, the joint workspace of Charles University, the Czech Academy of Sciences and the University of the State of New York. In addition, he has four specialisations from Johns Hopkins University (online) in data analysis and statistics with the application of the programming language R (including the application of machine learning technologies). He is an author of computer software (financial software) that automatically analyses holdings in different industries. He has also authored several books in different languages (three of them are written fully autonomously by the computer software he creates).

Iryna Shepelenko has a PhD in sociology and is Associate Professor in Kiev. She is a member of the International Sociological Association and an independent researcher working with Support Ukraine Now!.

Richard Simmons is Professor in Public and Social Policy, and Co-Director of the Mutuality Research Programme at the University of Stirling. Over the last decade or so he has led an extensive programme of research on voice and cooperation in public policy. This includes four studies funded by the Economic and Social Research Council/Arts and Humanities Research Council, a Single Regeneration Budget-funded study, and work for the National Health Service, Scottish Executive, National Consumer Council, Carnegie Trust, Organisation for Economic Co-operation and Development, World Bank, Co-operatives UK, Nesta and the Care Inspectorate. He is currently working on an EU (H2020) project working with local municipal governments and schools to improve the quality of primary school meals through better procurement. He writes widely on these issues for academic, policy and practitioner audiences. His book, *The Consumer in Public Services*, is published by Policy Press. As well as a series of journal articles in high-quality international journals such as *Social Policy and Administration*, *Policy and Politics*, *Annals of Public and Co-operative Economics* and *Public Policy and Administration*, Richard has written a number of policy oriented publications and professional journal articles for a practitioner audience. His research interests are broadly in the field of user voice, the governance, delivery and innovation of public services and the role of mutuality and cooperation in public policy. The Mutuality Research Programme has acquired an international reputation as a centre of excellence for research, knowledge exchange and consultancy on these issues.

Richard Smith has enjoyed various senior management positions in both public and private sectors. Qualifying as a barrister in 1978 he initially worked within GEC-Marconi and then was appointed as Director of Contract Services (1988) and Head of Businesses (1991) for Portsmouth City Council where he was instrumental in the introduction of the council's internal market (1991–1995). He founded 'Public Sector Plc' in 2006, a private sector organisation utilising a new and innovative legal framework based on a cultural relationship between partners forming in advance of formal legal commitments.

In 2019, he established the Centre for Partnering (CfP) as a new organisation initially bringing together five universities. CfP is focused on developing and introducing the idea of *relationalism* and in evidencing the relational dividend that arises from its application. An aim of CfP will be to accredit organisations and individuals in the use of *relationalism* utilising a knowledge base compiled from the CfP's *Exemplar Projects Initiative*. Richard is an honorary professor at the University of Stirling and chairman of Centre for Partnering.

Emilie Søyseth holds a bachelor's degree in child welfare and child protection in a multicultural society from the University of South-Eastern Norway, and has further education in special pedagogy with focus on challenging behaviours from Folkeuniversitetet.

She has experience working with adults and children in various challenging life situations through her work in schools, nurseries, and the child welfare sector.

Currently, Emilie is employed at The Salvation Army's emergency centre for refugees in Kongsberg, where she is responsible for working with refugees with special needs. This includes refugees from particularly vulnerable or at-risk groups, individuals, and families residing at the centre.

Her work with refugees also includes areas such as human trafficking and the exploitation of vulnerable people on the run.

Joanna Szostek is Senior Lecturer in Political Communication at the University of Glasgow, and an associate fellow of the Chatham House Russia and Eurasia Programme. She has conducted extensive research in Ukraine and Russia, with a focus on the media and public opinion. Her research is published in leading peer-reviewed journals, including *Perspectives on Politics*, *International Journal of Press/Politics*, *New Media and Society*, *Post-Soviet*

Affairs and *European Security*. She has also given numerous interviews about Russia's war on Ukraine to national and international media, including BBC Newsnight, BBC Scotland, France 24 and the *New York Times*. Joanna's professional experience includes several years at BBC Monitoring and many years of living and working in Russia and Ukraine. She has also spent time on secondment with the UK Foreign and Commonwealth Office, and she holds a doctorate in politics from the University of Oxford.

Ivor Telfer had a career in merchant banking before being ordained in 1984. Latterly he served as Territorial Commander of The Salvation Army (TSA) in Pakistan until retirement and now works part-time as the Ukraine Response Unit Coordinator at International Headquarters. His experience covers church and community work in Northern Ireland during the Troubles, director of an Afghan refugee programme in Pakistan caring for 120,000 refugees, international development throughout Africa, Latin and South America in coordination with the Canadian government non-governmental organisation division and head of business for TSA in the UK and Ireland. His master's dissertation was 'Linking Relief and Development: A Framework for The Salvation Army'. He is happily married to Carol and has three children, three grandchildren and lives in Scotland.

Lada Tesfaiie lives in Ukraine and is a journalist, TV presenter and communications manager, with a PhD in political science. She works as a journalist for different editions. She is the author of social projects. The spheres of her interest are social themes, charity and psychology. She was a TV host of news on All-Ukrainian Channel 'Ukraine24'. Her specialisation in journalism is interviewing. She has done more than 1,000 interviews with famous people.

Lada is communications manager in the international project 'Support Ukraine Now'. This initiative is for foreigners who want to help Ukrainians and don't know how to do this. This project is a multifunctional resource with different ways of helping Ukrainians.

Also, she was a communications manager in an inclusive bakery, Good Bread from Good People. The main goal of Good Bread is to give people with mental disabilities – autism, intellectual disability and Down's syndrome – a chance to realise themselves in society. Now the bread of this bakery is given to soldiers of the Armed Forces and Territorial Defense, the police, people on the liberated territories, and those who live in destroyed houses.

She is author of scientific articles and research on political science. In her works, she investigates electoral behaviour, the electoral process and communication in electoral process.

Olly Thorp is Director for Research and Development in The Salvation Army. He has had various roles in the movement since 2008, as well as a brief time with the Scout Association. He has an MA in youth work and community development and has held a variety of volunteer roles in local churches, supporting with community work and in leadership.

Emma Tomalin is Professor of Religion and Public Life at the University of Leeds. Her research and teaching focuses on the role of faith actors in the public sphere in a range of interconnected areas, including humanitarianism, international development, peacebuilding, environmental justice and gender equality. Her most recent book is the *Routledge Handbook of Religion Gender and Society* (2022), co-edited with Caroline Starkey.

Bohdana Tymoskyshyn is a teacher of English language. She worked and is still contracted to work in a primary school in Ukraine, but now displaced to the UK. She trained at Vasyl Stefanyk Precarpathian National University, following studies at Kolomyia Organisation of The Red Cross Society. She maintains her academic studies on a yearly basis at IvanoFrankivsk Institute of Postgraduate Pedagogical Education.

Foreword

Cornelius Katona

It is both a pleasure and a privilege to write the Foreword to this important and wide-ranging book which is part of a series addressing the impact of major world challenges such as austerity, climate change, the COVID-19 pandemic and (in this volume) war on mental health and wellbeing.

I worked closely with the editor, Adrian Bonner, between 2003 and 2008 when we were both based at the Kent Institute of Medicine and Health Sciences at the University of Kent. By then, Adrian already had a senior role within The Salvation Army, heading up its research work into addictive behaviour and social exclusion. It was already clear how skilful and forward-looking he was in combining rigorous scientific research with a spiritual perspective. This approach informs and illuminates the structure and perspectives within the present volume, which starts from (and justifies) the strong premise that war is inherently wicked.

I am a psychiatrist; for the past 20 years I have specialised in the field of refugee and asylum mental health. I am based at the Helen Bamber Foundation (https://helenbamber.org), which works with people seeking sanctuary in the UK after suffering extreme human cruelty such as torture or human trafficking. My day-to-day work involves assessing the mental health of such people and preparing expert reports that help inform decisions as to their entitlement to protection. In practice this means assessing people who have suffered the consequences of war and political oppression in their countries of origin and (all too often) suffered further trauma during long and complicated journeys towards a potential host country. These people's experiences often provide, in particular and individual form, a representation of the recent and evolving history through which they have lived, and which has scarred them – both mentally and physically. In the past 18 months I have also been part of the Commission on the Integration of Refugees (https://refugeeintegrationuk.com/), which brings together Commissioners from multiple backgrounds with a particular emphasis on faith-based and interfaith expertise in enabling refugees to integrate effectively. The Commission's perspective is strikingly similar to that of this book.

This book provides a larger-scale account of some of that recent history, with a focus on the recent conflicts in Ukraine and in Israel/Palestine. It addressed the consequences of these conflicts for health (particularly mental health) and wellbeing within Europe and worldwide, and of how the resultant challenges can be faced. Though the majority of the authors are UK-based, there are contributions from several European countries as well as from Africa and Australia. Their academic and professional backgrounds (and the content of the book's chapters) are wide-ranging, incorporating political, educational, economic and religious as well as health perspectives.

This book makes it all too clear that history never stops, that new conflicts emerge well before the impact of their predecessors has ended, and that conflicts have effects well beyond the countries directly involved in the fighting. The health and wellbeing of those already vulnerable, such as children and older people, is at particular risk. I was particularly struck by the chapter on the long-term outcomes of the Balkan conflict and of the terrible potential it describes for intergroup conflicts to be perpetuated rather than resolved. However, as is also made clear, it is possible for relatively durable solutions to emerge, as has been the case for the past 25 years in Northern Ireland. I was also struck by the evidence the book provides on how complex (but largely positive) the economic impact of war-driven migration on host countries can be – a crucially important point at a time when attitudes towards migration (and particularly forced migration) have become so hostile in many European countries, not least the UK.

There is much else in the book that is positive. One is the close relationship between the United Nations Sustainable Development Goals and key social determinants of health. Another (which forms the focus for Part III of the book) is the potential for 'relationalism' (that is, for governments and local authorities to work together with faith-based organisations and other charities) to generate a positive response to crises. The descriptions of local responses to the influx of people from Ukraine (in the UK, Ireland and Norway) and the equally 'relationist' and very successful attempt to address homelessness in Finland are inspiring.

I would, however, add that the latter is in stark contrast to the recent surge in homelessness among people newly granted refugee status in the UK – which, though a possibly unintended consequence of government policy to clear asylum accommodation more quickly, also reflects a lack of relationalism in the UK government's current approach, and an attitude to new refugees which has become anything but welcoming. On the other hand, as is clear within this book, the UK's Homes for Ukraine initiative, like other such initiatives across Europe, has been a beacon of relationalist good practice in which different localities have found appropriate ways of working together and generating locally appropriate responses.

Europe is often seen as having been relatively peaceful since the end of the Second World War. Sadly, this is no longer the case. War is in any case a global phenomenon with complex global impacts. Professor Bonner and the authorial team he has brought together should be commended. They have provided an invaluable guide on how war wickedness impacts on health and wellbeing, and on how we can work together to mitigate that impact and to strive for a more peaceful world.

Introduction: Changes in the nature and impact of wicked issues post-2020

Adrian Bonner

In the previous volume in this series (Bonner, 2023) the impact of a global pandemic and climate change were reviewed from the perspectives of health and social care, local authority institutions, social policy and business/management research, the third sector, the private sector and the legal profession. Understanding the nature of COVID-19, climate change, and the related issues of housing, homelessness and other interconnected and interrelated domains was viewed through the lens of the *'rainbow' model of social determinants of health*. Issues such as poverty, which can undermine effective education, nutrition and the economic status of the family, were considered to be interlinked and interdependent 'wicked issues' (Bonner, 2018). The *Conceptual Framework for Action on the Social Determinants of Health*, proposed by the World Health Organization (WHO) in 2010, is used as the structure around which this volume has been developed (see Figure I.1). This conceptual framework provides an operational approach to focus on people who are least likely to have resources and resilience to respond to challenges such as war and climate change. The *structural determinants* of social class, gender and ethnicity are mapped in this framework, onto which interventions can be described as *intermediate determinants* of health and wellbeing.

Health and wellbeing

The WHO's constitution states that 'health is a state of complete physical, mental and social wellbeing and not merely the absence of disease or infirmity'. With respect to mental health, this is more than the absence of mental disorders, it is an integral part of health; there is no health without mental health. Mental health is determined by a range of socioeconomic, biological and environmental factors. These include the strategic development of public health aimed at 'promoting, protecting and restoring mental health' (Anon, 2023a).

The concept of health, based on this WHO definition, is therefore highly complex and requires an understanding of the structure of societies and the complex social interactions which are influenced by societal norms, cultures and values. The Commission on Social Determinants of Health, established by the WHO to unpick and understand this complexity, has highlighted the need to understand and (cost) effectively procure services and resources as reviewed in earlier publication of this series, *Local Authorities and the Social Determinants of Health* (Chapters 2, 4, 9 and 13). Contributors in that volume reviewed the aspects of management and leadership approaches which contribute to an effective public health system which was lacking, in the UK and other countries, prior to the global challenges of COVID-19.

The Commission on Social Determinants of Health highlighted the distinction between the levels of causation, focusing on the emergence and maintenance of social hierarchies and the resulting conditions in which people live. This is fundamental to the resilience of people mitigated by *structural* and *intermediate* social determinants, as depicted in Figure I.1.

Historically 'technically-based medical care and public health interventions have gradually been complemented by an understanding of health as a social phenomena'. This Policy Press series on social determinants of health provides an arena for the discussions of a numbers of related issues with a focus on health equity (the absence of unfair and avoidable or remediable differences among social groups) and social justice. This perspective leads to a consideration of human rights frameworks: 'frameworks and instruments associated with human rights guarantees are also able to form the basis for ensuring the collective wellbeing of social groups' (CSDH, 2010).

Psychosocial approaches, social production of disease/political economy of health, and eco-social frameworks are the three main theoretical discourses reviewed by the Commission on Social Determinants of Health. These theoretical discourses are based on, social selection or social mobility; social causation; and life course perspectives. In this Commission on Social Determinants of Health framework the *structural* and *intermediate* determinants are reviewed with respect to the *social position* of people. Social position can be understood in relation to 'mechanisms of health inequality'. Diderichsen identified the following mechanisms for health outcomes:

> *Social contexts* – include the structure of society or social relations in society, creation of social stratification and the assignment of individuals to different social positions.
> *Social stratification* – in turn engenders *differential exposure* to health-damaging conditions and differential vulnerability, in terms of health conditions and material resource availability. Determines *differential consequences* of ill health for more and less advantaged groups (including economic and social consequences). (Diderichsen, 1998, emphasis in original)

The linkage between social economic and political mechanisms, noted in Figure I.1, results in a series of socioeconomic positions and a stratification

Figure I.1: Book chapters mapped onto the final form of the Commission on Social Determinants of Health's conceptual framework

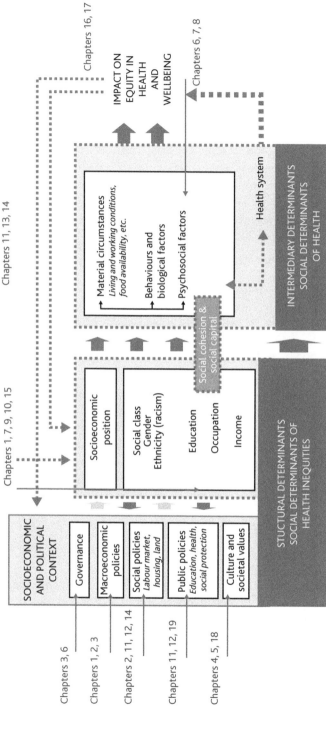

Source: WHO (2010)

3

in income, education, occupation, gender, race/ethnicity and other factors. Here, *interaction* and *interdependence* of these domains (identified in the rainbow model of social determinants of health [Dahlgren and Whitehead, 1991]) occur, for example, in the case of illness having an adverse impact on a person's social position by limiting employment opportunities and reducing income. This was exemplified in the COVID-19 epidemic by its effect on social, economic and political institutions, with the greatest impact on vulnerable groups such as the elderly and minority Black and ethnic groups. Social factors such as wealth inequality, housing, nutrition, clean water and air are critical to good health. War brings not only direct injury and death, but destroys housing, disrupts supplies of food, energy and water and causes large numbers of people to be displaced. The consequences for both displaced people and for the host countries raises critical challenges with a wide range of interrelated complexities, some of which are addressed in this book.

The post-COVID-19 period

A summary of the timeline showing deaths from COVID-19 was presented in 2019 in the Appendix of *Local Authorities and the Social Determinants of Health* (Bonner, 2022) and was continued in this series until March 2023 in *COVID-19 and Social Determinants of Health: Wicked Issues and Relationalism.* (Bonner, 2023). Although medical advances in monitoring, preventing and treating people infected by COVID-19 and related viruses continue to be developed, this and other global challenges will continue and will possibly be exacerbated by genetic mutations of the viruses, changes in transmission by insects (due to environmental events related to climate change) and the movement of people across the world (due to holidays, business travel, legal and illegal migration). The ever-mutating COVID-19, SARS viruses and other infectious diseases will continue to be transmitted from country to country, and disproportionately affect people at the lower end of the social gradient.

Climate change

Almost daily, there are media reports of climatic events, affecting the lives and livelihoods of people in many countries. Robust evidence for climate change and the need for a global response to limit global temperatures from rising more than 1.5°C above preindustrial levels by 2100, is being presented in ongoing intercontinental consultations from the United Nations Framework Convention on Climate Change. The latest meeting was held in Baku, Azerbaijan, 11–22 November 2024 in November–December 2023 (Anon, 2023b). These politically sensitive consultations are underpinned by data from the UN Intergovernmental Panel on Climate Change (Anon,

2023c). An accessible dynamic visualisation of the various data sources related to climate change is being collated and updated by leading climatologists managed by the University of Reading (see Anon, 2023d).

The lockdown period during the COVID-19 pandemic raised awareness of people across the world of the environmental benefits of reduced car and aircraft use and industrial pollution. This appeared to be an opportunity for political change to promote a less polluted world and potentially offset rising climatic temperatures. However, the negative impact of COVID-19 on economic development, resulting in a cost-of-living increase for people across the world, together with local and national pressures to resist changes in, for example, car use, have thwarted this political opportunity. This is evidenced by the problems of the local communities reacting against such changes proposed by local authorities, described for a local London Council in *COVID-19 and Social Determinants of Health: Wicked Issues and Relationalism* (Abellan, 2023).

Local and national budgets have been impacted by a second decade of economic challenges, necessitating austerity budgeting, as reviewed by Burton in Chapter 1 in this volume. The socioeconomic impact of the war in Europe following on the challenges of COVID-19 are presented in Part I of this volume, in which the *structural* drivers of change and stability are reviewed. Geopolitical reflections on the post-pandemic era and current global threats are reviewed from perspectives of the Czech Republic and Finland in Chapters 2 and 3. The *structural* determinants of culture and societal values (see Figure I.1) are considered in Chapters 4 and 5.

War in Europe

Since the emergence of early civilisations, warfare has been a human activity which has shaped the geopolitical nature of countries and continents, led to national identities, and promoted technological developments in the strategic planning and implementation of regional wars. The First and Second World Wars were global wars. Although the number of deaths in the First and Second World Wars were not a great as earlier global epidemics, an international response to global conflict was the establishment of the *United Nations* (UN), formed by the collaboration of 50 nations signing the Charter of the United Nations in 1945. This was an attempt to prevent future wars, initiated by the 26 Axis powers, endorsing the Atlantic Charter (USGov, 2023), see Table I.1 and Appendix A.

Since 1945 'the UN still works to maintain international peace and security, and provide humanitarian assistance to those in need, protect human rights, and uphold international law'. Extending its initial objectives to maintain peace and security, the UN has agreed on sustainable development goals for 2030, 'in order to achieve a better and more sustainable future for us all'.

Table I.1: Number of deaths in recent wars compared to deaths due to global epidemics

Wars	Epidemics
First World War (1911–1918): 6–13 million (Anon, 2023e; 2023f)	The Black Death (1347–1351): 200 million
Second World War (1940–1944): 85 million (Vergun, 2020).	Spanish Flu (1918–1919): 40–50 million
Bosnia and Herzegovina (1992–1995): 90,000–105,000 (UN, 2023a)	AIDS/HIV (1981–present): 25–35 million (Anon, 2023g)
Post-9/11 conflicts: 3.6–3.8 million	COVID-19 (2019–present): 3 million (WHO, 2023)

These global ambitions formed the basis of climate change action to limit global warming (UN, 2023b). A comparative review of the UN sustainability goals and social value was presented in the previous volume of this series by Whiteman et al (2023).

Despite the energies and resources brought together by this international organisation, regional wars in countries such as Iraq, Afghanistan, Yeman and Syria and Pakistan continue. The scale of death, physical, mental disabilities, adverse impacts on children and families, and negative effects on the life course result directly and indirectly from war. Since the 9/11-related conflicts, 432,093 civilians have died violent deaths. It has been estimated that 3.6–3.8 million died indirectly and more than 7.6 million children under five are suffering malnutrition. War-related deaths from malnutrition and a damaged health system and environment far outnumber deaths from combat (Anon, 2023h). Historically, responding to the human casualties of war has led to significant developments in medicine and health. However, the impact of war on educational development of children is major casualty affecting future generations (Schlein, 2023).

The impact of the wars in the Balkans (Chapter 6) and on women and children in Ukraine (Chapters 7, 8 and 9) are presented in Part II of this book. The immediate and cumulative effects of adverse life events, including war, on development and ageing are reviewed in Chapter 10.

The wicked issues of war

Collaborations between nations and between civic authorities and communities, promoted by the UN and the WHO are important in addressing the complex range of apparently intractable issues which lead to conflict and the complexity of multiple approaches to addressing the direct and indirect effects of conflict. Part III provides a *relational* perspective on the responses of countries supporting the displacement of people who become

Table I.2: Ten criteria which could be used to describe a 'wicked issue' (Rittel and Webber, 1973)

	Responding to conflict: a sociopolitical perspective. A wicked issue?
1	It does not have a definitive formulation
2	It does not have a 'stopping rule', that is, it does not have an inherent logic that signals when it is solved
3	There is no way to test the solution to this wicked problem
4	It cannot be studied by trial and error. The solution is irreversible, every trial counts
5	The solutions are not true or false, only good or bad
6	There is no end to the number of solutions or approaches to this wicked problem
7	This wicked issue is essentially unique
8	This wicked problem can always be described as the symptom of other wicked problems
9	The way this problem is described determines its possible solutions
10	Planners, who present solutions to this problems, should not be wrong. They are liable for the consequences of the solutions which they generate; the effects can significantly affect people touched by these actions

homeless, and without employment, as a result of conflict and migration (Chapters 12 and 15), and the collaborative responses of countries and local authorities to supporting women and children (presented in Chapter 12). Issues in developing collaborative working between the civic authorities and voluntary faith-based organisations are discussed in Chapter 14.

Strategic planners at local and national levels have developed various approaches to tackling apparently intractable problems. Early strategies such as 'system-based' approaches have been considered by Rittel and Webber to be inappropriate. The wickedness of these problems is identified by the ten characteristics listed in Table I.2. This concept was explored in the previous volume with regard to the COVID-19 pandemic and climate change, which were described as quintessential wicked issues (see Bonner, 2023, chapter 1; Chapter 18 in this volume).

Starting with a political perspective from a former UK government minister with extensive experience in conflict resolution, in the Introduction to Part IV, various lenses on the response to the war in Europe are provided by international and European approaches to war in Europe by the international faith-based organisation, The Salvation Army (Chapters 16 and 17). The involvement in causation and responses to war by faith-based actors is critically evaluated in Chapter 18, from a social justice perspective. This will include an initial reflection on the Israel–Palestine conflict.

Although the chapters in this book primarily focus on the health and wellbeing of people, the economic damage caused by the war on the agriculture industry in Ukraine (Case Study 15.2) is having a wider global impact on food and energy prices, impacting on the most vulnerable people in many countries. This is highlighted by their 'social position' as shown in Figure I.1.

The chapters in this book are mapped onto the *structural* and *intermediate* determinants of health identified in the conceptual framework proposed by the WHO and shown in Figure I.1.

This book lays the foundation for a further volume, currently being developed, from an international perspective on climate justice at this time of changing world order.

References

Abellan, M. (2023) UK local council strategies post-COVID-19: the local economy, climate change and community wellbeing. In A. Bonner (ed), *COVID-19 and Social Determinants of Health: Wicked Issues and Relationalism.* Bristol: Policy Press, pp 100–113.

Anon (2023a) Mental health. The Global Health Observatory, WHO. Available at: https://www.who.int/data/gho/data/themes/mental-health

Anon (2024) UN Climate Change Conference Baku November 2024 Available at: https://www.norden.org/en/event/un-climate-change-conference-cop29

Anon (2023c) Climate change reports. UN. Available at: https://www.un.org/en/climatechange/reports#:~:text=The%202023%20report%20finds%20that,consistent%20with%202°C

Anon (2023d) ShowYourStripes. Institute for Environmantal Analytics, University of Reading. Available at: https://showyourstripes.info

Anon (2023e) World War 1 casualties. Available at: http://www.100letprve.si/en/world_war_1/casualties/index.html

Anon (2023f) Word War I casualties, Reperers. Available at: https://www.census.gov/history/pdf/reperes112018.pdf

Anon (2023g) The global HIV and AIDS epidemic. HIVGov. Available at: https://www.hiv.gov/hiv-basics/overview/data-and-trends/global-statistics/

Anon (2023h) Costs of war: civilians killed and wounded. Watson Institute, Brown University. Available at: https://watson.brown.edu/costsofwar/costs/human/civilians

Bonner A. (ed) (2018) *Social Determinants of Health: An Interdisciplinary Approach to Social Inequality and Wellbeing.* Bristol: Policy Press.

Bonner, A. (ed) (2022) *Local Authorities and Social Determinants of Health.* Bristol: Policy Press.

Bonner, A. (ed) (2023) *COVID-19 and the Social Determinants of Health: Wicked Issues and Relationalism.* Bristol: Policy Press.

CSDH (2010) *Final Form of the CSDH Conceptual Framework.* WHO. Available at: https://apps.who.int/iris/handle/10665/44489

Dahlgren, G. and Whitehead, M. (1991) *Policies and Strategies to Promote Social Equity in Health*. Stockholm: Institute for Futures Studies.

Diderichsen, F. (1998) Towards a theory of health equity. Unpublished manuscript.

Rittel, H. and Webber, M. (1973) Dilemmas in a general theory of planning. *Policy Sciences*, 4: 155–169.

Schlein, L. (2023) Education also becomes a war causality for Ukrainian children. *VOA*. Available at: https://www.voanews.com/a/education-also-becomes-a-war-casualty-for-ukrainian-children/7247580.html

UN (2023a) International Criminal Tribunal for former Yugoslavia. UN. Available at: https://www.icty.org/en/search-results?as_q=number+of+deaths

UN (2023b) UN and sustainability. UN. Available at: https://www.un.org/en/about-us/un-and-sustainability

USGov (2023) The formation of the United Nations 1945. Office of the Historian, US Government. Available at: https://history.state.gov/milestones/1937–1945/un#:~:text=The%20Senate%20approved%20the%20UN,nations%20had%20ratified%20the%20Charter

Vergun, D. (2020) Significant events of World War II. US Department of Defence. Available at: https://www.defense.gov/News/Feature-Stories/story/article/2293108/

Whiteman, R., Reade, T. and Ayre, D. (2023) UN sustainability goals and social value: local authority perspectives. In A. Bonner (ed) *COVID-19 and Social Determinants of Health: Wicked Issues and Relationalism*. Bristol: Policy Press, pp 192–209.

WHO (2010) *A Conceptual Framework for Action on the Social Determinants of Health*. Available at: https://apps.who.int/iris/handle/10665/44489

WHO (2023) The true death toll of COVID-19. Available at: https://www.who.int/data/stories/the-true-death-toll-of-covid-19-estimating-global-excess-mortality

PART I

Drivers of change and stability

Introduction to Part I

Joanna Szostek

In the early hours of 24 February 2022, the Russian Federation launched its full-scale invasion of Ukraine, attacking simultaneously from the north, east and south, and launching massive missile strikes at targets across the country. Moscow's aim was to rapidly seize control of the Ukrainian capital, Kyiv, to decapitate (likely murder) the democratically elected Ukrainian government, then occupy most of Ukrainian territory and annex parts of it to Russia – thus destroying Ukraine's independent statehood (Zabrodskyi et al, 2022). This Russian plan for a short war of conquest failed, because Ukrainian resistance proved far stronger and more determined than most people – especially the Russian leadership – had expected. Ukrainian forces managed to repel the attack on Kyiv. Ukraine's government under President Volodymyr Zelenskyy remained in the capital, and, with support from international allies, Ukraine managed to take back substantial parts of the country that had initially been occupied by Russia during 2022.

Yet, this awful war, which has been ongoing at the time of writing for almost two years with no end in sight, has been massively destructive and caused immeasurable losses and hardships. Besides huge military causalities on both sides, tens of thousands of Ukrainian civilians have been killed or injured, while others have been captured and tortured.[1] The war has caused more than six million Ukrainians to flee the country as refugees, while over five million more have been internally displaced.[2] Infrastructure has been badly damaged across Ukraine, and access to water, electricity, heating, healthcare and education has been disrupted. In occupied areas, local people face ill-treatment, sexual violence and arbitrary detention.[3] As things stand in late 2023, Russia occupies about 18 per cent of Ukrainian territory, including Crimea and the parts of eastern Ukraine which it has controlled since 2014.[4] Ukrainians remain defiant, though, and determined to liberate their country rather than capitulate to Russian aggression.[5]

The consequences of Russia's war on Ukraine have been felt globally. First of all, countries around the world had to welcome and accommodate the Ukrainian refugees who sought safety abroad. Poland, for example, welcomed more than three million Ukrainians in just the first two months following the full-scale invasion (Lee et al, 2023). By 2023, the largest numbers of Ukrainian refugees were living in Germany, Poland and the Czech Republic, but other countries across Europe, including the UK, were each providing refuge for many tens of thousands of Ukrainians.[6] The challenge of providing appropriate accommodation for Ukrainian families and sufficient support with integration has been daunting, but civil society has helped governments to tackle these challenges with a lot of goodwill, generosity and compassion.

Meanwhile, the war has negatively impacted the global economy by pushing up the prices of energy and food. For many years, European countries relied heavily on imports of Russian oil and gas.[7] The war forced recognition in European capitals that reliance on Russian energy came with unacceptable security costs, as Moscow used revenue from oil and gas sales to fund its aggression against Ukraine. The European Union and G7 countries have introduced sanctions on the Russian energy sector,[8] and countries such as Germany have worked to reduce their consumption of Russian gas with considerable success.[9] However, the higher energy costs associated with these necessary policies have left businesses and households struggling with their bills, as inflation rates soared and interest rates also rose to counteract the inflation. Ukraine is a major exporter of grain and other vital agricultural commodities, so Russian attacks on Ukrainian ports and agricultural production have further contributed to food price inflation and economic difficulties worldwide.[10]

It is thus hard to overstate the impact of this war on the health, wellbeing and security of populations of Europe and beyond. Ukrainians have suffered the most grievous direct harm, but the indirect consequences of Russia's war on Ukraine have been felt by ordinary people across the world. The first section of this volume addresses some of the interconnected problems generated by the war, which together make the war itself a 'wicked issue' for public health and social policy – a long-term, highly complex challenge that will require well-informed and wide-ranging policy interventions.

In Chapter 1, Michael Burton discusses the war's economic impact in Europe. Burton's analysis explains how the escalation of the war exacerbated pre-existing socioeconomic and financial problems associated with the global COVID-19 pandemic. He observes that high rates of inflation since the Russian full-scale invasion have hit low-income European households particularly hard. At the same time, the war has strained public finances due to rising defence costs and increased demand for social support. The chapter looks particularly at the case of the UK, where the average standard of living has been stagnating for over a decade.

In Chapter 2, Alexander Shemetev and Martin Pělucha study how the Czech Republic responded to the overlapping challenges of the COVID-19 pandemic and Russia's war on Ukraine. Their analysis describes the country's macroeconomic performance, as well as the impact of the pandemic and war on the Czech population's everyday life.

In Chapter 3, Annalisa Sannino reflects on the heightened risk of a human-made global catastrophe following Russia's full-scale invasion of

Ukraine. Her point of departure is the decision of the *Bulletin of the Atomic Scientists* in early 2023 to move the hands of the 'Doomsday Clock' forward to just 90 seconds from midnight – the closest to the moment of catastrophe that the clock hands have ever been. The Russian Federation has one of the world's largest nuclear arsenals and the war has already seen dangerous fighting around the Zaporizhzhia Nuclear Power Station, which is now under Russian control. The war therefore raises the prospect of some form of nuclear escalation or nuclear disaster. Sannino's chapter examines the limitations of the Doomsday Clock as a driver of change to reduce nuclear risks via collective action.

In Chapter 4, Rebecca Harrocks examines religious dimensions of Russia's war on Ukraine. She notes that leading figures from the Russian Orthodox Church, including Patriarch Kirill of Moscow, have expressed staunch support for the Russian invasion. Meanwhile, many sites of religious significance in Ukraine have suffered severe damage. Harrocks asks whether religion could, nevertheless, play a role in long-term reconciliation and peacebuilding, as established theories suggest. She argues that religion could become a source of influence in diplomatic efforts to end the war, by engaging key actors and mapping religious drivers of war onto a path to peacebuilding.

In Chapter 5, Helen Froud considers how the war and its economic, social and environmental consequences have affected European social determinants of health. She maps the 2015 United Nations Sustainable Development Goals against social determinants of health, arguing that a 'values-based-approach' borrowed from healthcare can help to tackle some of the most intractable problems exacerbated by the war.

Overall, the contributions within this section of the book offer diverse insights into how Russia's war on Ukraine is affecting the health, wellbeing and security of people in different parts of Europe. While recognising the severity and scale of challenges created by the war, these contributions also suggest some approaches with potential to mitigate the war's indirect effects and improve conditions for human flourishing.

Notes

[1] https://www.ohchr.org/en/news/2023/09/ukraine-civilian-casualty-update-11-september-2023

[2] https://www.unrefugees.org/emergencies/ukraine/

[3] https://news.un.org/en/story/2023/10/1141872

[4] https://www.nytimes.com/interactive/2023/09/28/world/europe/russia-ukraine-war-map-front-line.html

[5] https://dif.org.ua/article/den-nezalezhnosti-ukraini-shlyakh-do-peremogi-identichnist-ta-tsinnist-derzhavi-na-tli-viyni

[6] https://data.unhcr.org/en/situations/ukraine

[7] https://ecfr.eu/article/conscious-uncoupling-europeans-russian-gas-challenge-in-2023/

8 https://eu-solidarity-ukraine.ec.europa.eu/eu-sanctions-against-russia-following-invasion-ukraine/sanctions-energy_en
9 https://www.theguardian.com/business/2023/sep/30/how-will-europe-weather-a-second-winter-without-gas-from-russia
10 https://www.kcl.ac.uk/has-the-invasion-of-ukraine-caused-our-food-prices-to-rise-over-the-past-year

1

The economic impact of the war in Europe

Michael Burton

Introduction

The American political scientist Francis Fukuyama famously coined the phrase 'the end of history' in a 1992 reference to the collapse of the Soviet Union and the assumed triumph of liberal democracy as the last stage in the evolution of ideology (Fukuyama, 1992). That assumption was arguably later unravelled by a series of dramatic events from 9/11 through to the rise and fall of Isis, the Syrian civil war, Brexit, the election of President Trump in 2016 and other populist leaders across the world, the COVID-19 pandemic in 2020 and more recently in 2022 the bloody invasion of the Ukraine by its neighbour Russia. For as former US secretary of state James Baker who was involved with the discussions around the dissolution of the Soviet Union, once commented: 'As you address the problems of one era, you're often planting the seeds for the next set of challenges. History doesn't stop' (Anon, 2022c).

This chapter looks at the economic consequences of that most recent event, the invasion of Ukraine, which brought war to Europe and directly impacted the lives of millions of Europeans due to the resulting soaring energy prices, inflation and sharp rises in public spending, taxation and the cost of living. The war also occurred just as the world was recovering from the COVID-19 pandemic whose global death toll was over six million and which had put huge pressure on European health systems and on their public finances through state financial intervention to help their citizens. The consequences of war in rocketing inflation and energy costs also starkly highlighted the pre-existing social determinants of health inequalities such as poverty, low wages, poor diet, inadequate housing, with the poorest households most negatively affected (see Figure I.1).

The invasion of Ukraine in February 2022, although in itself a shock for most Europeans, had long been on the horizon. Russia's President Vladimir Putin had never subscribed to the 'end of history' view that liberal democracy was finally and permanently triumphant. He regretted the break-up of the Soviet Union and the independence of former Soviet republics like Ukraine with its 40 million citizens, Georgia and even the Baltic states which he continued to regard as being within Russia's zone of influence. He saw the entry into the North Atlantic Treaty Organization (NATO) and the European Union (EU) of the former Central and East European states which had once been part of the Soviet empire as proof of expansionism by the West. He was especially concerned that Ukraine, whose long history was so entwined with Russia's, might also join the EU and move into the West's orbit and was determined to prevent it. But over the years, as Putin's regime became increasingly authoritarian, so European liberal democracy in turn became attractive to Ukrainians, particularly those in the more European western part of the country.

Putin's annexation of the Crimea in 2014, arguing that until 1954 it had been part of the Russian Soviet republic anyway, and the fostering of pro-Russian breakaway 'republics' in Ukraine's eastern regions was a wake-up call for Europe and the United States. In hindsight this was the first stage of a plan to ultimately bring Ukraine into the Russian orbit altogether but at the time NATO showed little appetite for military involvement. Indeed the European economies, especially Germany's, were closely tied up with Russia, a major exporter of gas and oil. As from 2011 the Nord Stream 1 gas pipeline ran directly from Russia to Germany while Nord Stream 2, a controversial project to double gas exports to Europe direct from Russia and financed by Russia's state energy firm Gazprom, was completed in 2021, though never opened due to the subsequent war. The Nord Stream 1 pipeline replaced gas transit lines across Ukraine which hitherto had provided Ukraine with lucrative transit fees. It was clear that Russia was already politicising energy. Ukrainian president Volodymyr Zelenskyy presciently insisted in August 2021 that the Nord Stream 2 gas pipeline, which Ukraine opposed, was a 'dangerous weapon', posing a threat not only to his country but to all of Europe (Anon, 2021).

In 2021 total Russian energy exports to the EU were 275.6 million tonnes. Russia's share in EU energy imports in the three years leading up to the first quarter of 2022 hovered between 26 and 27 per cent. Russia was the largest supplier of natural gas to the EU with a share of 39.3 per cent in 2021, followed by Norway (24.2 per cent) and Algeria (8.2 per cent) (Yanatma, 2023). According to a study from the European Central Bank in 2019, Russia's energy production accounted for 12 per cent of the global supply of oil, 5 per cent of coal and 16 per cent of gas. In 2021 the country was the largest supplier of energy commodities to the euro area, constituting 23 per cent of total energy imports. Russia accounted for 23 per cent and 43 per cent of euro area crude oil and coal imports respectively in 2020, which represented 9 per cent and 2 per cent of the euro area's primary energy consumption. The euro area was particularly dependent on natural gas imports from Russia, which in 2020 were 35 per cent of euro area gas imports and 11 per cent of the euro area's primary energy consumption. The European Central Bank's report said Germany and Italy had the highest dependence on Russian gas among the large euro area countries (Adolfsen et al, 2022).

None of this suggested that Europe was in any position to embark on a military conflict with Russia when it was so dependent on Russian energy. The chaotic withdrawal of US troops from Afghanistan in mid-2021 seemed to have provided final confirmation to the Kremlin that the United States and NATO also lacked the political will for further intervention. Even so, when Russian troops began massing on Ukraine's borders in early 2022 there was still disbelief in the West that Putin would go so far as to launch a war and also believe it could be easily won and a pro-Russian regime installed in Kyiv. Western sceptics were wrong: Putin's so-called 'special military operation' was launched on 24 February 2022.

The energy war and the cost of living crisis

Western powers, especially Europe and the United States, in contrast to their response to the annexation of Crimea, acted swiftly and decisively with tough sanctions and even military support. The immediate consequence – as predicted by Ukraine's President Zelenskyy – was an energy war as Western sanctions cut back imports of Russia's oil and gas to cripple its economy while in turn Russia deliberately cut back its gas exports to Europe to force up the price of energy and hurt Western households. Gas prices in Europe increased by 50 per cent on 24 February 2022, the day Russia launched its full-scale invasion of Ukraine (HoL, 2023). The EU introduced economic sanctions targeting the Russian energy industry, mainly the coal and oil sectors. The sanctions included a ban on EU exports of goods and technology used to develop the Russian oil and gas sectors while the EU prohibited the import of Russian coal in August 2022. At a special meeting of the European Council at the end of May, it was decided to stop most Russian oil imports (Adolfsen et al, 2022). Nord Stream 2, the controversial pipeline from Russia to Germany, was put on hold by Germany while in the first two weeks after the invasion, the prices of oil, coal and gas went up by around 40 per cent, 130 per cent and 180 per cent, respectively (Adolfsen et al, 2022). The price of electricity produced from gas increased in line with gas prices. Gas prices in Europe increased more than four-fold by October 2022 compared to 2021, with Russia cutting deliveries to less than 20 per cent of their 2021 levels (IMF, 2022a). The price of crude oil in the global market rose from around US$76 per barrel at the start of January 2022 to over US$110 per barrel by March 2022 (GEP.com blog, 2022).

The rise in energy costs fed through immediately into household budgets as the price of electricity and gas soared, creating a 'double whammy' since businesses, especially food suppliers, in turn put up their prices, driving up inflation to offset their own energy costs. In the UK, energy used in the home, like electricity, gas, heating oil, and so on made up 31 per cent of total final energy consumption in 2022 and gas was the largest source of domestic energy use, at 64 per cent, followed by electricity (25 per cent), oil (6 per cent) and renewables for heat (3 per cent). Households collectively spent GBP£30.2 billion on electricity in 2022, up by GBP£8 billion (36 per cent) on 2021 and the fifth record high figure in a row (HoL, 2023).

The poorest households were invariably the worst hit and 'the cost of living crisis' became a political issue. As an International Monetary Fund (IMF) report noted in April 2022:

> The main channel through which the war in Ukraine and sanctions on Russia affect the euro area economy is rising global energy prices and energy security. Because they are net energy importers, higher global prices represent a negative terms-of-trade shock for most European countries, translating to lower output and higher inflation. (IMF, 2022a: 1)

Six months later the IMF reported:

> The war is having severe economic repercussions in Europe, with higher energy prices, weaker consumer confidence, and slower momentum in manufacturing resulting from persistent supply chain disruptions and rising input costs. Adjoining economies – Baltic and eastern European states – have felt the largest impact, with their growth slowing sharply in the second and third quarters and their inflation rates soaring. (IMF, 2022b: 6)

A July 2022 IMF report concluded that in the euro area, inflation in June 2022 reached 8.6 per cent, its highest level since the euro was launched. In the United States, the Consumer Price Index rose by 9.1 per cent in June, compared with a year earlier, and by 9.1 per cent in the UK in May, the highest inflation rates in these two countries in 40 years. The IMF report added: 'The principal driver of global food price inflation – particularly prices of cereal, such as wheat – has been the war in Ukraine ... rising borrowing costs combined with high inflation and slowing growth have prompted comparisons to the 1970s and early 1980s' (IMF, 2022c: 4). A later IMF report in October 2022 commented: 'Inflation has soared to multi-decade highs, prompting rapid monetary policy tightening and squeezing household budgets. The euro area saw inflation reach 10% in September, while the UK saw annual inflation of 9.9%' (IMF, 2022a: 4). According to EU figures, while inflation in August 2022 averaged 10.1 per cent across the EU this masked wide discrepancies especially in the Baltic states nearest to Russia; Estonia's was 25.2 per cent, Lithuania's 21.1 per cent and Latvia's 21.4 per cent (Anon, 2023a).

Putin doubtless hoped that the impact on European households of inflation caused by energy price hikes would reduce public support for Ukraine and force European governments to cut military aid. A big fear was that a cold winter in 2022/2023, especially in Central and East Europe, would create a chronic energy shortage and an even greater escalation of prices.

In fact the increases in energy prices, as Russian supplies dwindled and Western economies sought alternatives, were so stark and so immediate that European governments were forced to intervene with financial help to households. A precedent had already been set during the COVID-19 pandemic with support to business and employees affected by government-imposed lockdowns. It was estimated that budgetary support for EU households and firms to offset energy hikes from the Ukraine war amounted to 1.3 per cent of the EU's entire gross domestic product (GDP) (IMF, 2023a). In June 2023 since the start of the energy crisis in September 2021, €651 billion had been allocated across European countries to shield consumers from the rising energy costs. Of this figure, €540 billion was in the EU, of which €158 billion was by Germany and €8.1 billion in Norway (Anon, 2023b).

Government support for households helped cushion the worst of the energy price hikes but it also ratcheted up public spending again just at a time when central banks had hoped that the phasing out of the COVID-19 pandemic would see a reduction in government deficits. Inflation, along with labour shortages, as economies recovered capacity after the pandemic, also pushed up wage costs. In July to September 2022 in the UK, regular wages rose by 5.7 per cent year-on-year, and total pay, which includes bonuses, rose 6.0 per cent, but this was way below the inflation rate of 9.6 per cent in October 2022 according to the UK's Office for National Statistics (ONS). As inflation continued increasing steeply during 2022, regular wage growth fell behind inflation in all industries except professional and scientific (ONS, 2020). Not surprisingly many households were struggling financially as the UK's ONS found in its regular report on social trends in November 2022. When asked about the issues facing the UK, 93 per cent of adults reported the cost of living as an important issue and 91 per cent reported their cost of living had increased from the previous year. The most common actions reported by all adults because of the rising cost of living were spending less on non-essentials (65 per cent) and using less fuel, such as gas or electricity in their homes (63 per cent). Around six in ten (56 per cent) adults reported that they were very or somewhat worried about keeping warm in their home during the coming winter (2022/2023) (Anon, 2022b). Even a year later in October 2023 the regular ONS survey still found that when asked about the important issues facing the UK, the most commonly reported continued to be the cost of living (89 per cent), along with the economy (72 per cent) while almost 40 per cent of those who paid energy bills said they were difficult to afford (ONS, 2023).

As of the first quarter of 2023, real hourly wages had decreased in 22 countries out of 24 in Europe over the previous year due to rises being lower than inflation according to a Euronews report later that year. The real hourly wage increased only in Belgium (2.9 per cent) and the Netherlands (0.4 per cent) between the first quarters of 2022 and 2023. The decline in real wages varied from 0.8 per cent in Luxembourg to 15.6 per cent in Hungary in this period. Hungary was followed by Latvia (−13.4 per cent), the Czech Republic (−10.4 per cent) and Sweden (−8.4 per cent) (Anon, 2023c).

In the first quarter of 2023, despite the pick-up in nominal wages, the difference between nominal annual wage growth and inflation was −3.8 per cent on average across the 34 Organisation for Economic Co-operation and Development (OECD) countries with available data, with a negative difference observed in 30 countries. As the OECD report noted: 'The loss of purchasing power is particularly challenging for workers in low-income households, who have less leeway to deal with increases in the cost of living through savings or borrowing and often face higher actual inflation rates because a higher proportion of their spending goes to energy and food' (OECD, 2023: 13).

Inflation proved stubbornly hard to reduce. In order to squeeze inflation out of the economy and damp down pay pressures central banks increased their interest rates from their historically rock-bottom levels. The Bank of England increased interest rates 14 times between December 2021 and October 2023 to 5.25 per cent. The European Central Bank raised the rate it paid on bank deposits to 4 per cent in September 2023, the highest since the founding of the eurozone in 1999 as it battled to get inflation back down to its target of 2 per cent. Interest rate rises also pushed up the cost of government borrowing, taking a slice out of the already squeezed public finances. In the UK in April 2023 central government debt interest payable was GBP£9.8 billion, or GBP£3.1 billion more than April 2022 and the highest April figure since monthly records began in 1997 (ONS, 2023).

Fortunately, the winter of 2022/2023 was milder than feared, reducing expected demand on energy supplies, just as European states were finding other sources than Russia to provide oil and gas, and energy inflation began to decline, albeit slowly. The average annual price of Brent crude oil was US$79.75 per barrel in June 2023, around US$21 lower than the annual average in 2022 (Anon, 2023d). Wholesale gas and electricity prices on the spot market fell in autumn 2022 to levels below those at the start of the year. Employment also remained robust due to labour shortages and a pick-up in economic activity after the COVID-19 pandemic. The IMF reported in October 2023 that 'despite the disruption in energy and food markets caused by the war, and the unprecedented tightening of global monetary conditions to combat decades-high inflation, the global economy has slowed, but not stalled' (2023b: xiii). Nonetheless the IMF's outlook report warned that the poorest countries had been worst hit by the rise in energy and food cost (IMF, 2023b).

The economic impact of Ukrainian refugees

The invasion of Ukraine also produced a flood of refugees from the war-torn country into Europe on a scale not seen since 1945. Many of the countries, largely from East and Central Europe, which were sheltering refugees received help from the World Health Organization (WHO). Because the Ukraine government imposed martial law, no males between 18 and 60 were allowed to leave so refugees were primarily women, children and older people. The UN High Commissioner for Refugees recorded 5.8 million Ukrainian refugees in Europe and a further 392,000 outside Europe.

In a report detailing its response to the refugee crisis the WHO found that some 1.56 million Ukrainian refugees were registered for temporary protection in Poland as of 16 January 2023; however, more than nine million cross border crossings from Ukraine had been recorded since 24 February 2022. The Polish healthcare system provided refugees the same health benefits and services as Polish citizens but the impact on the Polish health system was 'considerable with the increased burden of TB, HIV/AIDS, chronic diseases, patients that need emergency medical evacuation services, and a high population of women and children that need health care' (WHO, 2023: 25).

By mid-December 2022, almost one million Ukrainian refugees had crossed the border into Bulgaria alone, with some staying and others passing through, according to the WHO study. In the year since February 2022 the Czech Republic sheltered around 500,000 Ukrainian refugees, and 433,781 were currently recorded by March 2023 as granted temporary protection status, with up to 25 per cent of those residing in the capital city of Prague.

As of 31 December 2022, 34,248 refugees from Ukraine registered for temporary protection in Hungary. Between 24 February 2022 and 29 January 2023, almost 1.9 million border crossings from Ukraine into Romania were recorded, though most were heading to other countries with only 111,000 remaining in Romania. Over 100,000 refugees from Ukraine had registered for temporary protection in the Slovak Republic as of 31 January 2023, although more than a million border crossings from Ukraine had been registered since 24 February 2022. Even in the tiny country of Moldova between 24 February 2022 and 31 January 2023, 755,368 border crossings from Ukraine were recorded, while 108,824 were registered as refugees, mainly women, children and the elderly (WHO, 2023). In the UK around 174,000 Ukrainians moved there as at May 2023 although 228,300 visas were issued (MOO, 2023). In Germany as at March 2023 there were 1.1 million and in Spain 186,000 (Anon, 2023e).

Some reports suggested that the arrival of Ukrainian refugees provided a boost to host country economies which were experiencing labour shortages and ageing populations, offsetting the extra costs from public spending on health, housing and schooling. A European Central Bank report commented:

> The increase in labour supply that results from the influx of Ukrainian refugees could slightly ease the tightness observed in the euro area labour market. If they can find jobs without a lengthy integration process, Ukrainian refugees could help the market to respond to the currently buoyant demand for labour and address worsening skill shortages. (Botelho, 2022: chart B)

More cautious was an IMF report in April 2022, noting that: 'In the short term, refugee arrivals will strain local services, including for shelter and health care. In the longer term, the dispersion of a large number of refugees across the European Union will have important social and economic effects, increasing labor supply but potentially exacerbating anti-immigrant sentiment' (IMF, 2022d: 12).

According to the Centre for Economic Policy Research (CEPR), Ukrainian migrants drove an initial short-term boost to retail trade and private consumption during 2022, especially in Poland and Estonia. The centre quoted data from the National Bank of Ukraine, saying that spending by Ukrainians abroad in 2022 was US$2 billion a month in 2022, three times the amount of the previous year, as migrants initially drew on their own bank accounts until they began to earn local currency in their host countries. Once migrants were able to work they could pay taxes. According to estimates by the Center for Migration Research at the University of Warsaw, Ukrainians in Poland paid ten billion Polish zloty (around US$2.4 billion) in taxes. The CEPR March 2023 report, which quoted the figures, added: 'Although migrants create additional challenges for state finances in the short run, they are likely to make a positive impact on the budget and economy of recipient countries if migrants stay in these countries longer than several years and actively participate in the labour market' (Pogarska et al, 2023). The forecast, however, depended on how long the war would last, how many refugees would want to return to their country to help rebuild it once the war was over, and whether host countries were generous long-term in granting work visas and even citizenship.

The economic impact of higher defence spending

A key component of Europe and NATO's robust response to the invasion of Ukraine was the supply of military aid. Putin had gambled on the West's response being confined to limited sanctions such as it had been in the past with his other incursions in Syria, Georgia and the Crimea. The provision of Western military hardware from February 2022 and know-how for Ukraine stiffened its defences but the war also stimulated a reappraisal of defence strategy among NATO members which had previously ruled out any large-scale military conflict in Europe. The net result was a substantial planned increase in defence budgets with a renewed commitment to meeting or even exceeding NATO's target of defence spending being at least 2 per cent of GDP. In 2021 defence spending in the EU amounted to 1.3 per cent of GDP. Germany announced in February 2022 that it would spend an additional €100 billion on defence; its share of GDP from 2008 and 2021 averaged 1.3 per cent, while Poland set a defence budget of 2.4 per cent of its GDP for 2022 (Anon, 2022b). According to the UK's defence ministry the UK's share of its GDP was 2.3 per cent in 2021/2022 and it had the world's third largest defence budget in cash terms, higher than Russia's, though still about a tenth that of the United States (MOD, 2022).

According to the Stockholm International Peace Research Institute (SIPRI), which analyses military spending, military expenditure in Europe saw its steepest year-on-year increase in at least 30 years in 2022, driven mainly by Ukraine and Russia. The sharpest increases were seen in Finland (+36 per cent), Lithuania (+27 per cent), Sweden (+12 per cent) and Poland (+11 per cent). The UK had the highest military spending in Central and Western Europe at US$68.5 billion, of which an estimated US$2.5 billion (3.6 per cent) was financial military aid to Ukraine. As an indication of the war's cost, Ukraine's military spending reached US$44 billion in 2022. A 640 per cent rise, this was the highest single-year increase in a country's military expenditure ever recorded in SIPRI data. As a result of the increase and the war-related damage to Ukraine's economy, its military spending as a share of GDP rocketed to 34 per cent in 2022, from 3.2 per cent in 2021 (SIPRI, 2023).

This was bad news for Putin, especially when Russia's neighbours, Finland and Sweden, announced they wanted to join NATO, but it was not without its challenges for Europe. Public finances were already under pressure from the cost of financial support for households during COVID-19 followed by the added support for households to offset energy price hikes due to the war in Ukraine and the impact of inflation. Defence was now jostling with other spending departments like welfare, health and education for a greater slice of the public spending cake.

Inflation was further eating into real-term increases in defence spending just as it was for other government services. In 2022 McKinsey estimated that for Europe's defence budgets, 'the cumulative loss of buying power could be close to €300bn under a scenario where inflation averages 5% from 2022 to 2026; in a more conservative scenario, with inflation averaging 3% over this period, the cumulative loss of buying power would be about €185bn' (Anon, 2022b). The imperative was therefore to reduce procurement costs through collaboration among the European NATO states, a longer-term strategy.

Conclusion

Russia's invasion of Ukraine in February 2022 was a huge economic blow for Europe, still recovering from the fiscal shock of the COVID-19 pandemic, which had long-term fiscal consequences. The immediate result of the invasion was a sharp rise in the cost of energy as the EU and the United States and other countries imposed sanctions and Russia in turn curtailed oil and gas exports in order to damage the economies of the EU and United States. Since the EU in particular was so dependent on Russian energy the latter's block on exports sent EU energy costs soaring, feeding immediately into household bills. Governments intervened either with financial support for poor households or caps on energy costs subsidised by the taxpayer to damp down the worst impact on household bills. Escalating energy costs pushed up inflation across all sectors, not only energy. In an attempt to squeeze out inflation central banks raised interest rates, adding further misery to homeowners with mortgages. Rising interest rates increased the cost of government borrowing, putting pressure on public finances, already feeling the pinch from inflation. Recession was narrowly averted because economic capacity was still increasing after the COVID-19 pandemic and the labour market was relatively buoyant, but inflation bore down heavily on European households, creating an ongoing cost of living crisis for the poor. Two years after the invasion of Ukraine with the war still raging there were still only limited signs that the cost of living crisis was moderating. Responses to this impact on the most vulnerable are reflected in intermediate factors in pre-existing *intermediate* social determinants of health inequalities, discussed in this book.

References

Adolfsen. J.F., Kuik, F., Magdalena, E.L. and Schuler, T. (2022) The impact of the war in Ukraine on euro area energy markets. *ECB Economic Bulletin*, 4.

Anon (2021) Ukraine insists Nord Stream2 is 'dangerous' despite German reassurances. Available at: https://www.politico.eu/article/ukraine-insists-nord-stream-2-is-dangerous-despite-german-reassurances/

Anon (2022a) Invasion of Ukraine: implications for European defense spending. *McKinsey and Company*, 19 December.

Anon (2022b) Public opinions and social trends, Great Britain 26 October to 6 November 2022. *Office for National Statistics*, 11 November.

Anon (2022c) There was no promise not to enlarge NATO. *Harvard Law Today*, 16 March.

Anon (2023a) Eurostat, 19 September.

Anon (2023b) National fiscal responses to the energy crisis. *Bruegel*, 26 June.

Anon (2023c) Real wages are down in Europe: which countries have seen the biggest changes in salaries? *Euronews*, 25 August.

Anon (2023d) Brent crude oil price annually 1976–2023. *Statista*, 29 August.

Anon (2023e) Number of Ukrainian refugees by country. *Statista*, 14 September.

Botelho, V. (2022) The impact of the influx of Ukrainian refugees on the euro area labour force. *ECB Economic Bulletin*, 4. Available at: https://www.ecb.europa.eu/press/economic-bulletin/focus/2022/html/ecb.ebbox202204_03~c9ddc08308.en.html

Fukuyama, F. (1992) *The End of History and the Last Man*. London: Penguin.

GEP.com blog (2022) 5 July.

HoL (2023) Domestic energy prices. House of Commons Library, 13 September.

IMF (2022a) *Countering the Cost-of-Living Crisis*. World Economic Outlook. Washington, DC: IMF.

IMF (2022b) *War Sets Back the Global Recovery*. World Economic Outlook. Washington, DC: IMF.

IMF (2022c) *Gloomy and More Uncertain*. World Economic Outlook Update. Washington DC: IMF.

IMF (2022d) *War Sets Back the Global Recovery*. World Economic Outlook. Washington, DC: IMF.

IMF (2023a) *A Rocky Recovery*. World Economic Outlook. Washington, DC: IMF.

IMF (2023b) *Navigating Global Divergences*. World Economic Outlook. Washington, DC: IMF.

Lee, A.C.K., Khaw, F.M, Lindman, A.S. and Juszczyk, G. (2023) Ukraine refugee crisis: evolving needs and challenges. *Public Health*, 217: 41–45.

MOD (2022). *UK Defence in Numbers 2022*. UK Ministry of Defence.

MOO (2023) *Ukrainian Migration to the UK*. Oxford: Migration Observatory.

OECD (2023) *Artificial Intelligence and the Labour Market*. Organisation for Economic Co-operation and Development's Employment Outlook 2023.

ONS (2020) *Professional and Scientific Industry the Only One Where Pay Continues to Match Rising Prices*. Office for National Statistics.

ONS (2023) *Public Sector Finances*. Office for National Statistics.

Pogarska, O., Tucha, O., Spivak, I. and Bondarenko, O. (2023) How Ukrainian migrants affect the economies of European countries. Centre for Economic Policy Research, 7 March.

SIPRI (2023) World military expenditure reaches new record high as European spending surges. *Stockholm International Peace Research Institute*, April.

WHO (2023) *WHO's Response to the Ukraine Crisis: Annual Report*. Copenhagen: World Health Organization, Regional Office for Europe.

Yanatma, S. (2023) Europe's 'energy war' in data: how have EU imports changed since Russia's invasion of Ukraine? *Euronews*, 24 February. Available at: https://www.euronews.com/green/2023/02/24/europes-energy-war-in-data

Zabrodskyi, M., Watling, J., Danylyuk, O.V. and Reynolds, N. (2022) Preliminary lessons in conventional warfighting from Russia's invasion of Ukraine: February–July 2022. RUSI Special Report. Available at: https://rusi.org/explore-our-research/publications/special-resources/preliminary-lessons-conventional-warfighting-russias-invasion-ukraine-february-july-2022

2

Geopolitical and post-pandemic factors influencing the social perspective of individuals and families: a case study of the Czech Republic in a national and regional context

Alexander Shemetev and Martin Pělucha

Introduction

The social and resilience outlook of individuals and families in the Czech Republic is influenced by a variety of factors, including economic conditions, ethical norms, access to healthcare and the impact of geopolitical events. Economic indicators such as gross domestic product (GDP) per capita and unemployment rates shape the livelihoods of families, affecting their financial stability and access to basic necessities including digital services and possibilities of the digital economy. Ethical norms and societal values play a crucial role in determining social attitudes, behaviours and expectations, influencing issues such as gender roles, family dynamics and social mobility. Access to education, digital inequalities and healthcare further influences social outlooks by shaping opportunities for personal development, career advancement and overall wellbeing. In addition, the impact of geopolitical events, such as the war in Ukraine and the influx of refugees, adds another layer of complexity to the social landscape, influencing perceptions of security, identity and community cohesion. By comprehensively examining these factors, we gain valuable insights into the dynamics of social perspectives in the Czech Republic, which can inform policy interventions aimed at promoting inclusive growth and societal wellbeing.

This chapter explores the complex interplay between international factors, social justice and healthcare dynamics in the Czech Republic. It begins by explaining the country's reliance on assessing global trends for economic growth and political stability, using a Politics, Economy, Society, Technology, Environment and Law (PESTEL) analysis framework to comprehensively understand the external environment. It then introduces the innovative Gridded Uncertainty Impact Matrix (GUIM) approach, developed to address the challenge of representing and prioritising the vast array of health indicators. While the World Health Organization (WHO) has provided indicators and typologies, the GUIM is the first tool to effectively grid these indicators and highlight the most pressing issues and potential trends in healthcare. Through detailed analysis and graphical presentation, the GUIM provides valuable insights into the complex dynamics of health systems, enabling policy makers to identify critical issues and formulate effective strategies for societal wellbeing. By demonstrating its application in the Czech Republic, the GUIM demonstrates its potential to revolutionise health assessment and provide a pathway to improved health outcomes and equitable access to services. In addition, the chapter examines the impact of economic instability and the war in Ukraine on the Czech Republic, shedding light on trade disruptions, energy dependence, investment confidence and the refugee crisis. Through careful analysis and empirical evidence, this chapter provides a comprehensive overview of the multiple factors shaping health and socioeconomic dynamics in the Czech Republic, paving the way for informed policy interventions and sustainable development strategies that build the resilience of individuals and families.

International factors and social justice

The Czech Republic relies on assessing international factors for economic growth, attracting foreign investment, ensuring political stability and shaping European Union (EU) policies. This involves monitoring global market trends and geopolitical developments, and participating in international and regional organisations to safeguard national interests and promote cooperation. Conducting a PESTEL analysis provides a comprehensive understanding of the international factors influencing the Czech Republic's Politics, Economy, Society, Technology, Ecology and Environment and Law. We offer an approach of using a gridded PESTEL Uncertainty Impact Matrix (Figure 2.1) at the macroeconomic level, which offers advantages over traditional methods by improving the assessment of the international environment.

The gridded PESTEL Uncertainty Impact Matrix (Figure 2.1):

• Bottom sector (low to medium uncertainty, low potential impact): secondary elements that require attention after the core issues have been resolved.
• Upper left sector: highlights trends for the Czech Republic, including smart central banking, digitalisation, transparency, bureaucratic problem-solving, digital inequalities and online work.
• Top right corner (critical uncertainties): represents the highest risks, including trade in green technologies, the spread of military conflicts,

Figure 2.1: Gridded PESTEL Uncertainty Impact Matrix for the Czech Republic in 2023

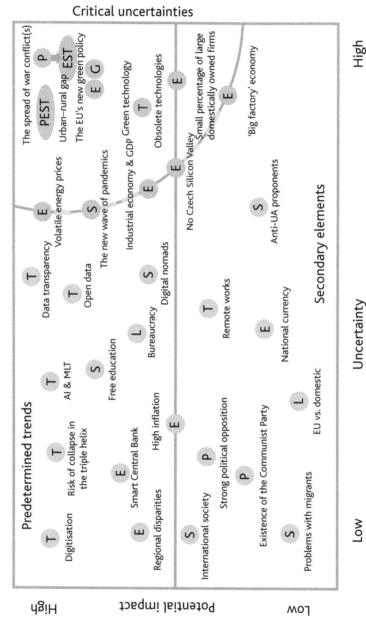

Note: Abbreviations: P: political factors; E: economic factors; S: social factors; T: technological factors; G: ecological (green) factors; PEST: political, economic, social, technological factors; EST: economic, social, technological factors.
Source: Own work. The method for constructing the matrix is derived from Schoemaker and van der Heijden (1992) and Tesch (2019: 219–224).

the urban–rural divide, volatile energy prices, pandemics, the declining importance of the industrial economy, the loss of domestic financial ownership and the challenges of the 'assembly economy'.

Assessing the healthcare landscape and trends: a comprehensive analysis using the WHO framework and the GUIM model

The WHO has introduced an innovative methodology for assessing the state of healthcare in countries, as outlined in its 2018 report (World Health Organization, 2018). This comprehensive approach, shown in Figure 2.2, provides detailed insights into health monitoring.

The main problem with the current methodology is the lack of a coherent framework for integrating indicators and assessing the overall state of the health sector, including its response to different shocks. We propose the adoption of a GUIM model specifically tailored for the health sector, building on the framework outlined in the previous section. This approach involves constructing two matrices for each health sector identified by the WHO (Health Status, Health Risk Factors and Health Service Coverage) comprising three indicators in two dimensions: static state and proposed trends resulting from shocks. To address key issues in impact assessment, we define impact as the potential negative influence on the health of society, with a focus on identifying critical issues within the national health system, such as those faced by the Czech Republic.

In addition, we use an expert judgement method to determine the placement of each healthcare element within the GUIM and to identify the direction and strength of associated trends.

Figure 2.2: Framework for health status assessment: a World Health Organization perspective

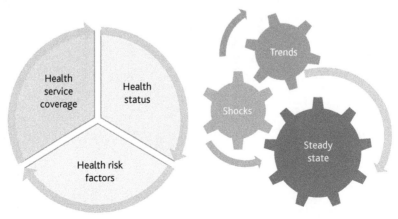

By using this approach, researchers can develop a robust model capable of effectively representing complex healthcare phenomena through concise graphical representations. The application of the GUIM in the Czech Republic serves as a first step, with the potential for future studies to extend this methodology to other countries and levels of healthcare, providing valuable insights for further research in this area.

Figure 2.3 illustrates the key issues in the health status of the Czech Republic. The main concern is the fertility rate, which is below the minimum required to maintain the current population size (F1). Morbidity challenges include a relatively high prevalence of hepatitis (M2) and cancer (M1). In terms of mortality, a relatively high suicide rate (C1) and deaths due to air pollution and household activities (C2) are of major concern.

The current shocks between 2020 and 2024 have the potential to significantly alter the healthcare landscape in the Czech Republic over the next decade (Figure 2.3). On the one hand, the influx of refugees from Ukraine could have a positive impact on the demographic situation (F1) by adding people with similar cultural backgrounds to the population. However, there are concerns about potential challenges related to adolescent fertility (F2) due to differences between the fertility rates of the refugee population and those of the Czech Republic, highlighting the need for careful monitoring. While the impact on morbidity indicators (M1 and M2) remains uncertain and requires further investigation, mortality indicators (C1, C2 and C3) are likely to be more challenging due to the shocks and require urgent attention from policy makers to mitigate any adverse effects.

The GUIM analysis (Figure 2.3) identifies key environmental and health risk factors in the Czech Republic. Urban air pollution (E1) emerges as a major concern, reaching up to a third of the global maximum (WAQI, 2024), particularly affecting eastern regions and metropolitan areas. Ongoing Green Deal initiatives hold promise for improving air quality in the country over the next decade. In addition, high per capita alcohol consumption (D1) is a key non-communicable disease issue. Nutrition-related factors pose several health risks, including low rates of breastfeeding up to six months (N1), high incidence of low birth weight (N2), potential problems with malnutrition in children under five (N3), and high levels of anaemia in both children under five (N4) and women of reproductive age (N5). Although these indicators do not pose an immediate threat, they will require considerable attention from policy makers in the coming years.

The forecast for the next decade (Figure 2.3) suggests changes in several health risk factors in the Czech Republic. The problem of breastfeeding (N1) may improve with new waves of immigration from countries with higher rates of breastfeeding up to six months. In addition, the influx of qualified medical personnel from these regions could improve antenatal

Figure 2.3: Dynamics of health status and risk factors in the Czech Republic: a comprehensive analysis

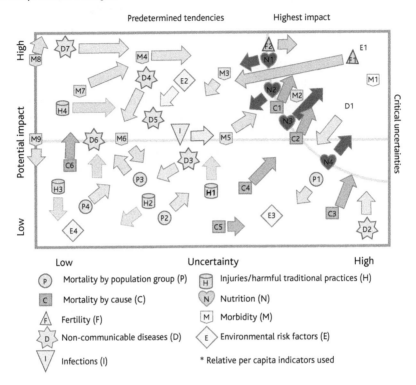

Note: This combined figure presents a comprehensive analysis of health status and risk factors in the Czech Republic, covering both the static state and trends due to shocks. Elements marked with capital letters PCFM provide insights into the health status landscape and its authors' projected dynamics (arrows), highlighting key issues such as fertility rates (F), morbidity challenges (M) and mortality concerns by population (P) and cause (C).

Elements marked with capital letters N (nutrition), E (environment), I (infections), D (non-communicable diseases), H (harmful practices/injuries) explore health risk factors, identify environmental and lifestyle factors that contribute to health risks, and project potential changes (arrows, authors' projections) over the next decade.

The numerical values in the figure reflect the urgency of each health problem in the Czech Republic's health system:

• F1: Fertility rate (births per woman) of 1.8 (2022)
• F2: Adolescent fertility rate (5 times [2022] the global minimum)
• M1: Cancer incidence (75.2% [2023] GM*)
• M2: Hepatitis (26.5% [2020] GM*)
• M3: Cancer mortality (66.25% [2022] GM*)
• M4: Data not available for all categories of morbidity
• M5: HIV/AIDS mortality (0.003% [2023] GM*)
• M6: COVID mortality (5% [by 03.2024] GM*)

Figure 2.3: Dynamics of health status and risk factors in the Czech Republic: a comprehensive analysis (continued)

- M7: Infant syphilis (0.4% [2022] GM*)
- M8: 0%(2020) malaria mortality
- M9: 0%(2020) diphtheria death rate
- C1: Medium suicide rate (16.9% [2023] GM*)
- C2: Household and air pollution mortality (10.6% [2020] GM*)
- C3: Sanitation/water mortality (0.3% [2021] GM*)
- C4: Road traffic deaths (8.3% [2022] GM*)
- C5: Tuberculosis mortality (0.01% [2021] GM*)
- C6: Maternal mortality (0.3% [2021] GM*)
- P1: Infant mortality (2.6% [2023] GM*)
- P2: Adolescent mortality (2.7% [2022] GM*)
- P3: Life expectancy (87.4% [2023] GM*)
- P4: Adolescent mortality (4.5% [2018] GM*)
- N1: 8% breastfeeding up to six months (2022; L**)
- N2: 7.8% low birth weight (2023; M**)
- N3: 19% anaemia in children aged <5 years (2020; H**)
- N4: 21.1% anaemia in women of reproductive age (2020; H**)
- E1: 30–35% of global peak urban air pollution (2024; M**)
- E2: 89.7% of population with access to safe sanitation (2023; M**)
- E3: 98% of population with access to safe drinking water (2023; M**)
- E4: 100% of the population will use clean fuels (2022; H**)
- I: HIV prevention
- D1: 10–14 litres/year of pure alcohol consumption (per capita, 2020–2023; H**)
- D2: 13g of salt per person per day (2024; H**)
- D3: ≈1/3 of the population is physically inactive (2017; H**)
- D4: 89.7% of the population will have access to safe sanitation (2023; M**)
- D5: 29.9% of the population will smoke (2023; M**)
- D6: Obesity***: 30.72% AM, 7.42% CM, 23.1% AF, 4.36% CF (2023; M**)
- D7: 7.1% of the population have diabetes (2023; M**)
- H1: 43% of children will have fought at school in 2019 (H**)
- H2: 14 rapes per 100,000 inhabitants in 2023 (M**)
- H3: 2.6% of women will experience violence in 2023 (L**)
- H4: 16% of children will be bullied in 2019 (M**)

* GM: Of Global Maximum (by year, per capita [if applicable])

** H: above world average; L: below world average; M: relatively close to world average

*** C: Children; A: Adults; M: Males; F: Females

Source: Reputable organisations such as the Czech Statistical Office, WHO, UN, World Bank, Our World in Data and private studies, providing a nuanced understanding of health dynamics in the country.

care and possibly reduce the incidence of low birth weight babies (N2). However, the proportion of children under five who are stunted (N3) may become a more pressing issue due to migration from regions with higher rates of child malnutrition. On the positive side, alcohol consumption (per capita, D1) is expected to decrease, partly due to a government campaign on temperance and an increase in the proportion of female migrants, who tend to consume less alcohol. However, salt consumption (D2) may increase with the arrival of refugees accustomed to a diet high in salted products, requiring proactive government action to mitigate the associated health risks.

The GUIM analysis (Figure 2.4) highlights urgent issues in healthcare provision in the Czech Republic. The most pressing concern is the need for more efficient alcohol dependence treatment facilities (H1) to address the high per capita consumption of alcohol. There's also a need for improved facilities for the prevention and treatment of drug dependence (H2), and for effective mass publicity campaigns (H3) to combat peer pressure to drink. There's also a need for better facilities and resources to deal with cases of severe alcohol poisoning (H4). Coverage of essential health-related services (H5), while slightly lower in priority, remains an area for potential improvement. These challenges are compounded by a moderate level of suicides (M1), indicating a need for improved psychological and psychiatric support services to prevent mental health crises and save lives.

Projected trends over the next decade (Figure 2.4) suggest some improvements in alcohol and drug treatment facilities (H1, H2), due to an influx of qualified medical personnel in the face of geopolitical shocks and the easing of the impact of COVID-19. This could also increase the overall coverage of medical services (H5). However, peer pressure on the drinking culture could increase, leading to higher rates of alcohol (and drug) related deaths (H3, H4). The current economic, political, social and spiritual upheavals may exacerbate depression rates, making it a prominent health service issue (M2) in the coming years. In addition, geopolitical tensions, post-pandemic recovery and economic shocks could increase suicide rates, requiring an advanced psychological and psychiatric infrastructure in the Czech Republic (M1).

Dynamics of the macroeconomic indicators and the quantitative ethics index in the Czech Republic during the shocks of 2020–2024

While macroeconomic indicators reflect temporary phenomena, enduring economic strength lies in people and their ethics (Stiglitz, 2005). We have developed a unique approach to the quantitative measurement of ethics

Figure 2.4: Dynamics of healthcare coverage in the Czech Republic: a comprehensive analysis

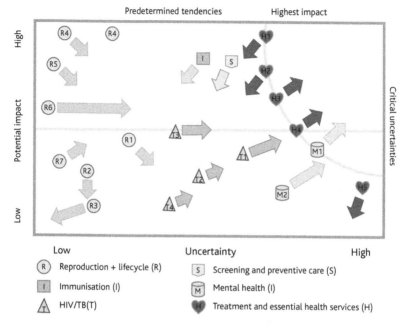

Note: The numerical values in the figure reflect the urgency of each health problem in the Czech Republic's health system:

• H1: Men consume 21–22 litres of pure alcohol per year, women 5–6 litres (2020; H*)

• H2: 1.05 drug-related deaths per 100,000 population (2020; M*)

• H3: More than 3/4 of adults drink alcohol (2018; H*)

• H4: 2.89 alcohol-related deaths per 100,000 population (2020; M*)

• H5: 84% coverage of basic health services (2022; H*)

• M1: 9.5 suicides per 100,000 inhabitants (2023; M*)

• M2: 3.84% of population with major depression (2023; M*)

• I: 95%–100% of children immunised (2023; H*)

• S: National Cervical Cancer Screening Programme (2015–2024); Most commonly used method: Cytology (from 2021)

• T1: 0.06% of adults living with HIV (2020–2022; L*)

• T2: 0.7% of tuberculosis patients with HIV (2023; L*)

• T3: 12% of HIV-positive people are women (2022; L*)

• T4: 0% of children under 5 have HIV (2020; L*)

• R1: Over 90% antenatal care coverage (2022; H*)

• R2: Good coverage (>80%) of reproductive services (2022; H*)

• R3: 99.8% of births attended by skilled health personnel (2018; H*)

• R4: 1.4 diarrhoea deaths per 100,000 population per year (2020; L*)

• R5: 15–17 adult + 2–3 child pneumonia deaths per 100,000 population per year (2021; M*)

(continued)

Figure 2.4: Dynamics of healthcare coverage in the Czech Republic: a comprehensive analysis (continued)

• R6: 54% contraceptive prevalence rate among women of reproductive age (2020; M*)

• R7:1-year postnatal care coverage (2024; H*)

* H: above world average; L: below world average; M: relatively close to world average

(by year, per capita [if applicable])
Source: Authors' calculations, relative per capita indicators used with projection of potential changes (arrows, authors' work) over the next decade. Data sources: WHO, UN, World Bank, Our World in Data.

(Shemetev, 2022; Shemetev and Pělucha, 2023). Figures 2.5 and 2.6 show the long-term potential of the Czech Republic compared to other countries in the world (Ethics Perception Index [ETPI]) and the differences within the Czech regions (regional ETPI).

The Czech Republic has a relatively high level of ethics compared to other countries, which should ensure its long-term prosperity. Thus, the core problems of the Czech Republic are not related to ethical issues, but to economic parameters and their sustainability in the face of negative shocks.

Impact of the period of economic instability (2020–2022) on the daily life of the population: national and regional perspective

The increase in GDP per capita alongside a decrease in GDP per capita PPP (at purchasing power parity) in the Czech Republic (Table 2.1) may be influenced by currency fluctuations, inflation rates, changes in the composition of the economy and statistical discrepancies.

An increase in gross fixed capital formation signals increased investment activity, the progressing process of digitisation of the economy following the possibilities of industry 4.0, which increases productivity, employment, infrastructure and attracts foreign investment.

A decline in household final consumption expenditure indicates an economic slowdown, affecting demand, sales, employment and government revenues, and may be influenced by various factors such as pandemics, government policies, territorial digital inequalities (especially in the urban-rural dimension) and external economic conditions.

The expansion of broad money points to an expansionary monetary policy aimed at stimulating economic activity, but requires vigilance to manage inflationary pressures and asset price bubbles.

The increase in net borrowing implies a larger deficit relative to GDP, which may reflect efforts to stimulate the economy, but requires careful fiscal management to maintain macroeconomic stability.

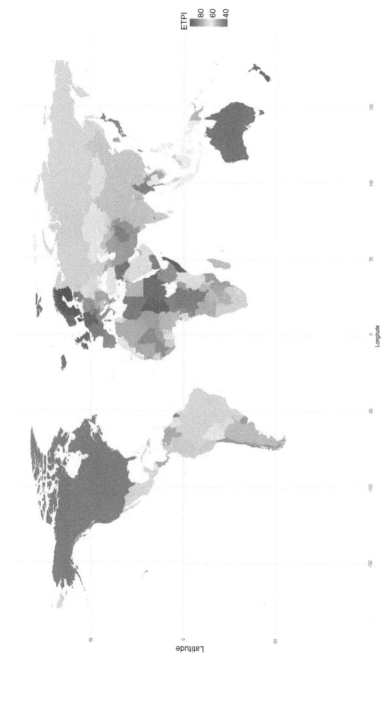

Figure 2.5: The Czech Republic in the Global Ethics Perception Index among 170 countries, 2023 (data to August 2024)

Source: Own elaboration in R; the methodology is based on Shemetev (2022).

Figure 2.6: Regional Ethics Perception Index rescaled to the Global Ethics Perception Index in the 14 regions of the Czech Republic, January 2022 (data to August 2024)

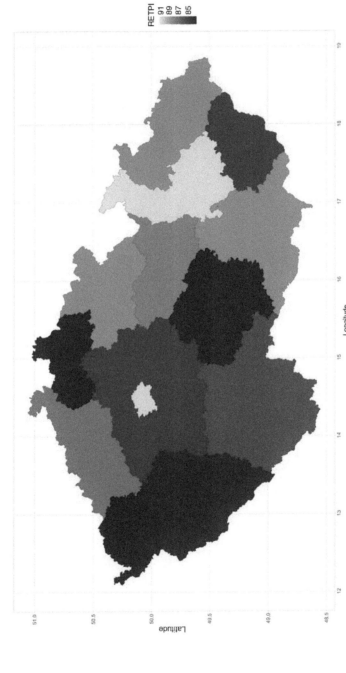

Note: The ethics parameter is related to education, human development, low corruption, freedom of enterprise and speech, human rights, negative impact on ecology for the sake of economic prosperity, and general interest in ethical issues (measured by internet search activity).
Source: Own elaboration in R; the methodology is based on Shemetev (2022) and Shemetev and Pělucha (2023).

Table 2.1: Dynamics of macroeconomic indicators in the Czech Republic, 2020–2022 versus 2011–2019

Name	Mean 2011–2019	Std.dev.	Min.	25%	Median	75%	Max.	Mean 2020–2022
GDP per capita (current US$)	20,655	1,999.62	17,829.70	19,870.80	20,133.17	21,871.27	23,664.85	24,907***
GDP per capita, PPP (constant 2017 international $)	36,519	2,838.26	33,661.47	34,002.19	36,168.42	38,824.89	40,989.73	18,638****
Gini index	25.71	0.59	24.9	25.3	25.9	26.1	26.5	26.2
Consumer price index (2010=100)	108.6	4.35	101.92	106.78	107.48	110.87	116.48	129.51***
Current health expenditure per capita (current US$)	1,517.63	176.19	1,284.05	1,387.41	1,516.56	1,554.51	1,803.05	2,119.8***
Imports of goods and services (% of GDP)	80.63	68.78	84.03	80.41	82.18	78.33	79.45	66.71
Exports of goods and services (% of GDP)	81.16	73.07	84.45	79.57	80.28	80.53	80.63	75.89
Net lending(+)/net borrowing(−) (% of GDP)	−1.21	1.48	−3.85	−2.25	−1.21	−0.32	0.68	−6.11***
Population, total (millions)	10.562	0.060	10.496	10.514	10.546	10.594	10.672	10.602*
Unemployment, total (% of total labour force) (national estimate)	4.77	2.04	2.02	2.89	5.05	6.71	6.98	2.67**
Urban population (% of total population)	73.5	0.26	73.18	73.29	73.48	73.67	73.92	74.14***

Note: Own elaboration in R (table), Excel and Google documents (design and final t-testing of differences between the periods).

*p<0.1;**p<0.05;***p<0.01 [2 tails]. Tested by common t-test. The borders values can have small shifts in both directions due to rounding. The data sources are Český statistický úřad (2024) and World Bank (2022), based on the Czech national statistics (where this selection is possible).

The data in the 'Mean 2020–2022' column are not included in the calculations for the following columns: Mean 2011–2019, Std.dev., Min., 25%, Median, 75%, Max.

The war in Ukraine and its economic impact on the Czech Republic

The war in Ukraine has had a moderate impact on the Czech economy, with indirect effects compared to neighbouring countries. The main effects include:

1. Trade disruption: The Czech Republic faces declining exports to Russia and Ukraine as war disrupts trade flows. Economic hardship and trade barriers in both countries have dampened demand for Czech goods and services, potentially affecting economic growth and specific industries (see Figure 2.7 for shifts in Czech exports to Russia).

Exports to Russia (Figure 2.7) peaked at around US$6 billion in 2013, halved in 2015–2016 following the events in Crimea and Donbass, and partially recovered over five years without fully reaching pre-2015 levels. They fell by around US$1.6 billion in 2022 (US$731.3 in 2023).

2. Energy dependence: Historically, the Czech Republic has relied heavily on Russian natural gas and oil transported through Ukrainian pipelines for its energy needs (Figure 2.8). However, significant changes have taken place since 2023–2024. The country has diversified its energy sources and now imports liquefied natural gas on a large scale from the United States, Azerbaijan, Kazakhstan and Arab countries. This shift has reduced dependence on Russian resources, easing concerns about energy security and potential disruptions from geopolitical conflict.

About nine out of every ten US dollars paid to Russia for imports between 2013 and 2022 were for mineral fuels (72.62 per cent in 2023, or US$2.52 billion [Trading Economics, 2024]), which have volatile prices, making the graph (Figure 2.8) look volatile. The highest prices for mineral fuels between 2013 and 2023 were in 2022, resulting in a high value of imports of US$11,370,818,689.00.

3. Investment and economic confidence: The political and military tensions in Ukraine have created uncertainty in the wider European region, affecting investor confidence. This uncertainty could lead to a decline in foreign direct investment into the Czech Republic, as investors become more cautious due to perceived geopolitical risks. Sectors such as manufacturing, services and infrastructure development could be affected. Parameters are estimated from the net investment position, using a rescaling formula for the rating (1):

$$\text{Re } scaled \ Rating_t \in [0;1] = \frac{Rating_t - \min(Rating_t)}{\max(Rating_t)};$$
$$\min(Rating_t) < 0; \max(Rating_t) \neq 0$$

The Eurostat (2023) methodology assigns Greece the lowest initial rating (−147 per cent of GDP, rescaled to 0 using formula [1]), while the Netherlands receives the highest rating (85 per cent of GDP, rescaled to 1 or 100 per cent using formula [1]). However, for time series analysis, adjustments are needed to ensure comparability across all periods by aligning with the global minimum and maximum values.

As of January 2023, the Czech Republic has a negative net investment position of −19.7 per cent of GDP (Figure 2.9), indicating that its foreign liabilities exceed its foreign assets (Eurostat, 2023; Trading Economics, 2023a). This implies a higher degree of foreign ownership of Czech assets, with potential implications such as capital outflows affecting local investment and economic stability. The negative position underscores the vulnerability to external shocks, highlighting the importance of maintaining stable external balances and effective debt management. Policy makers can consider strategies such as attracting foreign direct investment, encouraging domestic savings, promoting exports and prudent external debt management. While a negative net investment position isn't inherently harmful, vigilant monitoring is essential for financial stability and long-term economic resilience.

4. Sanctions: The Ukraine conflict has led to sanctions against Russia, affecting Czech companies with ties to Russia. Russian counter-sanctions, such as import restrictions, affect sectors such as agriculture. Further analysis of these sanctions and their interaction warrants separate studies.
5. Refugee crisis: The conflict in Ukraine has led to an influx of refugees into Europe, affecting the Czech Republic (Figure 2.10).

At the beginning of the conflict in Ukraine, the Czech Republic experienced an unprecedented influx of refugees, with the highest number per capita (around 4.5 per cent of the population) among EU countries (Maucorps et al, 2023: 8). By July 2023, over 530,000 Ukrainians had been granted temporary protection status in the country, with almost 350,000 in active status (UNHCR, 2024). Despite these challenges, the Czech response has shown remarkable regional and local flexibility. Looking forward, it is crucial to conduct a dedicated study to assess the impact of COVID-19 on this crisis and potential shocks to sectors such as the automotive industry and the wider economy.

Building on our previous research efforts, which examine the nuanced effects of COVID-19 on individual and family mobility in the Czech

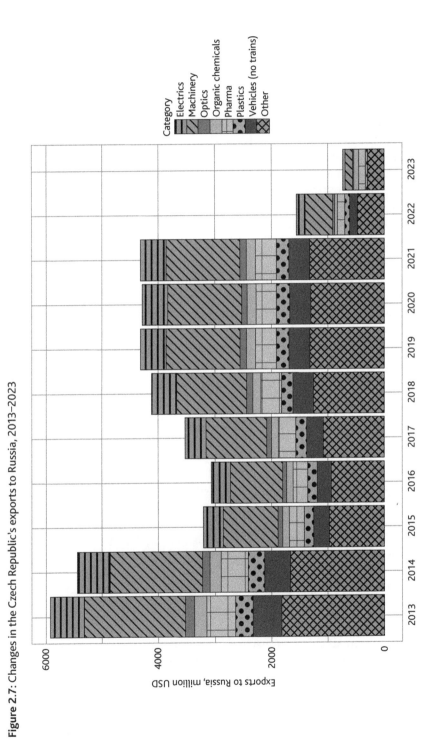

Figure 2.7: Changes in the Czech Republic's exports to Russia, 2013–2023

Figure 2.7: Changes in the Czech Republic's exports to Russia, 2013–2023 (continued)

Note: Own work in R based on statistical data from Český statistický úřad (2024), verified with the Trading Economics database (Trading Economics, 2023b) for 88 categories:

Electrical: electrical and electronic equipment (10%)

Machinery: machinery, nuclear reactors, boilers (about a third of total exports)

Optics: optical, photographic, engineering, medical equipment (2.4%)

Organic chemicals: organic chemicals (3.7%)

Pharmaceuticals: pharmaceutical products (8.7%)

Plastics: All types of plastics (5.3%)

Vehicles: Vehicles other than trains and trams (8.5%)

Other: including articles of iron or steel (2.2%), rubber (2%), beverages, spirits and vinegar (1.9%), toys, games, sports equipment (1.7%), dairy products, eggs, honey, edible products (1.7%), glass and glassware (1.6%), ceramic products (1.4%) and other miscellaneous items (18.1% in 74 categories).

Figure 2.8: Changes in the Czech Republic's imports from Russia, 2013–2023

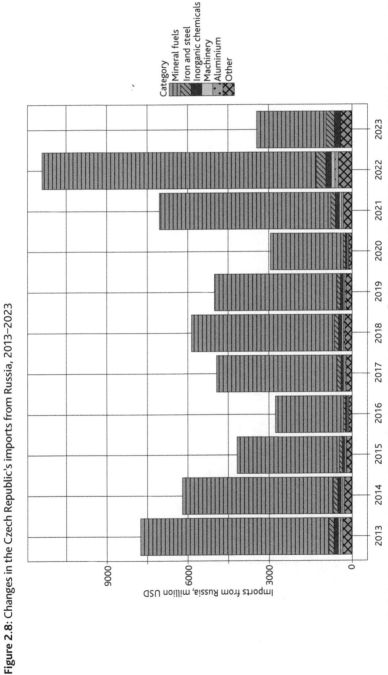

Note: Data are derived from own analysis conducted in R using statistical data from Český statistický úřad (2024), cross-checked with the Trading Economics database (Trading Economics, 2023c). The analysis includes information from 87 categories, including mineral fuels, iron and steel, inorganic chemicals, machinery, aluminium and other miscellaneous categories.

Figure 2.9: Rating of net investment positions in the European Union

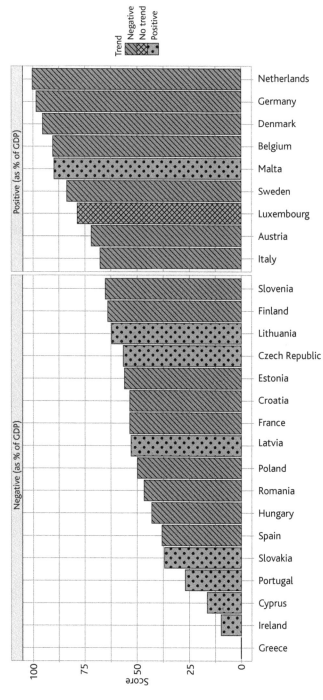

Note: Negative values indicate the negative percentage of the original index estimated by Eurostat (Eurostat, 2023) relative to GDP, while positive values indicate the positive percentage of the original index relative to GDP. The 'Trend' column indicates the actual trend observed between July 2022 and January 2023, with positive values indicating an increase, negative values indicating a decrease and 'no trend' indicating no change.

Source: Own work in R. Data are derived from Eurostat (2023) and verified with the Trading Economics database (Trading Economics, 2023a).

Figure 2.10: Countries with largest number of refugees from Ukraine, percentage of total refugees (up to August 2024, if data available; if not, then latest available date)

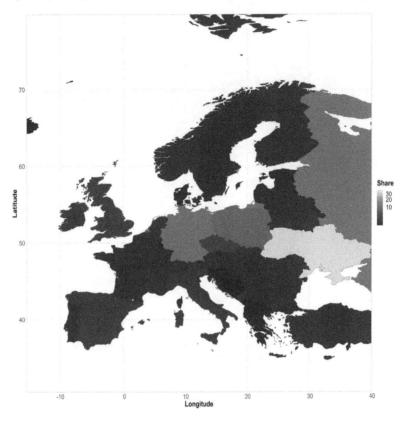

Note: Own work in R. The methodology combines data from various sources, including the European Commission (2023), Statista (2024) and United Nations Refugee Agency (2023), which have been rescaled into percentages. However, the statistics for Russia are outdated, with no data available after 3 October 2022. Data for the other countries, except Luxembourg, are recent and dated 2023. The distribution of refugees from Ukraine between Kosovo and Serbia is approximated as two-thirds in Serbia and one-third in Kosovo due to limited data. The total number of people in Serbia and Kosovo is consistent with data from Statista (2024) and the United Nations Refugee Agency (2023).

Republic from 2020 to 2021 (Shemetev et al, 2021), our investigation expands to explore the potential positive economic impact of stay-at-home policies during pandemics on county-level consumption and employment dynamics in the United States (Shemetev and Pělucha, 2022).

Conclusion

In examining the dynamics of health policy and social wellbeing in the Czech Republic, this chapter highlights the multiple factors that shape the social and resilience outlook of individuals and families. Economic indicators, including GDP per capita and unemployment rates, as well as ethical norms, access to healthcare and the impact of geopolitical events, such as the war in Ukraine and the influx of refugees, all influence the social outlook of Czech citizens. By comprehensively examining these factors, policy makers gain invaluable insights into the nuanced dynamics of social outlooks, enabling them to design targeted interventions aimed at fostering inclusive growth, resilience and societal wellbeing. The introduction of innovative tools such as the GUIM further enhances policy makers' ability to prioritise health indicators and address pressing issues in the Czech Republic's complex social landscape. By using this comprehensive understanding of the factors influencing social outcomes, policy makers can advance the overarching goals of social justice, equity and sustainable development in the Czech Republic and beyond.

Acknowledgements

This particular chapter was funded by the Czech Science Foundation (GACR), Grant:20–17810S 'Rural resilience in the context of trends in urban-rural digital divide'.

References

Český statistický úřad [Czech Statistical Office] (2024) Metainformation System Available at: https://www.czso.cz

European Commission (2023) *Romania: Report on the National Response to Those Displaced from Ukraine*. Available at: https://ec.europa.eu/migrant-inte gration/library-document/romania-report-national-response-those-displa ced-ukraine_en#:~:text=According to official figures%2C as,from Ukraine registered in Romania

Eurostat (2023) *International Investment Position Statistics – Statistics Explained*. Available at: https://ec.europa.eu/eurostat/statistics-explained/index. php?title=International_investment_position_statistics

Maucorps, A., Moshammer, B., Pindyuk, O., Tverdostup, M., Gorzelak, G., Khrapunenko, M., Kaldur, K., Zavarska, Z. and Castelli, C. (2023) *The Use of Cohesion Policy Funds to Support Refugees from Ukraine: STUDY Requested by the REGI Committee*. Available at: https://www.europarl.europa.eu/ RegData/etudes/STUD/2023/747249/IPOL_STU(2023)747249_EN.pdf

Schoemaker, P.J.H. and van der Heijden, C.A.J.M. (1992) Integrating scenarios into strategic planning at Royal Dutch/Shell. *Planning Review*, 20(3): 41–46.

Shemetev, A. (2022) The quantitative estimation of ethics: the regional and national index of ethics (the Ethics Perception Index [ETPI]). *DETUROPE – The Central European Journal of Regional Development and Tourism*, 13(3): 73–97.

Shemetev, A. and Pělucha, M. (2022) Are pandemics and stay-at-home orders economic factors? An analysis of their impact on employment and consumption in the USA. *Forum Scientiae Oeconomia*, 10(3): 169–188.

Shemetev, A. and Pělucha, M. (2023) Cultivating prosperity and resilience: a holistic approach to societal progress through moral-ethical growth indices. *DETUROPE – The Central European Journal of Regional Development and Tourism*, 15(3): 32–77.

Shemetev, A., Feurich, M. and Mitwallyova, H. (2021) Regional disparities in Covid and mobility in the Czech Republic (with patterns for employment). In V. Klímová and V. Žítek (eds), *24th International Colloquium on Regional Sciences: Conference Proceedings*. Masaryk University of Brno, pp 204–213. https://doi.org/10.5817/CZ.MUNI.P210-9896-2021-25

Statista (2024) *Estimated Number of Refugees from Ukraine Recorded in Europe and Asia since February 2022 as of May 9, 2023, by Selected Country*. Available at: https://www.statista.com/statistics/1312584/ukrainian-refugees-by-country/

Stiglitz, J.E. (2005) The ethical economist. Growth may be everything, but it's not the only thing. Review essay of 'The Moral Consequences of Economic Growth by B.M. Friedman', Knopf, 2005. *Foreign Affairs*, 84(6): 128–134.

Tesch, J.F. (ed.). (2019) *Business model innovation in the era of the Internet of Things: Studies on the aspects of evaluation, decision making and tooling* (2nd ed.). Cham: Springer.

Trading Economics (2023a) *Czech Republic: Net International Investment Position*. Available at: https://tradingeconomics.com/czech-republic/net-international-investment-position-eurostat-data.html

Trading Economics (2023b) *Czech Republic Exports to Russia*. Available at: https://tradingeconomics.com/czech-republic/exports/russia#:~:text= Czech Republic Exports to Russia was US%241.56 Billion during,updated on June of 2023

Trading Economics (2023c) *Czech Republic Imports from Russia*. Available at: https://tradingeconomics.com/czech-republic/imports/russia#:~:text= Czech Republic Imports from Russia was US%2411.37 Billion during,updated on June of 2023

Trading Economics (2024) *Czech Republic Imports from Russia (2023)*. Available at: https://tradingeconomics.com/czech-republic/imports/russia

UNHCR (2024) *Czech Republic*. Available at: https://www.unhcr.org/countries/czech-republic

United Nations Refugee Agency (2023) *Ukraine*. Available at: https://reporting.unhcr.org/operational/operations/ukraine#:~:text=At the end of October,of them women and children.

WAQI (2024). *World's Air Pollution: Real-Time Air Quality Index for More than 10,000 Stations in the World*. World Air Quality Index Project. Available at: https://waqi.info/#/c/26.313/16.13/2.5z

World Bank (2022) *World Bank Open Data.* Available at: https://data.worldb ank.org/

World Health Organization (2018) *Global Reference List of 100 Core Health Indicators (Plus Health-Related SDGs)*, edited by R. Schürch, 1st edn. World Health Organization. Available at: https://score.tools.who.int/fileadmin/ uploads/score/Documents/Enable_data_use_for_policy_and_action/ 100_Core_Health_Indicators_2018.pdf

3

Why is the Doomsday Clock not working? Rethinking the characteristics of effective drivers of change

Annalisa Sannino

Introduction

During the same weeks in the spring of 2023, when Finland joined the North Atlantic Treaty Organization (NATO) in response to the war in Ukraine, the Science and Security Board of the *Bulletin of the Atomic Scientists* moved the hands of the Doomsday Clock to 90 seconds before midnight, the closest to nuclear winter ever. This chapter delves into the contradictions of collective action urgently needed in response to the most acute wicked challenges of our time. The Doomsday Clock is aimed at stimulating reflexivity on the urgency of limiting arms and enhancing disarmament by mutual consent (Mathur, 2020).

Over the years, the Doomsday Clock has become the emblematic stimulus explicitly meant to awaken humanity to take action to avert reaching the point of no return. The drawing of what became the iconic Doomsday Clock was produced in 1947 by artist Martyl Langsdorf, upon the request of the so-called Chicago atomic scientists who worked in the Manhattan Project. Langsdorf was actually married to a scientist who worked in the project, directly exposed to the anxieties and concerns of these scientists in the aftermath of the atomic bombs that were dropped on Hiroshima and Nagasaki. The drawing was made with the specific aim to convey the scientists' concerns about the risks of nuclear technology for life on the planet and to foster citizens' mobilisation and engagement to influence the political leadership.

Change, understood as major reforms and organisational transformations, is inevitably linked with the economy and the market. Such a link is no longer a tendency or a deliberate priority. Globally it represents the very nature of dominant perceptions of change and development in contemporary societies. As a consequence, change efforts that reveal tangible transformative potential and might even take momentum from the self-organising ability of local communities tend to remain outside the frame of 'significant reforms'. In spite of this asymmetry, the literature makes it clear that drivers of change competing with this dominant focus on economics and market-based principles, when persistent and resilient, can eventually influence the directions of significant change and strengthen social determinants of health. The following statement by comparative public management scholar Lois Recascino Wise (2002: 564) is an example:

> One side is likely to dominate the other at a given point in time, but the balance is bound to shift. Both sets of reform drivers remain present, despite the fact that one is more influential than the other. The dominance of rational determinants of change foretells the return to influence of alternative drivers of change such as social equity, democratization, and humanization.

While hopeful and encouraging, these considerations raise the issue of how the affordances of alternative drivers can be enhanced to become more impactful and influential, especially against the background of the urgency to support life on our planet.

The chapter attempts to contribute to discussions on drivers of change and stability and social determinants of health, by examining why the Doomsday Clock has not generated the outcomes it was designed to attain. The analysis focuses on the specific affordances of the Doomsday Clock and their particular limitations as potential drivers of change by means of collective action. The analysis builds on a cultural-historical perspective which offers conceptual instruments for rethinking the characteristics of effective drivers of change.

Is the Doomsday Clock failing to drive change?

In analyses of crises of nuclear pacifism, the low capacity for sustained mobilisation has been typically attributed to inadequate collective leadership structures, decentralised decision-making as well as to underdeveloped indirect institutionalisation and social invention. The latter two resources, in particular, have been considered as holding the greatest promise of support and policy impact for nuclear pacifism (Wehr, 1986).

Since its creation, the Doomsday Clock has been adjusted 25 times. The resetting is determined upon deliberation of an expert panel including 18 Nobel laureates who consider initiatives from different countries on nuclear weapons, also in connection with the climate crisis and novel technological developments. Midnight symbolically represents the end of the world. References to 'the failure of international institutions to respond to the ticking clock' (for example, Beard et al, 2023: 15) are not rare. It is therefore warranted to ask why the Doomsday Clock might have failed to drive the change it was designed to attain.

The notion of drivers of change has been in scholarly and policy use for several decades across the most diverse scientific domains. In life sciences, for instance in the field of hydrobiology, drivers of change are defined as the human factors that cause modifications in the ecosystems and biodiversity on which the wellbeing of humans themselves and of other species depend (Gutiérrez et al, 2023). Human intervention has reached a point at which it has irreversibly affected the basic life-supporting equilibrium. In turn, underpinning resources and processes are also gravely affected. These include resources such as clean water and raw materials for safe consumption, regulating dynamics such as climate, decomposition and water purification, and cultural benefits of cognitive, aesthetic and spiritual kind, for instance.

The literature distinguishes between triggers and drivers of change and also direct and indirect drivers. From a political economic perspective of welfare states, Guiraudon and Martin (2012) refer to triggers of change as drastic global turns which cannot wait to be addressed, concerning, for instance, population trends, economic production and inequalities. The authors point out that triggers of change differ from drivers of change in that the latter are deliberate initiatives by actors and interest collectives. With this characterisation, the notion of drivers of change can be understood as applying to times in which 'emergency' factors pertaining to the triggers of change are not in place. Assuming that such times would be globally still an option today, drivers of change would involve power struggles and strategising.

Direct drivers of change are both natural and anthropogenic factors which exert pressure on biodiversity or ecosystem processes (Babai et al, 2021). Climate change is an obvious example. Changes in traditional land-use systems for agricultural production and indigenous sociocultural activities are also examples of direct drivers of change. Indirect drivers are factors such as economics and demographics which impact direct drivers as well as formal and informal social institutions.

The Russia–Ukraine war, along with the destruction, displacement and suffering typical of all wars, entails grave dangers of military escalation. The Eisenhower Media Network (2023) in a statement commenting on the war recalled the words of President John F. Kennedy as being crucial for survival:

> Above all, while defending our own vital interests nuclear powers must avert those confrontations which bring an adversary to a choice of either a humiliating retreat or a nuclear war. To adopt that course in the nuclear age would be evidence only of the bankruptcy of our policy–or of a collective death-wish for the world.

Yet, according to the Network, profits from weapons sales represented a major factor behind the NATO expansion.

Affordances and limitations of the Doomsday Clock

The announcement of the Doomsday Clock being set at 90 seconds to midnight came on 24 January 2023. The resetting of the clock was due largely to the Ukraine war and the possibility of nuclear escalation. In the press release, Mary Robinson, Chair of The Elders and former UN High Commissioner for Human Rights, stated the following:

> The Doomsday Clock is sounding an alarm for the whole of humanity. We are on the brink of a precipice. But our leaders are not acting at sufficient speed or scale to secure a peaceful and liveable planet. From cutting carbon emissions to strengthening arms control treaties and investing in pandemic preparedness, we know what needs to be done. The science is clear, but the political will is lacking. This must change in 2023 if we are to avert catastrophe. We are facing multiple, existential crises. Leaders need a crisis mindset. (Quoted in Spinazze, 2023)

In the arts, critical theory, literature and philosophy, clocks have not been typically portrayed in a very good light and as serving emancipatory and liberatory ends. On the contrary, they have come to symbolise capitalist forms of control and domination and for this reason they rarely appear as resources in participatory or activist endeavours:

> When trying to imagine a new time, a transformed time, a way of living time that is inclusive, sustainable or socially just – a liberatory time – it is unlikely that a clock will spring to mind. If anything, the clock has become the symbol of all that has gone wrong with our relationship to time. (Bastian, 2017: 41)

An exception to this is a clock described in a classic sociocultural experiment, originally conducted in Germany in the laboratory of Kurt Lewin, and then taken up by Lev S. Vygotsky as a prototypical example of how will arises (Sannino and Engeström, 2023). Ongoing discussions within sociocultural and cultural historical approaches to collective transformative agency (Sannino, 2022; Hopwood and Sannino, 2023) often refer to this Lewinian/ Vygotskian clock example as a potentially emancipatory and liberatory use of such an artefact. This specific use of a clock will be discussed in this chapter.

Barad's (2017) philosophical conceptualisation of human engagement by means of a clock starts by comparing the Doomsday Clock and the Hiroshima Peace Clock as two different ways of articulating time. The Doomsday Clock is synchronised to the apocalypse, whereas the Hiroshima Peace Clock is synchronised to peace. Both clocks serve the purpose of counteracting nuclear destruction. Also they function in similar ways, by being reset when there is a war or a nuclear test. The main difference between these two clocks lies in their specific epistemological orientation, towards destruction in the case of the Doomsday Clock and towards a future of peace in the case of the Hiroshima Peace Clock.

The idea of the end of civilisation is part of humanity's cultural heritage across its history. The prophecies of the apocalypse are an example (Vidal, 2015). Today, as studies from environmental sciences announce in journals such as *Nature* that the end is close with an irreversible collapse of Earth's ecosystems (Fortelius et al, 2012), 'the only difference between previous eras and our own is that the forecasting sciences and theories have come to replace prophecies' (Vidal, 2015: 175). As they typically offer no concrete alternative course of action, prophecies and forecasts alone are notoriously ineffective as drivers of change. This may also largely explain the apparently meagre impact of the Doomsday Clock.

Transformative agency as a new perspective

Understanding processes of collective agency formation is necessary to respond to today's acute learning and development challenges. As the discussions on social determinants of health amply demonstrate, these challenges are increasingly also challenges of equity and social justice which require multi-agency initiatives across sectoral and hierarchical boundaries. They require the mobilisation of the whole society with its organisations and neighborhoods. Cultural-historical scholarship on transformative agency in the learning sciences may contribute to these discussions (Sannino, 2022). Vygotskian perspectives on how human beings may become able to transform their circumstances is at the core of this perspective.

Originally described by Vygotsky (1997/1931), transformative agency (more accurately, transformative agency by double stimulation, or TADS for short) is a process by which individuals or collectives can intentionally break out of conflicts of motives and change their circumstances by turning to artefacts (also called second stimuli). The process goes as follows: A challenging situation triggers a paralysing conflict of motives (also called first stimulus). In trying to cope with a challenge, people may turn to an artefact (for example, a clock) and decide to rely on this when specific instances of the challenging situation reoccur. Each new instance of the challenging situation is cognitively and emotionally critical in that it reactivates the conflicting motives. When people actually put into use the second stimulus, this implementation helps them to gain control of and to transform the challenging situation into one that is more understandable and manageable.

The repeated implementation of the second stimulus strengthens their understanding of the challenge and capacity to take further actions. As a result, the challenging situation is transformed into one that can be actually dealt with.

In this agency process the second stimulus is an artefact that serves as support for transformative action. In Vygotsky's (1997/1931) description of an experiment originally realised in the research group of Kurt Lewin (Sannino and Engeström, 2023), participants were asked to take part in an experiment but found themselves in a room in which nothing was happening. Torn between the motive of remaining in the room where nothing was going on and the motive to move on with their lives, the participants would use the clock on the wall as a second stimulus. One would say, for instance, 'When the clock strikes two, I will leave', and then the person would actually leave when the clock struck two. By so doing, people would break out of the paralysing conflict of motives and exert wilful initiatives with the support of the artefact.

Vygotsky (1997/1931) used this 'waiting' experiment as a paradigmatic example of the transformative agency process. My research group replicated the experiment after Vygotsky's description, first with 25 individuals and then with 30 collectives of three to four participants (Sannino and Laitinen, 2015; Sannino, 2016). The results are in line with the original description by Vygotsky of the process of transformative agency.

A wide range of artefacts may be used as second stimuli depending on the challenging situation and available resources. They can be, for instance, material things (a clock, a calendar, a cup of coffee, a string tied around a finger) or discursive entities (a discussion on a specific topic, a set of questions, a song). What makes these artefacts second stimuli is that people deliberately take them up to face the conflict of motives triggered by the challenging situation. In the experiment participants amidst the uncertainty of the experiment used the clock as a resource to find the courage to leave the room.

We may think of a clock or an artefact as an anchor (Sannino, 2022). Anchors are commonly understood as stabilising devices to prevent a vessel from moving. However, not all anchors have this function. Beside the heavy-weight anchors, there are also kedge anchors serving the purpose of 'warping', that is, pulling the anchor once it has settled on the ground, for moving the vessel away from the problem area, for instance when the vessel has to be moved against the wind. Anchoring by stabilising devices to prevent a vessel from moving can be contrasted with 'anchoring forward' which requires movement into the unknown, dealing with uncertainty.

This type of anchoring or warping does not only consist of a movement forward. This would be inconceivable in turbulent waters. Tendentially it is a movement forward which nevertheless cannot exclude stabilising episodes. Similarly transformative agency is a process of step-by-step material grounding in the attempt to transcend troubled 'waters'.

Actions of throwing the kedge anchor are made in the attempt to find suitable ground. These are search actions. However, only when the kedge anchor hits the ground the crew gains control of the situation and is able to pull the vessel out of harm's way. These are taking-over actions: the vessel is still in the troubled area, but the crew is able to manoeuvre it. Breaking-out actions occur when the vessel is moved away from the problem area.

In our experiments all participants displayed search actions involving artefacts, that is, the throwing of kedge anchors was initiated in the attempt to find suitable ground. However, only when the participants put the adopted artefact into actual use, for instance by making a decision to leave when the clock would strike a certain hour, they would gain control of the challenging situation and be able to pull themselves out of the stall.

In the experiments, the participants turned to material means to search for a suitable ground for gaining control over the situation. In the large majority of these cases the participants reported experiencing conflicts of motives which were overcome by means of finding support in artefacts, including the clock on the wall of the experiment room.

The demands set by a challenge and related conflict of motives may lead to the use of a single artefact or to combine multiple artefacts. This is an aspect of transformative agency which still requires further investigation. However, it is clear that some challenging situations are of such nature that they require breaking out of established habitual or conventional patterns and acquiring new ones. For this, a single process of transformative agency by double stimulation is naturally insufficient and multiple reiterations are necessary.

The Vygotskian clock is deliberately adopted by individuals and collectives as means for action, signalled by the clock striking a certain hour. The Doomsday Clock, instead, represents stimuli signalling that it is too late to act. Vidal (2015: 178) describes very clearly how these stimuli, signalling that we are heading towards a known catastrophic end point, disorient and divert from action rather than afford agency.

> [F]rom a socio-cognitive perspective, besides exalting the power and domination of the modern man (only a few political decisions and a few eco-citizen efforts can change the outcome of our planet), as well as the thrilling notion of an imminent and unprecedented death … effectively carrying a new and techno-scientific Sword of Damocles over our heads, the Doomsday Clock contributes largely to usurping the power that, up until now, was intended for only the highest elite of professionals.

This way the Doomsday Clock might work against its own purpose. When it is not altogether ignored, it displays affordances that divert the public from adopting it as a mediator for emancipatory action. Vidal (2015) interprets the functioning of the clock as conducive to paralysis between anxiety and alarmism. This applies also to other timely variations of doomsday alarms.

> Psychologists and communications experts have demonstrated that fear can also lead to disengagement. … Actors are not only reflecting accurate climate science but also engaging in emotional rhetoric. The discourse of fear that presents climate change itself as the main threat to human rights, moreover, contributes to framing climate change primarily as a physical and scientific problem and obscures other important dimensions of climate change. (Saab, 2023: 113)

From the perspective of the cultural-historical theory of transformative agency adopted here, the Doomsday Clock does not even provoke a paralysis of the will. The stimuli of anxiety and alarmism do not lead to clashing motives that create productive tension conducive to transformative action.

Rethinking the characteristics of effective drivers of change

Time marked by a clock in its connection to mature capitalism in Western societies is dominated by exchange value. This goes to the extent that time is permeated with an artificial sense of urgency (Albright, 2023). The saying *time is money* conveys precisely that we need to make the most of the limited time we have for profit. Capitalist logics of time tend to operate this way at all levels, from the individual who throws plastic waste in the ocean to major corporations and political actors who depend on them. The politics of time, today more than ever, call for actionable collective awareness for reshaping our engagements with time. This means resisting and designing alternatives to the emphases of capitalist clock time: 'Time is to be maximized for profit, often leading to worker exploitation. … Time within a capitalist structure is transferred into monetized exchange units, and capitalism is about the minimal inputs producing maximized outputs' (Albright, 2023: 6–7).

Bastian's critical cartography perspective (2017) argues that, like maps, also clocks can serve the purpose of agentive initiatives for just and sustainable change. In line with this 'horology' view, the cultural-historical conceptual framework adopted here explores the functioning of the Doomsday Clock against the background of discussions on drivers of change, by starting from the assumption that clocks have the potential to be redesigned for opening new horizons within the politics of time.

The editor of the *Bulletin of the Atomic Scientists*, John Mecklin, in the introduction to the 2018 issue, 'Good news in perilous times', lamented that accusations of fear-mongering have occasionally reached the bulletin. Instead, atomic scientists should be praised for doing exactly the opposite:

> The magazine, its editors, and its authors could more accurately be charged with hope-mongering, having for more than 70 years aggressively pushed the idea that humans can control the technology they create and use it for the benefit of humanity, rather than its destruction. We are mongering that hope again, very purposely. (Mecklin, 2018: 1)

For the past 75 years, the Doomsday Clock has played a role in public discussions globally on the trade-offs of the benefits and risks of science and technology, advantages for enhancing life and serious danger. However, from the conceptual perspective adopted here, trade-offs are not enough to foster transformative action, as long as the stimuli that the clock affords do not trigger conflicts of motives, that is, a context of forward-looking productive tension.

The heterogeneity of geopolitical contexts calls for an exploration of diverse ways in which drivers of change may actually have impact. Drivers of change meant to operate at a global scale have been found to fulfil this promise only to a rather limited extent. Referring to agriculture, for instance, Hazell and Wood (2008) point out the limited value of global drivers. Although these offer a broad perspective, their contribution is far from significant when it comes to the actual design of sustainable strategies when food surpluses and widespread hunger coexist and agricultural growth in many ways leads to environmental degradation, due to unsustainable farming systems and country-specific economic contexts.

The limitations of global drivers point at the role local actors can play in influencing specific drivers at country and local scales, and are key structural determinants of health (see Figure I.1 in the Introduction). The role of frontline practitioners as policy makers in their own right is too often equated with protests and strikes only. Within a perspective of street-level bureaucracy (Lipsky, 1980), however, the specific ways in which individuals and collectives can foster just policies in public services may be much more potent when they translate into the situated actions of their own activities. It is at this level that actual resistance, reduction of the severity of reckless political decisions, as well as novel solutions and innovations, can be realised. When sufficiently grounded in the collective activities of the civil society with persistence and resilience, these 'policy-making actions from below' eventually do reach the heights of formal powers.

When decisions which owe to be urgently made in the interest of the commons are delayed or, worse, not even considered, it is easy to lose faith in change. History demonstrates, however, that science and activism together with capable progressive politics can make a difference (Chomsky, 2022). Eventually it is only up to those who really care to reach out to others for exploring grey areas of possibilities and act accordingly with coherence and determination.

Conclusion

In *Disaster Politics: Surviving End Times*, the sociologist Steve Matthewman builds a potent perspective based on lessons learned in Aotearoa New Zealand, one of the most disaster-prone countries globally and, more specifically, Ōtautahi Christchurch. This is a city that for decades has already seen it all, with earthquakes, floods, wildfires and a terrorist attack. Following the earthquake that struck New Zealand in 2011, part of the city had to be entirely rebuilt on the ruins of its historical central area.

> In liberal democracies the ultimate determinant is the electoral cycle. The climate crisis compels major transformation if our species, and indeed all others, are to prosper. For the privileged populations of the world this necessitates a radical politics of the other, prioritising those in entirely different spatial, temporal and social locations. And it entails a massive expansion of the democratic imagination, as it means that those in the Global North must cede to those in the Global South, who will suffer the most from climate heating. It means thinking about those yet to be born in order to enact inter-generational justice, and it means thinking about non-human others. (Matthewman, 2023: 3)

The approach conveyed here can be crystallised in the expression: 'There is nothing more practical than a theoretical approach to disasters' (Alexander, 2013). Theoretical reflection on the politics of existential threats and the hard choices they entail remain indispensable (Zala, 2023), precisely because this can foster the productive tension of conflicting motives referred to earlier. The framework of transformative agency by double stimulation (TADS), briefly introduced in this chapter, may be regarded as an additional theoretical resource in the service of practical transformations.

Referring to the legally binding international agreement of the Treaty on the Prohibition of Nuclear Weapons (Ruff, 2021) against which actions and inaction relating to nuclear weapons are measured, Jo-Ansie van Wyk (2021) from the South African Institute of International Affairs reminds us that the next phase of disarmament diplomacy needs to include multilateralism, global civil society and nuclear norm 'antipreneurs'. Voices from the global south, such as van Wyk's (2021), are of paramount importance to listen to as they are filled with the power of collectives actually striving for life – collectives we ought to join forces with.

The World Health Organization's (2010) *Conceptual Framework for Action on the Social Determinants of Health* includes an important section on social participation and empowerment. The report points out that 'in contrast to other progressive intellectual currents dominated by voices from the global north, groundbreaking work on empowerment and gender emerged from the south' (WHO, 2010: 59). The report further states that 'the increased ability of oppressed and marginalized communities to control key processes that affect their lives is the essence of empowerment as we understand it' (WHO, 2010: 59). These statements are *de facto* a call for nurturing collective transformative agency as a precondition and driving force for significant improvements in social determinants of health. The emphasis on communities locates the transformative potential at the ground level, in common people's policy-making actions from below.

When collectives design and perform policy-making actions from below, they may benefit from reflecting on three lessons stemming from studies based on the TADS framework. First, to generate transformative agency, we need to identify and make explicit the conflict of motives that paralyses those whose actions could make a difference. Second, to overcome the paralysing conflict of motives, we need to construct suitable artefacts or kedge anchors that will serve as support for transformative action. Third, we need to adopt and put into practice the artefactual resource time and again, in multiple iterations, so that new patterns of emancipatory action stabilise and gain generative power to spread and multiply.

References

Albright, T. (2023) A teacher residency's entanglement with time: 'we always say we will get to it, but we never do'. *Educational Philosophy and Theory*, 55(13): 1487–1500.

Alexander, D. (2013) Talk no. 1: there is nothing more practical than a theoretical approach to disasters. Available at: http://emergency-planning.blogspot.com/2013/05/talk-no-1-there-is-nothing-more.html

Babai, D., Jánó, B. and Molnár, Z. (2021) In the trap of interacting indirect and direct drivers: the disintegration of extensive, traditional grassland management in Central and Eastern Europe. *Ecology and Society*, 26(4): Article 6.

Barad, K.M. (2017) Troubling time/s and ecologies of nothingness: re-turning, remembering, and facing the incalculable. *New Formations*, 92(92): 56–86.

Bastian, M. (2017) Liberating clocks: developing a critical horology to rethink the potential of clock time. *New Formations*, 92(92): 41–55.

Beard, S.J., Rees, M., Richards, C. and Rojas C.R. (eds) (2023) *The Era of Global Risk: An Introduction to Existential Risk Studies*. Cambridge: Open Book Publishers.

Chomsky, N. (2022) *Chronicles of Dissent*. London: Penguin.

Eisenhower Media Network (2023) Russia-Ukraine War: the U.S. should be a force for peace. 23 May. Available at: https://eisenhowermedianetwork.org/russia-ukraine-war-peace/

Fortelius, M., Getz, W.M., Harte, J., Hastings, A., Marquet, P.A., Martinez, N.D., et al (2012) Approaching a state shift in Earths biosphere. *Nature*, 486(7401): 52–58.

Guiraudon, V. and Martin, C. (2012) Drivers for change. In B. Greve (ed), *Routledge Handbook of the Welfare State*. London: Routledge, pp 283–291.

Gutiérrez, M.R.V.A., Nicolás-Ruiz, N., Sánchez-Montoya, M.D.M. and Alonso, M.L.S. (2023) Ecosystem services provided by dry river socio-ecological systems and their drivers of change. *Hydrobiologia*, 850: 2585–2607.

Hazell, P. and Wood, S. (2008) Drivers of change in global agriculture. *Philosophical Transactions of the Royal Society B: Biological Sciences*, 363(1491): 495–515.

Hopwood, N. and Sannino, A. (eds) (2023) *Agency and Transformation: Motives, Mediation, and Motion*. Cambridge: Cambridge University Press.

Lipsky, M. (1980) *Street-Level Bureaucracy: Dilemmas of the Individual in Public Services*. London: Russell Sage.

Mathur, R. (2020) *Civilizational Discourses in Weapons Control*. Cham: Palgrave Macmillan.

Matthewman, S. (2023) Disaster politics: surviving end times. *E-International Relations*. Available at: https://www.e-ir.info/pdf/100890

Mecklin, J. (2018) Introduction: good news in perilous times. *Bulletin of the Atomic Scientists*, 74(1): 1.

Ruff, T. (2021) Advancing the TPNW. *The Nuclear Ban Treaty*, 160–163.

Saab, A. (2023) Discourses of fear on climate change in international human rights law. *European Journal of International Law*, 34(1): 113–135.

Sannino, A. (2016) Double stimulation in the waiting experiment with collectives: testing a Vygotskian model of the emergence of volitional action. *Integrative Psychological and Behavioral Science*, 50(1): 142–173.

Sannino, A. (2022) Transformative agency as warping: how collectives accomplish change amidst uncertainty. *Pedagogy, Culture & Society*, 30(1): 9–33.

Sannino, A. and Laitinen, A. (2015) Double stimulation in the waiting experiment: testing a Vygotskian model of the emergence of volitional action. *Learning, Culture and Social Interaction*, 4: 4–18.

Sannino, A. and Engeström, Y. (2023) In search of an experiment: from Vygotsky to Lewin and Dembo and back to the future. In P. Marsico and L. Tateo (eds), *Humanity in Psychology: The Intellectual Legacy of Pina Boggi Cavallo*. Cham: Springer, pp 159–177.

Spinazze, G. (2023) Press release: Doomsday Clock set at 90 seconds to midnight. 24 January. Available at: https://thebulletin.org/2023/01/press-release-doomsday-clock-set-at-90-seconds-to-midnight/

van Wyk, J.-A. (2021) 100 seconds to midnight: what could be done to bolster nuclear disarmament globally? *South African Institute of International Affairs (SAIIA)*. Available at: https://saiia.org.za/research/100-seconds-to-midnight-what-could-be-done-to-bolster-nuclear-disarmament-globally/

Vidal, B. (2015) Doomsday Clock: the apocalypse and the scientific imaginary. *A Journal of the Social Imaginary*, 6(4): 171–183.

Vygotsky, L.S. (1997/1931) Self-control. In *The Collected Works of L. S. Vygotsky: The History of the Development of Higher Mental Functions*, Vol 4. New York: Plenum, pp 207–219.

Wehr, P. (1986) Nuclear pacifism as collective action. *Journal of Peace Research*, 23(2): 103–113.

WHO (2010) *A Conceptual Framework for Action on the Social Determinants of Health*. Geneva: World Health Organization.

Wise, L.R. (2002) Public management reform: competing drivers of change. *Public Administration Review*, 62(5): 556–567.

Zala, B. (2023) 'No one around to shut the dead eyes of the human race': Sartre, Aron, and the limits of existentialism in the Nuclear Age. *Review of International Studies*: 1–18.

4

The role of religion in long-term Ukrainian–Russian reconciliation

Rebecca Harrocks

Introduction

For centuries, Ukrainians and Russians have been bound together by Eastern Orthodoxy, a common religious tradition that has dominated both countries for over 1,000 years, with almost three-quarters of Russians (71 per cent) and Ukrainians (77 per cent) identifying as Eastern Orthodox Christians (Pew Research Center, 2017). Until recently the official seat of Orthodoxy for both countries was the Moscow Patriarchate, but the Russian invasion of Ukraine has wrought havoc on this long-standing religious unity. Not only has religion played a significant part in the history of the close relations between the two countries, but it has continued to play a key role in the current conflict. Patriarch Kirill, the head of the Russian Orthodox Church (ROC) since 2009, has cast Putin's invasion as a holy war – causing widespread condemnation across the Christian world – while the Ukrainian response has been to attempt to outlaw the Ukrainian arm of the ROC in Ukraine.

Despite the bleak headlines that have dominated reporting from the region there remains hope of an end to the conflict, and when that time comes there will be extensive work to be done to ensure the long-term peace and stability of the region. Just as religion has been used in fanning the flames of the Russia–Ukraine war, so will it play an essential role in supporting post-war efforts. Established theories of peacebuilding and reconciliation emphasise how religious actors can be powerful agents in post-conflict reconciliation, evidenced by examples from across the globe. Therefore, religion – a structural determinant among the social determinants of health, according to the World Health Organization's Commission on Social Determinants of Health conceptual framework – has the potential to be routed towards reconciliation and used as a source of power and influence in supporting diplomatic efforts towards conflict resolution, restoring relationships and peacebuilding.

Kyivan Rus': the historical significance of religion

The Russo-Ukrainian war is inseparable from the formal origins of Christianity in the region. Kyivan Rus' was the first East Slavic state, existing from the mid-9th to mid-13th centuries CE and covering areas of modern-day Belarus, Ukraine and western Russia. It is traditionally believed to have been Christianised in or around 988 CE following the baptism of Volodymyr the Great, its leader from 980 to 1015 CE, who converted to Christianity in preparation for his marriage to Anna, sister of Basil II, Byzantine emperor, in a union intended to seal their diplomatic allegiance. Despite the obvious political advantages that resulted from Volodymyr's conversion there is evidence of a genuine and active Christian faith, and it is impossible to accurately determine his true motivation, especially given the value of the Christianisation of Kyivan Rus' in achieving his political ambitions.

Not merely a strong military leader who had consolidated Kyivan Rus' through a series of campaigns to secure and expand its territory, Volodymyr realised that its long-term stability was reliant on more than this. As such, and following earlier aborted attempts to unite his people through the promotion of shared pagan deities, after his wedding to Anna in 989 CE he instigated mass baptisms in Kyiv and the other major cities of Kyivan Rus' such as Novgorod (Zernov, 1950). At his command, pagan idols were removed and Christian churches built, and he began a programme of social and economic regeneration rooted in Christian concern for the poor (Obolensky and Woodbury, 1993).

Christianity (as well as Judaism and Islam) was already known in Kyivan Rus' (Ware, 2015) but Volodymyr's intentional programme of Christianisation as a political policy marked its formal beginning there. As with all obligatory 'conversions', the depth and authenticity of Christian belief across Kyivan Rus' is questionable and was not without opposition, some of which (such as at Novgorod) was crushed violently. Nonetheless, the implementation of a common theological framework ultimately served Volodymyr's purpose of unifying and stabilising the region, at least during his reign (Martin, 2009).

This use of religion for national unification, shared identity and the cohesive stability that can result from this is an important tactic still used today. As we shall see, today's entwining of religious and national identities in the *Russkiy Mir* ('Russian world') concept can trace its roots back to Volodymyr the Great's Christianisation of Kyivan Rus' and is crucial in understanding not only the role of religion in the ideology constructed around the Russian invasion of Ukraine but also – consequently – in how hopes of both short- and long-term reconciliation in the region are dependent on the cooperation of religious actors.

Religious history in the region

When speaking about 'religion' in Ukraine and Russia it is easy to assume that this is limited to Eastern Orthodoxy but both countries also contain small numbers of many other religious groups. Among the larger ones are other forms of Christianity, representing approximately 14 per cent of the population in Ukraine, of which around half are members of the Ukrainian Greek Catholic Church (Brylov et al, 2023). In Russia the percentage of non-Orthodox Christians is much lower at around 2 per cent, and there is also a notable Muslim population (mostly concentrated in Chechnya) of around 7 per cent (Levada Center, 2023); the Muslim population in Ukraine is much smaller, representing around 1 per cent or less (USDOS, 2022). Regardless, it is undeniable that Eastern Orthodoxy dominates faith and religious culture across Ukraine and most parts of Russia, and thus its role in the war between these two countries cannot be ignored. Although impossible to do justice to the complex and eventful religious history of the region within the confines of this chapter, some key events should be noted.

First, despite maintaining ecclesial relations with the churches at both Rome and Constantinople, the earliest church of Kyivan Rus' sat under the authority of the Patriarchate of Constantinople, indicative of the region's long-standing leaning to the east. Over time the Metropolitan moved his base from Kyiv to Volodymyr (1299 CE), and finally to Moscow (1325 CE), where it has remained ever since. After a couple of centuries of power struggle between Moscow and Constantinople, Moscow declared autocephaly in 1448, and this was formerly recognised by Constantinople in 1589. It is from this period that the theological concept of Moscow as a 'third Rome' has its roots following the falls of Rome and Constantinople, initially envisioned predominantly with guardianship responsibilities to safeguard the Orthodox faith, but additionally in later centuries with imperialist notions of expansion (Poe, 2001). Closely associated with this is the idea of 'Holy Rus', a theological vision of a Kingdom of Heaven on Earth encompassing Russia, Ukraine and Belarus (Brylov et al, 2023).

After several decades of further bold behaviour from Moscow, by 1722 the Metropolitanate of Kyiv had formally shifted from Constantinople's jurisdiction to become a diocese of Moscow's. This went alongside Peter the Great's abolishment of the position of Patriarch of Moscow and all Rus' in 1721, a position hitherto equal in power in the ecclesial realm to that of the Tsar in the political. In its place Peter the Great established the Holy Synod (or Ecclesiastical College), a council of 12 Church and monasterial figures that sat underneath the ultimate authority of the emperor. This shift saw the church effectively demoted to become 'a department of State' (Ware, 2015). The 1917 Bolshevik Revolution would later bring about the separation of Church and state, and along with it the reintroduction of the position of Patriarch. The 20th century saw great fluctuation and volatility in how clergy and Christians in the ROC were treated by the Russian government, swinging dramatically between periods of persecution and revival.

Russkiy Mir

The concept of *Russkiy Mir* ('Russian world') relates to the politics, language, culture and religion of Russia, as well as the influence of this in the wider world. Despite its older roots, *Russkiy Mir* is a 21st-century 'attempt at conceptualising the identity of Russia and her place in the post-Soviet space' (Wawrzonek, 2021: 20), and for which in 2007 a government-sponsored foundation was set up at the decree of Vladimir Putin to promote Russian language and culture worldwide. The Russkiy Mir Foundation has since established dozens of overseas outposts that are ostensibly for the promotion of Russian language and culture, but that also have the potential to spread pro-Russian propaganda and nurture pro-Russian sentiment outside of its borders. A key tenet espoused in the *Russkiy Mir* worldview is the historical narrative of the USSR as liberators from the Nazis in the Second World War (Conley, 2015); it is against this that Patriarch Kirill's 2012 description of Putin's rule as 'a miracle of God' is best understood, framed as bringing relief from the preceding period that he likened to the 1941 Nazi invasion (Bryanski, 2012).

Russia's compatriot policy is also relevant to the *Russkiy Mir* ideology, with 'compatriots' understood as ethnic Russians or Russian speakers living outside of the borders of Russia, many (though not all) of whom are situated in countries that used to form part of the Soviet Union. The compatriot policy aims to develop and maintain ties with 'compatriots' residing outside of Russia's borders, supporting them in their right to preserve their Russian identity (Russian Federation, 2023). Although language was the founding concern of *Russkiy Mir*, evident for example in the Russkiy Mir Foundation's concerns to campaign for government-recognised bilingualism within countries of the former Soviet Union (Wawrzonek, 2021), it is inseparable from other dominant aspects of Russian identity, such as values, history and the ROC; for example, a stipulated aim of the compatriot policy is to support 'compatriots' in preserving their 'Russian spiritual and moral values' (Russian Federation, 2023). As such, understanding the close relationship of Church and state that is bound up in *Russkiy Mir* is vital to long-term Ukrainian–Russian reconciliation.

Religion, *Russkiy Mir* and the current conflict

The concept of *Russkiy Mir* and the associated compatriot policy – with its professed aims to protect the interests of Russia overseas – have been weaponised and used as justification for the 2014 annexation of Crimea and 2022 full-scale invasion of Ukraine. On the day of the 2022 invasion, Putin stated his aim as to 'protect people ... facing humiliation and genocide ... including ... citizens of the Russian Federation' (Putin, 2022). Although in the same speech he claimed that 'it is not our aim to occupy Ukrainian territory' the land does in itself form part of the sacred history of Eastern Orthodoxy in the region, with Kyiv as the traditional birthplace of the ROC, and both Russia and Ukraine laying claim to descendancy from Kyivan Rus' and Volodymyr the Great.

In 2008 the then-president of Ukraine, Viktor Yushchenko, established a national holiday with state celebrations to commemorate the Christianisation of Kyivan Rus'; this was also to become a national holiday within Russia in 2010. Patriarch Kirill, the ROC's head and mouthpiece, has described Kyiv as 'our common Jerusalem, that of the Orthodox faith' (Wawrzonek, 2021: 29), theologically mirroring Putin's political view that Ukraine is not a foreign state but a 'key part of the Russian civilization and sphere of influence in greater Eurasia' (Brylov et al, 2023). Kirill has also declared that 'the Russian world starts at the Kievan baptismal font' and 'it is impossible for us to separate Kiev from our country, as this is where our history began. The Russian Orthodox Church preserves the national consciousness of both Russians and Ukrainians' (Liik et al, 2019).

Even prior to the 2022 escalation of the conflict, this was seen as an alarming 'act of cultural and spiritual appropriation' by many Ukrainians (Mitchell, 2022: 591). Since then, just as the concept of *Russkiy Mir* has been used by Putin to justify Russia's invasion of Ukraine, so has its religious character been used for propagandist purposes. Patriarch Kirill has echoed the Russian narrative of the Ukrainians and Russians as 'one people' (Gudziak, 2023) and 'brothers ... in this fratricidal war' (Reuters, 2022). He has reinforced the compatriot policy by lamenting the 'suffering' of 'our brothers and sisters' in the Donbas and positioned the war as 'a struggle that has not a physical, but a metaphysical significance' (Patriarch Kirill, 2022; 2024). Six months into the 2022 invasion, he boldly declared that those who sacrificed their lives in the conflict would have their sins 'washed away' as a result (Reuters, 2022), repeatedly emphasising the centrality of Eastern Orthodox religion to the war rhetoric.

Church schism

The religionising of the conflict has, unsurprisingly, not been without wider impact on Eastern Orthodoxy. The Ukrainian Orthodox Church (UOC) has historically represented the Ukrainian branch of the ROC under the jurisdiction of the Moscow Patriarchate. However, in December 2018 the Orthodox Church of Ukraine (OCU) was established and following a request from the then president of Ukraine, Petro Poroshenko, its legitimacy was affirmed by a *tomos* of autocephaly granted by the Ecumenical Patriarch of Constantinople, formally recognising its status as autonomous and independent of the Russian Orthodox Church. At the time this symbolised an affirmation of Ukrainian identity in the face of Russia's annexation of Crimea and ongoing occupation of the Donbas, as well as a significant risk to the ROC of losing their 36,000 UOC parishes within Ukraine should they shift allegiance to the OCU (Liik et al, 2019). The ROC responded in anger, breaking off relations with the Ecumenical Patriarchate of Constantinople.

Meanwhile, on 27 May 2022 a UOC council voted to separate from their parent church in protest at Patriarch Kirill's support of the Russian invasion; although they have not yet (January 2024) declared autocephaly, they have cut administrative ties with Moscow. This split has been met with scepticism over the extent and authenticity of the split, and in late 2023 the Ukrainian government started to take steps towards trying to outlaw the UOC due to its suspected ongoing ties with Russia, accusations that the UOC denies. The OCU has appealed to the UOC for its priests to move themselves and their parishes over to their jurisdiction (Kalenychenko and Brylov, 2022).

Elsewhere in the Eastern Orthodox world hundreds of clerics and theologians signed the 2022 Volos Declaration, a statement rejecting the *Russkiy Mir* theology as ethnophyletist and heretical (Mitchell, 2022), and one of many condemnations of Russian aggression from the Eastern Orthodox world. Within the ROC there is not unequivocal support for the Russian invasion, as evidenced by those who have spoken out, and, for example, the punishment of dozens of ROC priests who have refused to lead compulsory prayers for the victory of Holy Rus (Trevelyan, 2024).

Linked to the ongoing battle over religious identity, it has been reported that a significant number of religious sites have been damaged by the war (Kishkovsky, 2022), either deliberately or as collateral damage. Varying numbers have been cited for the extent of the damage, with these as high as 700 churches by the end of 2023 (Whitaker et al, 2023). Many see this as part of a wider programme of cultural genocide that aims to eliminate Ukrainian identity and subsume the country into Russia though it has been countered that the religious element to this is nonsensical as Orthodox churches might be 'be claimed for Russia ... as elements of a common Orthodox Russian culture' (Mick, 2023: 144). Lending credence to this are reports suggesting that over a third of damaged religious sites belonging to Protestant and Jehovah's Witness churches (DESS, 2023).

In addition, the *Russkiy Mir* narrative of liberation from Nazism took a curious turn with a missile strike near to the Babyn Yar Holocaust Memorial just a week into the 2022 invasion. Whether intentional or not, the sensitivity of the site – commemorating a horrific massacre of 33,771 Kyivan Jews in September 1941 by occupying Nazi forces – caused particular outcry.

Alongside the uncomfortable juxtaposition of claims of denazification of Ukraine with the rule of its Jewish president, it is clear that religion has been a recurrent theme and played a central part in this conflict from very early on. With that in mind, might it also contribute to its resolution?

Peacebuilding and reconciliation

There are no simple resolutions to the current crisis in Ukraine, especially given its far-extending historical and ideological roots, and little doubt that the horrors of this war will echo down the generations. But as there is hope that one day the conflict will cease, so must we be hopeful in scanning the horizon to establish what tools could be used in peacebuilding and reconciliation, in anticipation of that day finally arriving. Established theories of peacebuilding and reconciliation emphasise how religious actors can not only exacerbate conflict but also be powerful agents in making inroads in its resolution and long-term conciliation; indeed, elsewhere in this book Tomalin remarks on the value of faith actors, faith spaces and prayer in faith-based peacebuilding, and touches on the importance of faith-based actors both in advocacy and soft diplomacy (Chapter 18, this volume).

Despite variations in the definitions and practices of peacebuilding (Barnett et al, 2007) as well as considerable crossover with peacekeeping and conflict prevention (UN, 2010), it is generally accepted that peacebuilding starts when the conflict ends (or even before) and is aimed at building long-term stability that promotes sustainable peace, minimising the possibility of future conflict by confronting its root causes and consequences (Hamber and Kelly, 2004). The first two years following a conflict are seen as a crucial window in which to commence peacebuilding tasks, though the efforts stretch far beyond this. Just as conflict itself can touch upon all parts of life and across a multitude of spheres (for example, culture, health, economy), so too must peacebuilding; as such, the actors involved are many and various. Peacebuilding is 'a national challenge and responsibility' (UN, 2010), supported by citizens as well as their politicians and other local, national and international leaders.

A cornerstone of peacebuilding is the work of reconciliation and – as with peacebuilding – it is not a quick task but involves ongoing processes containing multiple stages, and towards which there are many approaches. Reconciliation is 'the process of addressing conflictual and fractured relationships' (Hamber and Kelly, 2004) and cannot be imposed, but should be undertaken freely (International IDEA, 2003). Sánchez and Rognvik (2012) identify four elements essential to successful reconciliation which are inclusive national dialogue, political will, freedom of speech and security of movement, and a shared common vision of the nation's end state. Hamber and Kelly (2004) emphasise the need to acknowledge the past and changes in people's attitudes to one another. António Guterres, current Secretary-General of the United Nations, has also stressed the need for truth and justice for past crimes in order for reconciliation to succeed (UN, 2019), which may also lead to reparation (UN, 2010).

Religious actors

Although each post-conflict setting is different, religion is often a factor; we have seen it has been a central theme of the Russian invasion of Ukraine, and religious rhetoric has been repeatedly used to legitimise it. Religious actors can play a significant role in processes of reconciliation, and the religious undertones of the Russia–Ukraine crisis only underscore this potential. 'Religious actors' is understood here as an umbrella term that can include religious institutions and their leading representatives, faith-based organisations, and groups or individuals for whom peacebuilding is motivated by religion (Powers, 2010). They can operate on local, national or international levels, though Lederach underscores the strategic significance of middle-range actors who are usually well-networked and have the capacity to impact those both above and below at grassroots (Lederach, 1997). They can also include experts and practitioners whose theological expertise 'form and advance ... a specialised type of knowledge that shapes public understanding of religion' and who therefore constitute a powerful 'expert community [that] has an influence on multiple policy fields' (Sandal, 2017).

Religious actors should be proactive and not merely reactive (Kalenychenko and Brylov, 2022). They can give legitimacy to peacebuilding and thereby assist in winning public approval for the process, as well as being viewed as neutral and respected figures who are 'often uniquely positioned to reach out to both the grass roots and elites' (Bramble et al, 2023). They are, in short, essential to reconciliation processes, and even more so in conflicts that have been exacerbated by a religious narrative, as with the Russian–Ukrainian war. Those who have influence over public theological discourse of a conflict have real power in shaping the conversations both during a conflict, and in consequent peacebuilding and reconciliation processes. This is not merely hypothetical but has been borne out in other conflicts in which religion has played a prominent role, as seen in the following examples from Northern Ireland, Guatemala and Sierra Leone.

Sandal (2017: 20) lauds the indispensable role played by 'prominent religious leaders and religious civil society members in Northern Ireland that helped transform exclusive public theologies into inclusive ones, which ultimately contributed to the peace process'. Leading religious actors from the four main churches in the region (Roman Catholic, Presbyterian, Methodist and the Church of Ireland) helped to shape theologies of belonging through an inclusive vision of governance and citizenship embedded in their respective traditions, a horizontal theology that Sandal argues is a prerequisite to ensuring reconciliation of a divided society. Religious actors also emphasised the need for sacrifice to achieve lasting peace, while a common empathy borne of faith encouraged dialogues of reconciliation and justice (Maiangwa and Byrne, 2015).

In Guatemala, resolution of a 36-year civil war (1960–1996) was brought about with the involvement of the Catholic Church which was seen as a neutral and legitimate participant in the process due to its efforts to hold all parties to account and to stimulate a national dialogue including all sectors of society. As such, in 1989 Archbishop Rodolfo Quezada Toruño of the Guatemalan Episcopal Diocese was invited to preside over a Grand National Dialogue of the government-formed National Reconciliation Commission. This brought religious groups together to find 'a common voice and become an integrated sector', thus amplifying the influence of these religious actors in the processes of reconciliation and peacebuilding (Bramble et al, 2023).

Furthermore, in 1995 – even before an official commission had been established – the Archbishop's Office for Human Rights of Guatemala launched the project 'Recovery of the Historical Memory' to document repression, persecution and human rights violations that had occurred during the civil war, with the aim of giving voice to these experiences for the purposes of truth, justice and reconciliation (Sánchez and Rognvik, 2012). In addition, Christian churches were key in disseminating information about the conflict and consequent peacebuilding process as they already had an established presence across Guatemala, including in remote and rural areas.

Elsewhere, the Inter-Religious Council of Sierra Leone (IRCSL) is another example of the pivotal role that religious actors can play in conflict resolution and reconciliation; in this case, as in many others, their credibility came from being established as respected, neutral, fair and committed to their communities (Jafari, 2007). Following the civil war (1991–2002) the IRCSL played a significant role in reconciling the warring factions and the population. They were also critical to the initiation and support of the Lomé Peace Agreement of 1997, drawing on the spiritual resources of preaching and prayer when facing an impasse.

Inspired by the Inter-Religious Council of Liberia, Muslim and Christian leaders of the IRCSL sought peaceful resolutions to the conflict and condemned the violence as ungodly, thus making themselves and their religious institutions targets of vandalism, abduction and murder (Turay, 2000). They initiated dialogue with coup leaders, eliciting criticism from others by listening to the IRCSL's concerns and urging others to hear them, while also placing diplomatic pressure on coup leaders to return the country to civilian rule. As well as securing the release of abducted children, the IRCSL played a central role in truth commissions (Kelsall,

2005); reconciliation and reintegration programmes, especially of child soldiers (Bramble et al, 2023); distribution of thousands of copies of the peace treaty; and holding services of thanksgiving throughout the country after the restoration of the civilian government in 1998 (Turay, 2000).

Conclusion

Thus can religious actors be peacemakers, bridge builders, politicians and theological influencers, regardless of whether conflicts are fuelled by religious tensions, but especially in those that are. While there are multiple causes for the Russian invasion of Ukraine, a key one of these is Putin's ideological agenda (Blattman, 2023) embedded in the *Russkiy Mir* worldview. This has been deliberately imbued with motivations rooted in the Eastern Orthodox tradition. The aims of this are not only legitimation of the conflict but also endorsement and mobilisation of the ROC in support from Patriarch Kirill at its very top, down to the seven out of ten Russian citizens who profess Eastern Orthodoxy as their chosen religious tradition.

Therefore, just as religion has been used to stoke support within Russia as the tightening grip of sanctions continues to affect ordinary citizens (Korhonen, 2023), so must it be used in forging pathways to peace; reconciliation seems otherwise impossible. By mapping religious drivers of war onto a path to peacebuilding, as well as engaging key religious actors across all strata in addressing these, the religious narrative can be rerouted from conflict towards resolution, and religion used as a source of power and influence in supporting diplomatic efforts towards an ongoing process of long-term reconciliation. As the founding myth of Eastern Orthodoxy in Kyivan Rus' has been used to shape *Russkiy Mir* and justify the Russian invasion, so must it be redirected to forge theologies of peaceful and independent coexistence rooted in the bond of a common beginning.

References

Barnett, M., Kim, H., O'Donnell, M. and Sitea, L. (2007) Peacebuilding: what is in a name? *Global Governance*, 13(1): 35–58.

Blattman, C. (2023) *Why We Fight: The Roots of War and the Paths to Peace*. London: Penguin Random House.

Bramble, A., Kadayifci-Orellana, S. and Paffenholz, T. (2023) Religious actors in formal peace processes. United States Institute of Peace, October. Available at: https://www.usip.org/sites/default/files/PW_194_Religious_Actors_in_Formal_Peace_Processes_Bramble.pdf

Bryanski, G. (2012) Russian patriarch calls Putin era 'miracle of God'. *Reuters*, 8 February. Available at: https://www.reuters.com/article/uk-russia-putin-religion-idUKTRE81722Y20120208/

Brylov, D., Kalenychenko, T. and Kryshtal, A. (2023) *Peaceworks: Mapping the Religious Landscape of Ukraine*. Washington, DC: United States Institute of Peace Press. Available at: https://www.usip.org/sites/default/files/2023-10/pw_193-mapping_religious_landscape_ukraine.pdf

Conley, H.A. (2015) Putin's invasion of Ukraine and the propaganda that threatens Europe. Center for Strategic and International Studies, 3 November. Available at: https://csis-website-prod.s3.amazonaws.com/s3fs-public/legacy_files/files/attachments/ts151103_Conley.pdf

DESS (The State Service of Ukraine for Ethnopolitics and Freedom of Conscience) (2023) List of religious sites ruined in Ukraine as a result of Russia's full-scale attack February 24 2022 – January 26 2023, in cooperation with the Academic Religious Studies Workshop (ARS). Available at: https://dess.gov.ua/wp-content/uploads/2023/01/Perelik-na-2023-01-26_ENG.pdf

Gudziak, B. (2023) Russian Orthodox leader Kirill's unholy war against Ukraine. *Atlantic Council*. Available at: https://www.atlanticcouncil.org/blogs/ukrainealert/russian-orthodox-leader-patriarch-kirills-unholy-war-against-ukraine/

Hamber, B. and Kelly, G. (2004) Reconciliation: a working definition. Available at: https://cain.ulster.ac.uk/dd/papers/dd04recondef.pdf

International IDEA (2003) *Reconciliation after Violent Conflict: A Handbook*. Stockholm: International IDEA. Available at: https://www.idea.int/sites/default/files/publications/reconciliation-after-violent-conflict-handbook.pdf

Jafari, S. (2007) Local religious peacemakers: an untapped resource in US foreign policy. *Journal of International Affairs*, 61(1): 111–130.

Kalenychenko, T. and Brylov, D. (2022) Ukrainian religious actors and organizations after Russia's invasion: the struggle for peace. Berkley Center for Religion, Peace and World Affairs. Transatlantic Policy Network on Religion and Diplomacy Policy Brief #2, September. Available at: https://berkleycenter.georgetown.edu/publications/ukrainian-religious-actors-and-organizations-after-russia-s-invasion-the-struggle-for-peace

Kelsall, T. (2005) Truth, lies, ritual: preliminary reflections on the Truth and Reconciliation Commission in Sierra Leone. *Human Rights Quarterly*, 27(2): 361–391.

Kishkovsky, S. (2022) Ukrainian churches and places of worship devastated by war. *The Art Newspaper*, 15 July. Available at: https://www.theartnewspaper.com/2022/07/15/ukrainian-churches-destroyed-war-russia

Korhonen, I. (2023) Sanctions against Russia: what have been the effects so far? *Economics Observatory*, 22 June. Available at: https://www.economicsobservatory.com/sanctions-against-russia-what-have-been-the-effects-so-far

Lederach, J. (1997) *Building Peace: Sustainable Reconciliation in Divided Societies*. Washington, DC: United States Institute of Peace Press.

Levada Center (2023) Religious beliefs. Press release, 2 June. Available at: https://www.levada.ru/en/2023/06/02/religious-beliefs/

Liik, K., Metodiev, M. and Popescu, N. (2019) Defender of the faith? How Ukraine's Orthodox split threatens Russia. *European Council on Foreign Relations*. Available at: https://ecfr.eu/publication/defender_of_the_faith_how_ukraines_orthodox_split_threatens_russia/

Maiangwa, B. and Byrne, S. (2015) Peacebuilding and reconciliation through storytelling in Northern Ireland and the border counties of the Republic of Ireland. *Storytelling, Self, Society*, 11(1): 85–110.

Martin, J. (2009) From Kiev to Muscovy: the beginnings to 1450. In G.L. Freeze (ed), *Russia, A History*, 3rd edn. Oxford: Oxford University Press, pp 1–30.

Mick, C. (2023) The fight for the past: contested heritage and the Russian invasion of Ukraine. *The Historic Environment: Policy & Practice*, 14(2): 135–153.

Mitchell, J. (2022) Religion and peacebuilding in the Ukraine-Russia conflict. In J. Mitchell, S. Millar, F. Po and M. Percy (eds), *The Wiley Blackwell Companion to Religion and Peace*. Hoboken: John Wiley and Sons, pp 589–606.

Obolensky, A. and Woodbury, J. (1993) From first to third millennium: the social Christianity of St. Vladimir of Kiev. *CrossCurrents*, 43(2): 203–211.

Patriarch Kirill (2022) Patriarchal sermon on cheese fat week after the liturgy in the Cathedral of Christ the Saviour. 6 March. Available at: http://www.patriarchia.ru/db/text/5906442.html?fbclid=IwAR11tviU4WTuDWxmUYzV7Xf4_xd3yGvJayvum3iBDLyChu0uqvcko52JcWo

Patriarch Kirill (2024) Patriarchal speech after great vespers on the Feast of the Nativity of Christ. 7 January. Available at: http://www.patriarchia.ru/db/text/6092378.html

Pew Research Center (2017) Orthodox Christianity's geographic center remains in Central and Eastern Europe. 8 November. Available at: https://www.pewresearch.org/religion/2017/11/08/orthodox-christianitys-geographic-center-remains-in-central-and-eastern-europe/

Poe, M. (2001) Moscow, the Third Rome: the origins and transformations of a 'pivotal moment'. *Jahrbücher Für Geschichte Osteuropas*, 49(3): 412–429.

Powers, G. (2010) Religion and peacebuilding. In D. Philpott and G. Powers (eds), *Strategies of Peace: Transforming Conflict in a Violent World*. Oxford: Oxford University Press, pp 317–352.

Putin, V. (2022) Address by the President of the Russian Federation. 24 February. Available at: http://en.kremlin.ru/events/president/news/67843

Reuters (2022) Orthodox Church leader says Russian soldiers dying in Ukraine will be cleansed of sin, edited by Mark Trevelyan. 26 September. Available at: https://www.reuters.com/world/europe/orthodox-church-leader-says-russian-soldiers-dying-ukraine-will-be-cleansed-sin-2022-09-26/#:~:text=goes%20to%20do%20what%20their,that%20a%20person%20has%20committed.%22

Russian Federation (2023) The concept of the foreign policy of the Russian Federation. 31 March. Available at: https://mid.ru/en/foreign_policy/fundamental_documents/1860586/

Sánchez, E. and Rognvik, S. (2012) Building just societies: reconciliation in transitional settings. *United Nations*. Available at: https://www.un.org/peacebuilding/sites/www.un.org.peacebuilding/files/documents/12-58492_feb13.pdf

Sandal, N. (2017) *Religious Leaders and Conflict Transformation: Northern Ireland and Beyond*. Cambridge: Cambridge University Press.

Trevelyan, M. (2024) Russian Orthodox priest faces expulsion for refusing to pray for war victory. *Reuters*, 13 January. Available at: https://www.reuters.com/world/europe/russian-orthodox-priest-faces-expulsion-refusing-pray-war-victory-2024-01-13/

Turay, T. (2000) Civil society and peacebuilding: the role of the inter-religious council of Sierra Leone. *Accord*, 9: 50–53. Available at: https://www.c-r.org/accord/sierra-leone/civil-society-and-peacebuilding-role-inter-religious-council-sierra-leone

UN (United Nations) (2010) UN peacebuilding: an orientation. *Peacebuilding Support Office*. Available at: https://www.un.org/peacebuilding/sites/www.un.org.peacebuilding/files/documents/peacebuilding_orientation.pdf

UN (United Nations) (2019) Reconciliation must evolve to reflect growing complexity of today's conflicts, participants stress during day-long Security Council open debate. 19 November. Available at: https://press.un.org/en/2019/sc14024.doc.htm

USDOS (United States Department of State) (2022) *2022 Report on International Religious Freedom: Ukraine*. Available at: https://www.state.gov/reports/2022-report-on-international-religious-freedom/ukraine/

Ware, T. (2015) *The Orthodox Church: An Introduction to Eastern Christianity*. London: Penguin.

Wawrzonek, M. (2021) The 'Russian world' and Ukraine. In C. Noack (ed), *Politics of the Russian Language beyond Russia*. Edinburgh: Edinburgh University Press, pp 19–44.

Whitaker, B., Chasan, A., Abbott, H. and Scott, L. (2023) Ukrainian investigators preserve heritage as Russia targets its cultural legacy. *CBS News*, 12 November. Available at: https://www.cbsnews.com/news/ukraine-protecting-cultural-heritage-art-from-russia-60-minutes/

Zernov, N. (1950) Vladimir and the origin of the Russian Church. Part II. *The Slavonic and East European Review*, 28(71): 425–438.

5

Values, social determinants of health and the UN Sustainability Goals

Helen Froud

Introduction

There are many well-recognised critical issues facing global governments which affect population health and wellbeing. The Geneva-based World Economic Forum (WEF) non-profit identified five key short-term risks in its 2023 Global Risks Report (energy supply, cost of living crisis, rising inflation, food supply and cyberattacks on critical infrastructure) as the key and immediate threats to human flourishing. The WEF and others have also identified longer-term and horizon-based risks which are significant to individuals, commerce and civil governance over the next decade. Geoeconomic confrontation is also signalled as a risk in the WEF risk matrix. For many European nations, this currently includes issues arising from the proximity to the conflict in Ukraine, and the consequential impact upon economies, civil society and the environment.

At all population levels, the need to tackle the consequences of global and local issues has become pressing. Most current and future global crises will have a significant linkage to the social determinants of health, and many have a negative, compounding effect upon ill-health and wellbeing. While individual effort and engagement in tackling the world's contemporary 'wicked issues' (Introduction, this volume) is important, so is the long-term involvement of corporations, institutions and transnational entities. Political, economic and social pressures can sway governments (Krznaric, 2019) and business (Murray, 2021) and can drive decision-making into a pattern of short-term thinking. This behavioural habit reduces the effectiveness of otherwise influential actors and risks small issues developing into unsolvable, long-term problems. The presence of major armed conflict between Ukraine and Russia on the European mainland has served to highlight the importance of understanding risk management at nation-state level.

Aims

This chapter will examine the ways in which European social determinants of health are deeply affected by war in Ukraine. It will examine progress with the 2015 United Nations Sustainable Development Goals (UN SDGs) and will ask how this model has performed since it was launched. It will suggest that the SDGs model presents potential approaches to post-conflict recovery and reconstruction in the wake of the current conflict in Ukraine. This chapter will also co-map the SDGs alongside the policy priorities of the 2010 World Health Organization (WHO) social determinants of health model. In a case study, it will also consider how a relatively new concept from healthcare and management, the 'values-based' approach (Mohanna, 2017), can potentially add value and understanding to the social determinants of health model beyond the SDGs' quantitative metrics.

The chapter will also review early steps in post-Ukraine conflict recovery. It will advocate the use of evidence from all three approaches to assist European nations seeking to improve long-term population health and wellbeing in the wake of the Russia–Ukraine conflict.

Short-termism: a 'wicked issue' in itself?

One of the most difficult dimensions of current global crises is that many key risks are the consequence of issues which were on expert risk registers, but which were not high on many influential government agendas. Mackenzie (2016) affirms that short-term political agendas often influence election priorities in democracies, and lays some of the blame at the door of poor institutional design.

Many European governments were aware of the possibility of the global health risks surrounding COVID-19 or a similar pandemic becoming critical but either chose not to take immediate action to mitigate these risks or did not place them sufficiently high on their political agenda. The WHO began consulting on an International Treaty on Pandemic Prevention, Preparedness and Response in late 2021 but, arguably, sufficient investment in pre-existing international health protection machinery within the governance arrangements of many nations could have been equally effective. Short-termism within this context affected the degree of nation-state preparedness for pandemic within Europe.

The risks of the current conflict in Ukraine have been evident for decades, and the 2014 Russian annexation of the Russian-speaking Crimea and the continued conflict in the Donbas region of Ukraine provided a clear indicator of intent and capacity. It has been suggested (Vicente, 2022) that the conflict was potentially preventable – or at least containable, but that divergent political interests and a lack of an enforceable European security mechanism ensured that conflict prevention did not happen effectively. The short-termism inherent in European political and economic interests meant that institutional reform was not attempted.

The problems of political and institutional short-termism have been raised repeatedly in both the behavioural and political science literature. Gonzalez-Ricoy and Gosseries (2016) offer a critique of short-termism as a matter of intergenerational injustice, suggesting that short-termism is an affront against the interests of future generations. They suggest several ameliorating strategies to deal with the tendency to only deal in short-term timescales, some of which involve significant institutional and legal reform.

Long-term approaches: the United Nations Sustainable Development Goals

In 2015 the UN agreed the 17 SDGs, which it described as an 'urgent call to action' for all countries. The SDGs arose from a decades-long series of campaigns and carefully negotiated agreements, including Agenda 21, which was adopted in Rio de Janeiro by 178 countries in 1992, and the 2002 Johannesburg World Summit on Sustainable Development in 1992. The SDGs (see Figure 5.1) run from 2015 to 2030.

The UN, created in 1945 from the League of Nations after the Second World War, was itself the product of a mostly European and North American resolve to produce a global mechanism for peacekeeping and cooperation. However, as its own history outlines, the UN has had to pivot roles since its inception to cope with a much wider range of global threats than those

Figure 5.1: United Nations Sustainable Development Goals 2015

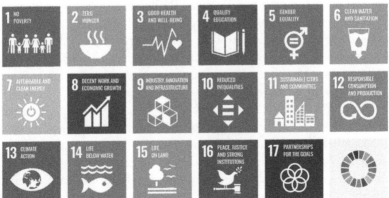

envisaged by its founders. This includes an enlargement of the scope of the UN's work into issues of climate change and environmental protection, which has itself been politically controversial.

The UN has reported annually (UN, 2023a) on progress with the SDGs since 2015, using detailed metrics derived from over 50 transnational organisations as well as from member state governments. The 2022 annual report outlines the combined impact of the COVID-19 pandemic, a sharp rise in refugee movements and the largest number of violent conflicts since 1946 which have put the Agenda for Sustainable Development with its SDGs in 'grave peril'. In July 2023, the UN published a Special Edition of the SDGs Report which suggested that the aims of the SDGs were in 'deep trouble' at their halfway point, with half the 140 metrics used to measure the targets 'severely off track', and over 30 per cent of the measures having 'seen no movement or regressed below the 2015 baseline'. In its foreword, the UN Secretary-General cited the war in Ukraine as part of the problem with progress, suggesting that this conflict had also created 'a global cost-of-living crisis affecting billions of people'.

Despite the disappointing lack of progress with the targets, the SDGs nevertheless represent a comprehensive attempt to summarise the key health and wellbeing issues facing UN member regions and nations. Their aim was to provide a quantitative measure of progress, and their comprehensive reporting has been successful to date even if the outcomes have been negative ones. This chapter will suggest that the SDGs already provide evidence that the conflict in Ukraine is impacting the wellbeing of global citizens beyond the borders of Ukraine.

Mapping the Sustainable Development Goals during conflict in Europe

All 17 of the SDG the goals are relevant to most European nations, although some measures are less significant in the European microstates because of issues of scale and breadth. However, the different starting points of each of the six UN SDG world regions makes global comparisons between regions more challenging. For administrative purposes at sub-regional level, the UN divides Europe into four, with many EU nations in each of the four sub-regions. Ukraine sits in the 'Eastern Europe' sub-region with many of the former Soviet bloc nations. Progress (or otherwise) on the indicators was by 2022 already beginning to show evidence of the impact of the conflict in Ukraine.

Probably the most comprehensive interpretation of the SDGs for mainland Europe is the European Union (EU)'s Eurostat version (Eurostat, 2023). This publication, which summarises the annual UN SDG progress, also features an online interactive dashboard. It should be noted that the Eurostat versions of the SDGs do not exactly match (but aim to track) the UN Goals. The

Eurostat data also excludes non-EU members such as the United Kingdom. Within Europe, falling 2022 indicators were SDGs 4, 5 and 10 (Quality Education, Gender Inequality and Reduced Inequalities), mostly due to the COVID-19 pandemic; and SDGs 6 and 15 (Clean Water and Sanitation, and Life on Land), mostly due to the impact of climate change. There is also a specific section of the Eurostat website devoted to what it calls 'military aggression against Ukraine' tracking key metrics relating to the conflict. The Eurostat report in 2023 also noted that the influence of conflict in Ukraine, especially the impact of refugee movement, was beginning to show on the SDG indicators, particularly for those EU nations which border or are close to Ukraine. These show at a European level in 2023 as reduced progress for SDG 16 (Peace, Justice and Strong Institutions) and SDG 15 (Life on Land). The SDGs are therefore sufficiently responsive, albeit lagging historical metrics which can capture the impacts of major conflict.

Mapping the metrics of European conflict

The UN and the EU work with each national government to ensure that the SDG data recorded and mapped is accurate. The task is easier at a continental level and is made simpler within the EU as several indicators are already harmonised between the 27 member states. Some data from the European Free Trade Association is also included in the Eurostat data.

It should be noted that data directly from Ukraine is not included in Eurostat, as the nation is not a member of any of the qualifying bodies for inclusion. Metrics evidencing the impact of the conflict are therefore not collected directly on Eurostat but would normally be collected by the UN as part of its 'Eastern Europe' sub-region. At UN level, data is still being captured for activity within Ukraine, but the UN is starkly honest in its 2023 country report that its work within the nation (UN, 2023b) since 2022 has comprised mostly humanitarian relief activity. Most of the current UN data held on Ukraine (UN, 2023) against the SDGs is therefore now historical.

The net effect of the conflict in Ukraine is to both severely reduce the evidence of data to the UN SDGs and to severely degrade the progress made by Ukraine in achieving elements of the goals. Until 2022, Ukraine had made significant progress with the SDGs, but it will clearly be a few years more before there is likely to be sufficient opportunity or national infrastructure to support any further detailed reporting. It may be that the SDGs will in future have the potential to assist with the measurement of reconstruction in a post-conflict scenario for Ukraine, and for longer-term evidence of the impact to be recorded.

Also evident is the indirect impact of the conflict on the nations of Europe. Since 2022 Eurostat has maintained a special statistical section on the impact of the war in the following areas:

- population and migration;
- energy and economy; and
- trade and agriculture.

These are mostly quantitative measures, from which the impact upon communities using the social determinants of health approach can only be inferred. Also missing from this analysis are the intangible cultural losses for Ukraine arising from the conflict, as unique communities, dialects, traditions, practice and faith expressions have been destroyed by war or have been displaced internally or externally. Some of these distinct elements are captured in Chapter 12 of this book.

Clearly, the conflict in Europe is not unique, and this continent is not the only area of the world where difficult health and humanitarian conditions pertain. The global mapping of the SDGs includes other areas of the world where war, civil unrest, climate change and outbreaks of disease have had a negative impact on progress. The UN Statistical Bureau relies on 169 targets which comprise the dataset for the SDGs, but in 2023 the UN was unable to secure sufficient data for 31 of these targets.

Mapping the Sustainable Development Goals to the social determinants of health

While the SDGs are useful quantitative measures of national progress, they have limitations as they do not attempt to discover causes. SDGs simply measure the direction of travel as percentages in either direction from the 2015 baseline. However, the SDG metrics are key pieces of evidence which can help illustrate the impact of the social determinants of health model. Table 5.1 maps the SDGs against the WHO 2010 version of the social determinants of health model. Using this pathway, it should therefore be theoretically possible to attempt to attach metrics for progress (or otherwise) from the SDG against each of the elements of the social determinants of health at a national level within Europe.

There are some shortcomings to this comparative approach, as well as some advantages. Both models were written at very different times, in different contexts and for differing purposes. The WHO model, drawn from the Dahlgren and Whitehead model (1991) version, is designed to explain the multi-layered and interdependent nature of health inequities, rather than to measure them. The UN SDGs are designed as metrics-based policy drivers with sufficient commonality to allow measurement of the conditions of human life in vastly different national contexts. Some of the UN SDGs could potentially appear several times to support or contest different dimensions of the social determinants of health, and this is shown in the mapping exercise in Table 5.1.

Table 5.1: United Nations Sustainable Development Goals mapped against the World Health Organization's social determinants of health model (2010)

Social determinants of health (WHO, 2010)	UN Sustainable Development Goals (2015) (goal numbers in brackets)
Structural conflict; social inclusion and non-discrimination	No poverty, zero hunger, reduced inequalities (1, 2, 10); Gender equality (5); Peace, justice and strong institutions (16); Partnerships for the Goals (17)
Food insecurity	Zero hunger (2); Reduced inequalities (10); Responsible consumption and production (12); Affordable and clean energy (7); Life on land (15)
Education and early childhood development	Quality education (4); Gender equality (5); Reduced inequalities (10)
Income, social protection and working life conditions	Good health and wellbeing (3); Gender equality (5); Decent work and economic growth (8); Responsible consumption and production (12); Industry, innovation, infrastructure (9)
Unemployment and job insecurity	Decent work and economic growth (8); Reduced inequalities (10); Responsible consumption and production (12)
Housing, basic amenities and the environment	Clean water and sanitation (6); Industry, innovation, infrastructure (9); Life on land (15); Life below water (14); Sustainable cities and communities (11); Peace, justice and strong institutions (16)
Access to healthcare services of decent quality	Good health and wellbeing (3); Gender equality (5); Peace, justice and strong institutions (16)

Individually, both models have been subject to criticism that they may be missing key elements which weaken any claim that they independently provide a comprehensive view of human health and wellbeing. The UN's measures appear to emerge from both a modernist and market-based approach to human flourishing which seeks to measure the performance of a nation, but which is unable to capture less visible aspects of life and wellbeing. The British Council (2020) suggests that the 'missing pillar' of the SDGs is culture, which also does not feature in the WHO model. The concept of 'intangible cultural heritage' defined and agreed by the United Nations Educational, Scientific and Cultural Organization in 2003 appears not to directly intersect with the UN's SDGs.

Rice and Sara (2019) have suggested that the missing element in the social determinants of health model is 'information and communication technologies' which are clearly measured in the SDG 9 indicator (Industry, innovation, infrastructure). The suggested co-mapping exercise therefore brings strength to each model, with clear evidence from the supporting SDG metrics to be attached to each dimension of the social determinants model. A whole-nation health reconstruction plan for Ukraine post-conflict could use the SDG/social determinants of health model as part of a framework with targets for recovery.

The co-mapping exercise, if extended into real metrics, would need to consider the weighting of SDG indicators which are repeated in several of the social determinants of health model.

This suggested approach is not the first time that an attempt has been made to attach values to the social determinants of health model. The US Department of Health and Human Services has a 'Healthy People 2030' campaign (Office of Disease Prevention and Health Promotion, nd) which seeks to group the SDH concept (without attributing it directly to particular authors) into five domains. This 'Healthy People' campaign has been running for longer than the SDG indicators, and a similar, albeit smaller, grouping of indicators has been chosen. The US model then ascribes values to each domain from existing US government data. In the same manner as the UN SDG measures, each measure shows an indicator of progress or otherwise. Figure 5.2 shows the domains:

- economic stability
- education access and quality
- healthcare access and quality
- neighbourhood and built environment
- social and community context.

Figure 5.2: US 'Healthy People 2030' model

Social Determinants of Health

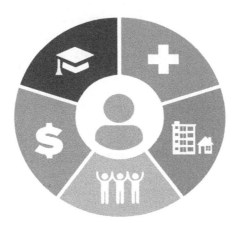

Social Determinants of Health
Copyright-free

Healthy People 2030

However, this mapping exercise has the same shortcomings as the co-mapping exercise between the social determinants of health and the UN SDGs earlier in this chapter. It does not contain any response to the criticism that culture is omitted from the model. It does, however, continue a series of long-term responses to key issues of health improvement campaigning through successive US political administrations which began in 1980. Each ten-year model has contained numerical targets which precede the UN SDGs, although the 2020 version is the first to contain such explicit reference to the concept of the social determinants of health.

Values-based approaches

Within the past two decades, an additional approach to capturing less tangible aspects of culture has emerged. Copeland (2014) suggests that the 'values-based approach' to leadership evolved from a concern in the early 1990s that ethical behaviour in Western organisational management had been found wanting. Other authors suggest that the approach developed in the intersection between medicine and philosophy, with the work of Fulford (1989) and others providing a catalyst for the adoption of values-based approaches within contemporary medical practice. Values-based approaches have transformed ethics, medicine, corporate culture and public governance. Crucially, values-based practice in any discipline sits alongside quantitative, fact-based measures and allows individual perspectives, culture and tradition to be heard and respected. In this manner, a values-based approach is entirely congruent with and provides additionality to the WHO model of the social determinants of health.

Values-based practice has moved successfully and established itself in several sectors and disciplines, including into faith-based organisations. In these communities, the intangible contribution of faith and the easy recognition of values-based practice has been advantageous. In Case Study 5.1, the application of a set of values and their association with the organisation's key objectives provides a useful model for suggesting a future approach to the shortcomings already delineated within the social determinants of health model and with the SDGs.

Case Study 5.1: The adoption of values-based practice in a faith-based institution – The Salvation Army UK and Ireland Territory

In 2022, The Salvation Army adopted a values-based approach to its work in the UK and Ireland. The Salvation Army in these nations is both a church and a charity, seeking to put faith into action across churches, residential and day centres and homelessness hostels, as well as in community support projects and specialist services provided under contract. It has been an active supporter of relief and outreach work towards displaced members of Ukrainian communities. Under the corporate aim of 'Love God, Love Others' it had during the previous year formally adopted a series of values which it calls its 'Five Missional Priorities'. This broad approach to faith-based practice originated from the Anglican Communion (Zink, 2017) via a 1984 Anglican Consultative Council document which was eventually called the 'Five Marks of Mission'. This model has also been adopted within the UK by the Church of Scotland and the Methodist Church, with some amendment to allow for denominational distinctives. The 'Five Missional Priorities' priorities renamed and adopted by The Salvation Army are:

- share the good news;
- serve others without discrimination;
- nurture disciples of Jesus;
- care for creation; and
- seek justice and reconciliation.

At a whole-organisation level, these five domains can be seen to mirror the US social determinants of health model for 'Heathy People 2030' or the nine community domains of the Dahlgren and Whitehead model. None of these domains of themselves imply any link with specific data sources or metrics, and at present, there is only early work underway to attach these domains to specific organisational outcomes.

Further development of the Missional Priorities work into application throughout The Salvation Army's UK and Ireland church and social work programmes took place during 2022. The aim was to examine the behavioural values sought by the organisation among its ministers, volunteers, staff and worshippers. The specific work was shaped and framed by the ideas of Woodhead (2021) who analyses key organisational value propositions in Western democracies, particularly in education. Her work is in turn inspired by Walsh (2016), who suggests that values are relational and contextual, and characterised by how people treat one another. Woodhead proposes the idea that the adoption of 'values' within entities and nations derived from a period in the late 20th century when Japanese corporate culture was in the ascendancy in the West, largely because of the economic success of Japanese business.

Additional support for the concept of a values-based approach within The Salvation Army came from the work of Smidt et al (2023). They suggest that systematic institutional failures to protect vulnerable people can be prevented (or their impact ameliorated) by high levels of what they call 'institutional courage'. Their work suggests that most people are dependent upon institutional integrity and competence, but that large-scale failures often occur unintentionally. They believe that the open and transparent values which are explicitly stated and tied to organisational behaviour can provide the encouragement to behave appropriately at an organisational level. Work on organisational values had been implicit from the faith-based origins of the organisation, and some early work on this had

Figure 5.3: The Salvation Army's values-based model, 2022

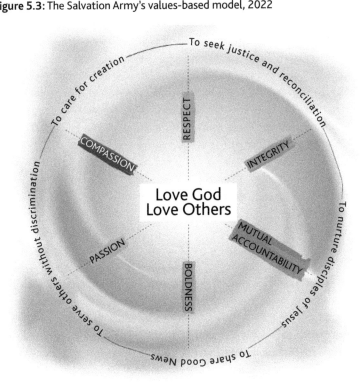

taken place in the early 2000s. The formal re-adoption and definition of The Salvation Army's values model also came following an internal organisational review published in 2018 which strongly recommended a reworking of its own process of cultural change.

The Salvation Army adopted a values-based model which fits within the framework of its 'Five Missional Priorities', placing them as spokes on the wheel of the organisation's purpose. The values are:

- boldness;
- compassion;
- passion;
- respect;
- integrity; and
- mutual accountability.

Each of the domains of the Five Missional Priorities is linked to two values which relate to their achievement. This is shown in Figure 5.3. For example, 'Caring for creation', which is The Salvation Army's environmental commitment, exemplified the values of

'Compassion' and 'Respect'. So far, there has not been a published commitment to how the values will be recorded or assessed, but there has been additional guidance issued which outlines the desired behaviours arising from the Values, and the organisational outcomes which are expected.

This case study illustrates how values can be explicitly linked to broad domains and indicators within an organisation. With slightly differing motivations, similar approaches have been successful at the nation-state level, with Behavioural Insights teams within many Western governments seeking to apply values-based human sciences to the implementation of policy and legislation. This work has an evidence-based track record of improving public health by ensuring that people receive the targeted information they need to encourage them to participate in positive healthcare initiatives; and assists policy makers by uncovering the cultural, behavioural and habit-based reasons why people do not behave as they claim to.

Using a values-based model to drive organisational change is not a novel approach, and has been thoroughly explored in many sectors. Branson (2008) cites this practice as an essential precondition to organisational change in the education sector. He notes that failures in organisational change often originate in a less than willing compliance among those affected by the change. Amis et al (2002) examine values-based organisational change in the voluntary sector and conclude that a values approach can be powerful where key individuals hold personal values congruent with the changes sought. Clearly, for The Salvation Army, using Christian-based values sets linked closely to Christian ethical practice is more likely to have effect, but this values-based approach is in its earliest stages of active use and a comprehensive monitoring framework will be necessary before this can be measured.

Building a values-based, multivariate approach to reconstruction

Ukraine is already well-engaged at an institutional and multinational level in political and economic initiatives to rebuild its economy and its society. The EU's Neighbourhood Policy and Enlargement Negotiations (EU, 2023) recommended that the European Commission open negotiations with Ukraine early in November 2023. By that date the EU was deeply involved in significant Cross Border Co-operation projects which are permitted by EU law to fund work in countries neighbouring existing EU members. The EU has very clear, published methodological frameworks for this funding and for the conduct and review of the projects. It is also clear that the rapid reconstruction of Ukraine is already underway – this represents both a political commitment to Ukraine by the EU, as well as an initiative which may build goodwill and trade between the participating nations.

The resumption of work on the SDGs will necessitate the provision of complete and accurate reporting from the government of Ukraine. In 2023 the UN will have allocated US$636.8 million to SDG achievement in Ukraine in specific funding streams (UN, 2023a), with the largest financial segment (US$112 million, or 17.6 per cent) going towards the achievement of SDG 16 (Peace, justice and strong institutions) and US$69 million, or 10.8 per cent, going towards SDG 9 (Industry, innovation and infrastructure). In 2024 the allocation switches dramatically, with 73.4 per cent being allocated to SDG 11 (Sustainable cities and communities). However, the main financial input towards ongoing Ukrainian reconstruction and capacity-building is likely to fall within other budgetary areas, including EU monies already outlined.

However, reconstruction of a nation following conflict is more than the rebuilding of homes, institutions and transport modes. It includes reconciliation between and within communities; restoration of cultural practices, including faith practices and other intangible cultural assets; and the return of the refugee diaspora. Volf (2019), who has written extensively on the aftermath of conflict in the Balkans at the end of the 20th century, describes post-war reconstruction and reconciliation as a movement to 'embrace' the other, which must be supported by 'pluralistic political arrangements' to ensure that the seeds of even more future conflict are not sown in the present. The UK parliament discussed its own perspective on Ukrainian reconstruction in June 2023 and agreed that the religious and cultural heritage of the nation were key issues which needed assistance with rebuilding. It is precisely this kind of scope which might conceivably give rise to a desire or need to adopt a values-based approach in government institutions in a future Ukraine. This approach might ensure that the intangible dimensions of public and community life are more adequately represented in the data.

Conclusion

The UN SDGs are an ambitious programme of long-term objectives designed to capture data on and promote positive stewardship of key quality-of-life indicators at nation–state level. Launched in 2015, the SDGs initially captured some of the significant progress has been made, as well as areas of the world where war, natural disaster and disease have impeded progress. Conflict in Ukraine has severely disrupted the progress made by that nation in the achievement of its SDG targets. The impact of the conflict and has spilled into surrounding parts of Europe where the achievement of SDGs has been impeded.

However, the Goals tend to be qualitative rather than quantitative, and this chapter has suggested that a more useful way to capture progress with both 'soft' and 'hard' indicators is to 'map' the SDGs onto the 1991 Dahlgren and Whitehead social determinants of health model. A version of this has been adapted by the US government. However, all the models fail to capture a broad perspective of intangible cultural assets which each nation possesses.

The use of a values-based model as outlined in Case Study 5.1 shows how values can be successfully 'mapped' onto a community outcome framework. Behavioural approaches like this which acknowledge the importance of human culture, faith and values are used successfully by many developed democracies. Similar work at national level could be applied to early reconstruction work within Ukraine, alongside the resumption of the measurement of the SDGs to track progress.

References

Amis, J., Slack, T. and Hinings, C. (2002) Values and organizational change. *Journal of Applied Behavioral Science*, 38(4).

Branson, C.M. (2008) Achieving organisational change through values alignment. *Journal of Educational Administration*, 46(3): 376–395.

British Council (2020) *The Missing Pillar: Culture's Contribution to the UN Sustainable Development Goals*. Available at: https://www.britishcouncil. org/sites/default/files/the_missing_pillar.pdf

Copeland, M.K. (2014) The emerging significance of values based leadership: a literature review. *International Journal of Leadership Studies*, 8(2): 105–135.

Dahlgren, G. and Whitehead, M. (1991) *Policies and Strategies to Promote Social Equity in Health*. Institute for Futures Studies, September. Available at: https://core.ac.uk/download/pdf/6472456.pdf

EU (2023) *EU Sustainable Development Goals Overview Dashboard*. Eurostat. Available at: https://ec.europa.eu/eurostat/web/sdi

Eurostat (2023) SDGs. https://ec.europa.eu/eurostat/web/sdi

Fulford, K.W.M. (1989) *Moral Theory and Medical Practice*. Cambridge: Cambridge University Press.

Gonzalez-Ricoy, I. and Gosseries, A. (2016) *Designing Institutions for Future Generations*. Oxford: Oxford University Press.

Krznaric, R. (2019) Why we need to reinvent democracy for the long-term. *BBC Future*, 19 March. Available at: https://www.bbc.com/future/article/ 20190318-can-we-reinvent-democracy-for-the-long-term

Mackenzie, M.K. (2016) Institutional design and sources of short-termism. In I. Gonzalez-Ricoy and A. Gosseries (eds), *Designing Institutions for Future Generations*. Oxford: Oxford University Press, pp 24–48.

Mohanna, K. (2017) Values based practice: a framework for thinking with. *Education for Primary Care*, 28(4): 192–196.

Murray, S. (2021) How to take the long-term view in a short-term world. *Financial Times*, 26 February.

Office of Disease Prevention and Health Promotion (nd) Healthy People 2030. https://health.gov/healthypeople

Rice, L. and Rachel, S. (2019) Updating the determinants of health model in the Information Age. *Health Promotion International*, 34(6): 1241–1249.

Smidt, A.M., Adams-Clark, A.A. and Freyd, J.J. (2023) Institutional courage buffers against institutional betrayal, protects employee health, and fosters organizational commitment following workplace sexual harassment. *PLoS ONE*, 18(1): e0278830.

UN (2023a) *The Sustainable Development Goals Report 2023: Special Edition Towards a Rescue Plan for People and Planet*. Available at: https://unstats.un.org/sdgs/report/2023/

UN (2023b) *United Nations in Ukraine, 2023*. https://ukraine.un.org/en/

Vicente, B. (2022) Why Europe slept? The failure to prevent the war in Ukraine. *European Leadership Network*, May. Available at: https://www.europeanleadershipnetwork.org/commentary/why-europe-slept-the-failure-to-prevent-the-war-in-ukraine/

Volf, M. (2019) *Exclusion and Embrace*. Nashville: Abingdon Press.

Walsh, F. (2016) Applying a family resilience framework in training, practice, and research: mastering the art of the possible. *Family Process Journal*, 55: 616–632.

WEF (2023) *Global Risks Report 2023*, 18th edn. World Economic Forum. Available at: WEF_Global_Risks_Report_2023.pdf

WHO (2010) *Social Determinants of Health*. https://www.who.int/health-topics/social-determinants-of-health#tab=tab_1

Woodhead, L. (2021) Values are the new religion. Edward Cadbury Lectures, University of Birmingham. Available at: https://www.birmingham.ac.uk/schools/ptr/departments/theologyandreligion/events/cadburylectures/2021

Zink, J. (2017) Five marks of mission: history, theology, critique. *Journal of Anglican Studies*, 15(2): 144–166.

PART II

Individuals and families: behavioural and psychological perspectives

Introduction to Part II

Kaia Rønsdal

Recognising vulnerable life conditions of our fellow human beings is normatively and ethically significant. It is not just a question of life conditions that make their way to media outlets, but everyday lives that sometimes make themselves visible to us.

Although the following chapters relate to statutory and voluntary practices, the concern of this introduction reflects phenomenologically on the universal responsibility for our fellow human being and non-instrumental approaches to this responsibility.

Using the term marginality presupposes that some are marginalised, implied by someone else. It is thus not a label placed on, or descriptive characteristic of someone, but a willed or subconscious marginalisation of someone by individuals or systems. This poses a challenge to society, and society starts at the level of the individual.

The Danish philosopher and theologian Knud E. Løgstrup (1999) wrote of a demand among humans, one that is given with life itself. This demand is present in human encounters: one never encounters another without holding pieces of their life in one's hand. In every encounter is an *unspoken* demand, regardless of the circumstances and character of the encounter (Løgstrup, 1999: 39). Furthermore, Løgstrup claimed that as our lives are created without our participation, whether in the sense that we did not set our own birth in motion or in the belief of a divine creator, it cannot be lived in any other way than by that a person surrenders more or less of their life in the hands of the other, whether in shown or desired faith (Løgstrup, 1999). What the parts of the other's life are is different, it can be something fleeting or their entire destiny (Løgstrup, 1999: 47).

This metaphorical holding of life has its roots in phenomenological thinking, where we are unavoidably and to a great extent interdependent (Løgstrup, 1999: 50). The metaphor emphasises that our encounters are tipping points. The emotional force of the metaphor emphasises the immediate power relations that arise in the encounter (Løgstrup, 1999).

In professional and voluntary practices among marginalised people, we are always in danger of making at least four mistakes. One is misinterpreting this demand as meaning something different for us, either that we have 'more' life in our hands, or more responsibility for it. Another is failing to consider or take seriously that our life is also in the hands of the marginalised. And third, that we, in our often professionally interpreted and understood perspectives of those we work with, do not let them present themselves and show us who they are. Even when we are acutely aware of our ethical responsibility as practitioners, we fall for the temptation to instrumentalise our approach. Løgstrup was clear in his reflections on the powerful situation of the ethical demand: there is an absolute rejection of the idea that caring can involve robbing the other of their independence. The responsibility of the other cannot be taking over their own responsibility (Løgstrup, 1999: 50).

In the wicked issue of war, when we are exposed to a spectacle of suffering, we are eager to act. In wars humans are marginalised, and sometimes peripheralised to the extent that they cross borders into new communities. We find ourselves in communities challenged and enriched by these humans. When we act, it should be our primary concern to not push to the margins, but to work for and trust our capacity to live together (Nahnfeldt and Rønsdal, 2021).

In our efforts to relieve suffering, we must strive to remember the ethical demand. Not merely in the sense that we are careful in encountering people we understand as being in vulnerable life conditions in ways that do not crush the life in our hand. Rather, that we consider in the encounter that we are in a trusting relationship where we revive and preserve shared life. Taking seriously the metaphor of holding each other's lives in our hands, we may be centring life itself. Løgstrup wrote that in the ways we relate to each other, we contribute to shaping each other's world. How I treat others decides the width and colours of their world (Løgstrup, 1999: 39).

Delving into the coming chapters, where incredibly important practices are described and discussed, my point is not to undermine these at all. Rather, my point is to reflect on how we as professional and volunteer agents must remember that we are never not humans living in interdependence. The human beings we encounter *also* need everyday community with fellow humans. In some Western societies, particularly those with strong welfare systems, migrants and refugees encounter a multitude of professionals, but often they do not encounter people without official purpose. As professionals we must remember that we too are neighbours. We are co-parents, strangers, friends and acquaintances, also with those in vulnerable life conditions (Nahnfeldt and Rønsdal, 2021). We need to find ways to allow for moments of sharing life, of remaining in encounters for the sake of the encounter, and for the sake of each other. These may be bare moments, but they may be tipping points where meaningful co-creating and shaping of life occur.

This part of the book offers insights into social, behavioural and psychological challenges confronting individuals and families affected by the previous wars in the Balkans, and the contemporary war in Europe. Issues of mental health in the post-conflict of the Balkan wars are reviewed in Chapter 6. This historical psychological aspects of 'post-conflict' label has to be extended well beyond the end of the war as the conflicts are kept alive mentally and socially, which serves political purposes while harming both individual and collective wellbeing.

Chapter 7 has been developed from interviews with mothers who have been displaced with their children from Ukraine. Psychosocial perspectives from Ukraine, the maintenance of cultural identity, through education and the nurturing of children, are provided from the personal and professional perspectives of a Ukrainian school teacher and a clinical psychologist, both mothers with their children in the UK, being supported and supporting the work with Ukrainian refugees in the London Borough of Sutton (see Chapter 12).

With reference to the role of mothers in providing protection and mitigation of the trauma to which children are exposed in the war zone and being displaced from their homes in Ukraine, Chapter 8 recognises the issues of language and integration, social support, finances, legal status and mental health as some of the key social determinants of health for both refugee adults and children. The issue of adverse childhood experiences is explored via a case study of displaced mothers and children being supported in Norway. The organisational aspects of this work in Norway are considered in Chapter 14.

Chapter 9 focuses on the perpetration of gender-based violence, particularly sexual violence, against women and girls, which increases during war and conflict. Reports of violence committed against women and girls by enemy forces, in the case of the Russian war in Ukraine, has been focused on Russian soldiers committing sexual violence against Ukrainian women and girls. However, less reported is a rise in cases of domestic violence and abuse committed by Ukrainian men against their Ukrainian wives or female partners. There are many accounts of women having 'perfect' relationships before the war, and then finding that as their husbands have returned from conflict, they have become violent towards them. This has been claimed to be related to rising stress, economic hardship, unemployment and trauma related to the conflict. The author of this chapter suggest that it should not be assumed that women fleeing Ukraine are automatically safe from domestic violence and abuse.

Chapter 10 provides a *life course approach* to ageing. Successful ageingiimpacted by the accumulated life events which, through a range of life challenges result in traumatic and chronic stress, affectmortality and later life burdens of disease.

References

Løgstrup, K.E. (1999) *Den etiske fordring* [*The Ethical Demand*] [first published in 1956]. Gjøvik: J.W. Cappelens Forlag A.S.

Nahnfeldt, C. and Rønsdal, K. (eds) (2021) *Contemporary Christian-Cultural Values: Migration Encounters in the Nordic Region*. Oxford: Routledge.

6

Impact of political instability and wars on mental health of people in European countries: lessons from the war in the Balkans

Marija Branković and Milica Ninković

Introduction

During the last decade of the 20th century, a series of violent interethnic conflicts occurred in what used to be the Socialist Federal Republic of Yugoslavia. Yugoslavia was a multiethnic socialist country on the Balkan peninsula, with six ethnic groups holding the status of constitutive nations: Bosniaks/Muslims, Croats, Macedonians, Montenegrins, Serbs and Slovenians (Čalić, 2013). Ethnic minorities were legally recognised, Albanians and Hungarians being the largest. However, following the rising levels of ethnonationalism in the 1980s and consequential wars in the 1990s, Yugoslavia dissolved along the borders of federated republics. During 1991 and 1992, four republics declared independence, and the federation formally broke into five independent states in 1992: Bosnia and Herzegovina, Croatia, Macedonia, Slovenia, and the Federal Republic of Yugoslavia (FRY) constituted of two republics – Serbia and Montenegro.

A series of armed conflicts (Yugoslav wars) followed the dissolution (Čalić, 2013). The most violent conflicts happened in Bosnia and Herzegovina and Croatia and were resolved by the end of 1995. After a few years of peace, the conflict between Serbs and Albanians in Kosovo escalated in 1998, leading to the Kosovo War and North Atlantic Treaty Organization bombing of FRY during the spring of 1999. The wars ended by signing the Ohrid agreement in 2001, after the insurgencies in Macedonia. In 2006, FRY peacefully broke into two independent republics (Serbia and Montenegro), and Kosovo declared independence in 2007.

The wars resulted in 140,000 people killed and almost four million displaced (International Center for Transitional Justice, 2009). Many of those who survived were traumatised, either as victims of rapes, ethnic cleansing or crimes against humanity (Antić, 2021). Additionally, the war resulted in enormous material damage (Vejvoda, 2004), followed by a deep recession (see Simon [2003] for a review).

Economic transition and health policies in post-conflict society

FRY was perceived as a major perpetrator in the Bosnian, Croatian and Kosovo wars. Thus, it was sanctioned by the United Nations first during 1992–1995, then again during 1998–2000, which contributed to the increasing poverty levels. Following the wars, the successor states started their transition from socialism and planned economy to a supposedly democratic market economy. In FRY, the transition began in 2000, after the ruling Socialist party of Serbia was overthrown (Čalić, 2013).

Due to their co-occurrence, the impact of war on public health is inseparable from the impact of economic changes, especially those in the healthcare system. Socialist Yugoslavia had a publicly funded healthcare system that granted universal healthcare. Shortly before the dissolution, this system was recognised by the World Bank as a role model for developing countries (Primary Health Care in Yugoslavia, 1992). Importantly, the system even identified psychotherapy as a promising paradigm to treat mental health issues, unlike the rest of Eastern Europe, where mental health was almost exclusively viewed through the biological lens (Savelli, 2018; Antić, 2021).

However, economic transition and the post-war recession had enormous impacts on the healthcare systems of the former Yugoslavian countries. Neoliberal economic policies promoted the privatisation of healthcare services, thus making them less affordable (Lazarevik et al, 2012; Đurić, 2021). Notably, economic inequalities in the Western Balkan countries are among the largest in Europe (Eurostat, 2023), further reflecting on healthcare inaccessibility. In Serbia, adequate mental health care is not accessible to all. Although psychiatric services are incorporated into the universal healthcare package, there is a lack of community mental health care services (Lečić Toševski et al, 2010), such as individual counselling and psychotherapy. A recent study indicated that around 40 per cent of Serbian citizens find psychological support too expensive (Psychosocial Innovation Network, 2022a). This finding is even more worrying, keeping in mind the long-lasting consequences of wars and recession on mental health: 16–35 per cent of Serbian citizens show clinically significant symptoms of psychiatric disorders (Marić et al, 2022; Psychosocial Innovation Network, 2022a).

In the following sections, we will discuss how wars and crisis affected mental health and then dive deeper into social psychological determinants of mental health in post-conflict society. In terms of the model of social determinants of health inequities (World Health Organization, 2010) we will focus our discussion on the culture and societal values as the structural determinants in this specific (post-)conflict context. We will also show how they link to the outcomes of the model, in particular the wellbeing and mental health of citizens of the region of the Western Balkans. As the issues we are tackling are inherently political our chapter has implications for the contested element of social cohesion, specifically, how social cohesion is being disrupted by the predominant values and exclusive social identities, and how this impacts the health-related outcomes in the region.

The impact of war on mental health: the seeable and less seeable

The devastating consequences of war on an individual's life are unquestionable, further aggravated by the sanctions and economic recession. The data from 2005–2006 shows that the levels of post-traumatic stress disorder (PTSD) in the whole region were high and correlated with the brutality of the war (Priebe et al, 2010). Prevalence of PTSD ranged from 11 per cent in North Macedonia, where the conflict never escalated enough to be labelled as a war, up to 35 per cent in Bosnia and Herzegovina, where the war was the most brutal. The observed frequency of PTSD symptoms in the region was substantially higher compared to countries without a recent experience of war (Priebe et al, 2013). Furthermore, almost one-third of Serbian citizens suffered from lifetime PTSD (Lečić Toševski et al, 2013). Currently, more than 20 years after the North Atlantic Treaty Organization bombing of FRY and 30 years after the onset of the Yugoslav wars, 11 per cent of Serbian citizens still meet clinically significant criteria for PTSD (Psychosocial Innovation Network, 2022a).

Such statistics get even more devastating, bearing in mind two factors: comorbidities of PTSD and barriers to seeking psychological support. Individuals suffering from PTSD are at heightened risk of alcohol misuse (Debell et al, 2014) and pathological gambling (Ledgerwood and Milošević, 2015). They are also more likely to develop high levels of symptoms of depression and anxiety (Spinhoven et al, 2014). Even individuals who suffer from subthreshold PTSD are at heightened risk of major depression and suicide (Marshall et al, 2001). In line with this, the results of a recent mental health screening in Serbia show that around 15 per cent of citizens have moderate to high levels of depressive symptoms, whereas 7 per cent suffer from high levels of anxiety (Psychosocial Innovation Network, 2022a). Moreover, 8 per cent of Serbian citizens satisfied the criteria for substance use disorders (Marić et al, 2022).

High levels of psychiatric disorders and mental health issues call for systemic and widely accessible mental health care. However, the public healthcare system is understaffed, especially in the domain of mental health. Lack of resources and stigmatisation of individuals who suffer from mental health issues are among the most prominent barriers to seeking psychological help (Psychosocial Innovation Network, 2022b). Citizens often recourse to unreliable methods of alternative medicine instead of seeking professional treatment (Budžak & Branković, 2022). At the same time, untreated mental health issues, especially PTSD, have numerous negative effects on the quality of life (Priebe et al, 2009). Moreover, research shows that the prevalence of symptoms of depression and anxiety is higher in the younger population that have faint, if any, memory of war (Psychosocial Innovation Network, 2022a). This implies that living in a post-conflict society bears additional mental health risks, and in the following, we will discuss them from a social psychological perspective.

Beyond the individual: social identities and the cultures of war

Social psychologists argue that a person's wellbeing often reflects the state of the groups that they see as important for themselves (Haslam et al, 2009: 5). The period of open conflict and war, followed by the period of transition and instability, entailed more than individual traumatisation and loss. These events and experiences also affected group-level or social identity processes within individuals. The social identity approach (Tajfel and Turner, 1986; Abrams and Hogg, 2006) builds on the idea that an important part of who we are reflects our belonging to different social groups. Social identity entails our knowledge about important groups we belong to and the value we attach to them. Put simply, social identity is the part of our identity through which we connect ourselves to our social surroundings so that something 'external' becomes something we see as a part of ourselves. Social identities imbue us with a sense of belonging, meaning that transcends ourselves, and, importantly, a sense of self-worth (Abrams and Hogg, 2006; Haslam et al, 2009).

In conflict and war, in addition to individual traumatisation and psychological harm, social identities also get hurt. Social identities are compromised on each side of the conflict, regardless of whether the specific group is the perpetrator or the victim, and further complicated by the fact that most groups assume both of these roles at specific points. Following the major social crises, individuals are thus challenged to re-evaluate and reinterpret their identities while preserving their sense of self-worth (Haslam et al, 2009). Even the individuals who did not actively contribute, for example, the generations born after the conflicts, also have to deal with these changes, as their social identities are inevitably connected to these experiences. This also applies to the communities as a whole, as these processes rarely depend on the individual but are subject to more collective efforts.

Collectively, the communities undergo a period of transformation during and in the aftermath of conflicts. The process of adaptation results in constructing a specific worldview – the ethos of conflict – in which the conflict becomes interpretable and meaningful (Bar-Tal, 2000; Bar-Tal et al, 2012). For instance, groups affected by conflict often tend to glorify themselves and belittle or even dehumanise their opponents. Ingroup cohesion becomes crucial so that any voices critical toward the conflict or violence are viewed as disloyal. The goals of one's group are seen as exclusively legitimate, while the opponent group is seen as the one fuelling the conflict. The group often resorts to history to legitimise its claims, regularly offering one-sided interpretations of historical events or the history of intergroup relations.

Research shows that, after the resolution of armed conflicts, the society in the Western Balkans has continued to spread and reinforce the ethos of conflict, keeping the conflict alive in people's heads (Turjačanin, 2014; Branković et al, 2017; Jovanović and Bermúdez, 2021). The polarised identities are utilised by the political elites to mobilise voters and secure their power (Milačić, 2022). A very good illustration is Bosnia and Herzegovina – here, the political system and the state structure are defined so as to reinforce ethno-religious divides (Turjačanin, 2014). To be a political subject, one has to be a Serb, a Croat or a Bosniak. Further, schools are divided into Serbian, Croatian and Bosniak schools. Although most of them are situated under the same roof, the students are typically discouraged from having contact with students outside of their group and are taught one-sided historical narratives.

These divisions have multi-layered consequences. Some can be thought of as general negative effects of deepening social divisions, namely, a disturbed societal cohesion (we will discuss this issue in more depth shortly). Second, constantly threatened social identities need to be defended, which requires psychological and social effort. As a result, the identities become less flexible and more exclusive (Branković et al, 2020), as well as more fragile. For instance, Serbian ethnic identity was severely affected by the perpetrator's role in the Yugoslav wars. The core of the dominant ethnic identity lies in a negation of responsibility for the role of the ethnic group in previous conflicts, coupled with fostering an uncritical patriotism and glorification of the heroic parts of the national history (Branković et al, 2017; Jovanović and Bermúdez, 2021), and even questioning the existence of other ethnic outgroups (Ninković, 2020). For instance, students are taught one-sided versions of history based on the idea that only one group (their ingroup) has legitimate interests and/or is legitimate and has, therefore, been persecuted and victimised. At the same time, ethnic identity is essentialised; that is, it is thought of as something a person is born into (for example, being a Serb is something you do not choose), thus becoming inseparable from the self. Consequently, to remain a part of the group, you must accept and defend the group uncritically (Branković, 2016). Defending the ethnic group becomes equated with defending the self. A fragile and overly defensive sense of identity does not afford a solid basis for wellbeing and mental health.

The psychodynamics of fear: terror management in the aftermath of war

The social dynamics of the post-conflict societies are characterised by constant retraumatisation and insecurity that negatively affect psychological equanimity. In addition, the local political elites in power reinforce the notion that the social and political order is constantly being threatened so as to present themselves as the guarantees of stability and peace (Milačić, 2022). Psychologically, this means raising the stress levels constantly and focusing on the imminent threats in the surroundings. The dominant affective orientation of post-conflict societies is fear (Bar-Tal, 2000; Bar-Tal et al, 2012), which is reflected by a high prevalence of anxiety-related disorders after the conflicts (Psychosocial Innovation Network, 2022a). Sensitivity to threats and a general defensive outlook have been captured quite accurately by the term 'siege mentality' (Bar-Tal and Antebi, 1992).

Terror management theory further clarifies these defensive psychological dynamics (Greenberg et al, 1986; Solomon et al, 2004). It suggests that individuals are fundamentally motivated by the need to achieve psychological equanimity, resolving the fear of personal mortality. To this end, individuals invest in building and maintaining symbolic worlds that provide meaning and security and strive to achieve their rightful place within these symbolic worlds. Ethnic and religious groups are particularly apt to provide this existential security and meaning, as these groups have relatively clear boundaries and values and a temporal continuity beyond an individual existence (Castano et al, 2002). In line with this, reminders of personal mortality have been experimentally shown to strengthen ethnic identification, positive image of the ethnic ingroup and perceptions of ingroup unity (Branković, 2016). Also, in post-conflict settings, presenting such reminders has decreased the preparedness for reconciliation, particularly when the threat concerns personal and group annihilation (Hirschberger et al, 2010). Clearly, the social and political context we described abounds in such reminders.

Reminders of personal and/or group mortality also heighten the proclivity to violence aimed at both individuals and groups (McGregor et al, 1998; Pyszczynski et al, 2006). Acceptance of violence is also characteristic of post-conflict societies (Bar-Tal, 2000). For instance, a study demonstrated that reminders of mortality heightened the proclivity to terrorism as a political means among otherwise peace-oriented Iranian students (Pyszczynski et al, 2006). At the same time, such reminders raised the support for violent anti-terrorist attacks among the students in the United States. Thus, intergroup dynamics provoking fear leads to support for violence on both sides of a conflict. In addition, the wider social context in such societies also tends to grow more aggressive and violent. Violence is not only reserved for the 'enemies' but directed towards political opponents and any critical voices in society, for example, the civil society striving for peace or reconciliation efforts (Kostovicova, 2006). Finally, as violence is legitimised and social divisions are heightened, it does not come as a surprise that interpersonal and family violence also thrives in such contexts (United Nations Development Program, 2022).

The role of religion for mental health

From a predominantly atheistic society of Yugoslavia, the most recent decades witnessed a religious awakening in the region. As many as 90 per cent of citizens today self-declare as religious in most of the countries (Dušanić, 2007; Blagojević, 2013; Branković et al, 2017), in particular among the youth (Popadić et al, 2019). However, according to research, religiousness takes different forms (Branković et al, 2017). For most people, declaring as religious is mostly related to following traditions of the (ethno-)religious group, thus being a sort of extended cultural identification. A much smaller number of people accept the core of the religious doctrine, while only a minor group actively practises religion (for example, going to church weekly).

Religious identity is most closely related to ethnic identity in the region, and they are typically perceived as interwoven (Branković et al, 2017), for example, Serbs are mostly Orthodox, Croats are mostly Catholic, and Bosniaks are mostly Muslim. As there are not many visible differences among the ethnic groups and as they share basically the same language, the religious identity and the related traditions became the most tangible characteristics on which the ethnic divides were based (Dušanić, 2007; Hronesova, 2012). After the wars, religious divides were also widened, and religious identities have become a factor of division rather than cohesion. The church has been recognised as a guardian of the traditional identities and one of the main channels through which the ethos of conflict is being spread and enhanced (Branković et al, 2017; Subotić, 2019). This role does not only apply to the formerly adversarial groups but to any groups that are seen as deviating from or challenging the dominant traditional identities (for example, feminists, LGBTQIA+ individuals, and so on).

Religiousness does seem to play at least some positive role in mental health. Although the research in the region is scarce, some studies established small positive correlations between intrinsic religiousness and life satisfaction, as well as a negative relationship with loneliness (Dušanić, 2007). However, this potentially positive role of religiousness can be easily diverted given its strict traditionalism, so, for instance, people not living in accordance with the traditional roles and stereotypes can feel excluded or ambivalent. Another potential negative impact is the fact that various religious practices and rites are seen as alternatives to professional medical advice or help (Lazarević et al, 2023). Research suggests that a large proportion of the population in Serbia, for instance, resort to prayer, visiting monasteries or using holy water to solve their medical issues (Lazarević et al, 2023). Similar treatments can also be used for mental health issues. Given the church's and clergy's spiritual authority, the role of religion is an important venue for future research. In particular, church officials promoting more inclusive identities and more tolerant attitudes toward outgroups would greatly contribute to reconciliation efforts (Pyszczynski et al, 2008).

The crisis of trust and solidarity

Wars and crises take their toll on the level of interpersonal relations and the sense of the common good, empathy and solidarity. Social divisions that stem from the wars and which are perpetuated trough the institutionalisation of the ethos of conflict are further aggravated by social inequalities that arose in much of the Western Balkans (Eurostat, 2023). Studies suggest that the region greatly suffers from a lack of trust. This lack of trust is observed at the institutional level, as a crisis of trust in institutions (Eurofund, 2013; Turjačanin et al, 2018), which is significantly lower compared to the mean of the other European countries. Citizens of the region do not trust the media, the political parties nor politicians, and particularly doubt the democratic institutions of parliament and government. The only (partial) exemption are the traditional institutions such as the church or military. Moreover, a severe lack of trust is also observable at the interpersonal level (Eurofound, 2013), even among the young (Popadić et al, 2019). For instance, youth trust only their most immediate family and to some extent close friends, while the level of trust steeply drops from there.

Further, political and economic transition introduced rising income inequalities, especially in Serbia (Eurostat, 2023). Studies show that inequality contributes to deepening group divisions in society, raised perceptions of threat, as well as negative intergroup stereotyping and hostility (Jetten et al, 2017; Jay et al, 2019). The threatened self of identity is an additional source of motivation to strengthen one's attachment to traditional identities (for example, ethnic identities), as well as the climate of social distrust (Jay et al, 2019). Thus, inequality disrupts social cohesion and solidarity (Jetten et al, 2017; Jay et al, 2019). Inequality exerts the most direct impact on the accessibility of mental health services and professionals (Psychosocial Innovation Network, 2022a). However, there are also more indirect consequences. For instance, a study shows that more loneliness is experienced by people who value hierarchical relations in society and competitiveness (Schermer et al, 2022).

The disturbed social cohesion has multiple harmful consequences for mental health. First, it constitutes a threat to wellbeing in its own right (Jovanović, 2016). For instance, it has been shown that in particular, the disruption of interpersonal trust contributes negatively to subjective wellbeing among participants in Serbia (Jovanović, 2016), while other studies also show that country-level social capital also has a negative impact on both health and subjective wellbeing (Elgar et al, 2011). A lack of trust and solidarity fosters a sense of isolation, breaches psychological safety, and adds to the prevalent fear and anxiety – if you do not trust your social surroundings, this means that you cannot feel safe and at ease. Second, they exert their negative influence in lacking social support and stigmatisation, especially related to mental health issues. Both mental and somatic health is dependent on social support and shared identities between the providers and receivers of care (Haslam et al, 2008; Jetten et al, 2014). For instance, studies we conducted in Serbia showed that a lack of trust in the medical system and healthcare providers, together with reported negative experiences with the healthcare system, predicted more intentional non-adherence to medical recommendations (Purić et al, 2023), as well as lower compliance to physicians' advice (Ninković et al, 2024).

Conclusion

In this chapter, we discussed the issues of mental health in a post-conflict region. Although war and its impact on the community is driven by a range of *structural issues*, mainly influenced by government policies, *intermediate issues* relating to the mental health of the population can benefit from analysis using the conceptual framework of the social determinants of health, with respect to historical time. As we have shown, the 'post-conflict' label is not psychologically accurate. In many ways, the conflicts are kept alive mentally and socially, which serves political purposes while harming both individual and social wellbeing. The social identity approach helps us elucidate how the characteristics of social context and relevant social identities impact on individual sense of self-worth and wellbeing. Social identity resources have been recognised as social cure (Jetten et al, 2014), however, they can become exactly the opposite. In post-conflict societies that are characterised by continuing traumatisation and insecurity, perpetuating the ethos of conflict thus has 'hidden' consequences. It is individuals who must tackle the implication of endangered social identities, which often leads to an overly defensive psychological dynamic: a chronic sense of fear, insecurity and uncritical clinging to the traditional identities that are based on conflicts. At the social level, this is coupled with lacking trust in others and a disturbed social cohesion. Therefore, as much as it is needed, provision of adequate individual mental health support and assistance is not sufficient. Communities and social identities have to be restructured to allow a more positive social psychological dynamic to take over. We believe that an essential issue is the possibility to confront the conflictual past in an open and rational manner, that is, recognising that one has the right not to support the violence and the crimes, but to take a critical stance as a base for a reformed social identification with the ethnic and religious groups. On a positive note, psychological and mental health professionals and researchers could provide the support and guidance needed in this process.

References

Abrams, D. and Hogg, M.A. (2006) *Social Identifications: A Social Psychology of Intergroup Relations and Group Processes*. Routledge, London.

Antić, A. (2021) *Non-Aligned Psychiatry in the Cold War: Revolution, Emancipation and Re-Imagining the Human Psyche*. Palgrave Macmillan, Cham.

Bar-Tal, D. (2000) From intractable conflict through conflict resolution to reconciliation: psychological analysis. *Political Psychology*, 21(2): 351–365.

Bar-Tal, D. and Antebi, D. (1992) Siege mentality in Israel. *International Journal of Intercultural Relations*, 16(3): 251–275.

Bar-Tal, D., Sharvit, K., Halperin, E. and Zafran, A. (2012) Ethos of conflict: the concept and its measurement. *Peace and Conflict: Journal of Peace Psychology*, 18(1): 40–61.

Blagojević, M. (2013) Savremena religioznost studenata i desekularizacija srpskog društva [Contemporary religiosity of students and desecularization of the Serbian society]. In M. Blagojević, J. Jablanov Maksimović and T. Bajović (eds), *(Post)sekularni obrt: Religijske, moralne i društveno-političke vrednosti studenata u Srbiji. [(Post)secular turnover: Religious, moral, and socio-political values of students in Serbia]*Institut za filozofiju i društvenu teoriju, Fondacija Konrad Adenauer, Centar za evropske studije, pp 11–61.

Branković, M. (2016) *Psychological Defenses from the Fear of Death* [Doctoral thesis]. Belgrade: Faculty of Philosophy.

Branković, M., Turjačanin, V. and Maloku, E. (2017) Setting the stage: research on national, ethnic, and religious identities after the recent violent conflicts in the Western Balkans. In F. Pratto, I. Žeželj, E. Maloku, V. Turjačanin and M. Branković (eds), *Shaping Social Identities after the Violent Conflicts: Youth in Western Balkans*. Cham: Palgrave Macmillan, pp 13–51.

Branković, M., Žeželj, I. and Turjačanin, V. (2020) How knowing others makes us more inclusive: social identity inclusiveness mediates the effects of contact on out-group acceptance. *Journal of Theoretical Social Psychology*, 4(3): 95–106.

Budžak, A. and Branković, M. (2022) Alternative ways to mental health: exploring psychological determinants of preference for CAM treatments. *Studia Psychologica*, 64(1): 118–135.

Čalić, M.-Ž. (2013) *Istorija Jugoslavije [The History of Yugoslavia]*. Belgrade: Clio.

Castano, E., Yzerbyt, V., Paladino, M. and Sacchi, S. (2002) I belong, therefore, I exist: ingroup identification, ingroup entitativity, and ingroup bias. *Personality and Social Psychology Bulletin*, 28(2): 135–143.

Debell, F., Fear, N.T., Head, M., Batt-Rawden, S., Greenberg, N., Wessely, S. and Goodwin, L. (2014) A systematic review of the comorbidity between PTSD and alcohol misuse. *Social Psychiatry and Psychiatric Epidemiology*, 49(9): 1401–1425.

Đurić, P. (2021) *Na šta mislimo kada kažemo … Novi zdravstveni sistem.* University of Belgrade, Institute for Philosophy and Social Theory. Available at: https://rifdt.instifdt.bg.ac.rs/bitstream/handle/123456789/2440/bitstream_8645.pdf?sequence=1

Dušanić, S. (2007) *Psihološka istraživanja religioznosti* [*Psychological Studies of Religiosity*]. Banjaluka: Filozofski fakultet.

Elgar, F.J., Davis, C.G., Wohl, M.J., Trites, S.J., Zelenski, J.M. and Martin, M.S. (2011) Social capital, health and life satisfaction in 50 countries. *Health & Place*, 17(5): 1044–1053.

Eurofound (2013) *Quality of life in enlargement countries: Third European quality of life survey – Serbia.* Available at https://www.eurofound.europa.eu/en/publications/2013/quality-life-enlargement-countries-third-european-quality-life-survey-serbia

Eurostat (2023) *Enlargement Countries: Statistics on Living Conditions.* Eurostat. Available at: https://ec.europa.eu/eurostat/statistics-explained/index.php?title=Enlargement_countries_-_statistics_on_living_conditions#Income_distribution

Greenberg, J., Pyszczynski, T. and Solomon, S. (1986) The causes and consequences of a need for self-esteem: a terror management theory. In R.F. Baumeister (ed), *Public Self and Private Self.* New York: Springer-Verlag, pp 189–212.

Haslam, S.A., Jetten, J., Postmes, T. and Haslam, C. (2009) Social identity, health and well-being: an emerging agenda for applied psychology. *Applied Psychology-an International Review-Psychologie Appliquee-Revue Internationale*, 58(1), 1–23.

Hirschberger, G., Pyszczynski, T. and Ein-dor, T. (2010) An ever-dying people: the existential underpinnings of Israelis' perceptions of war and conflict. *Les Cahiers Internationaux de Psychologie Sociale*, 3: 443–457.

Hronesova, J. (2012) *Everyday Ethno-National Identities of Young People in Bosnia and Herzegovina.* Frankfurt: Peter Lang.

International Center for Transitional Justice (2009) *Transitional Justice in the Former Yugoslavia.* International Center for Transitional Justice. Available at: https://www.ictj.org/sites/default/files/ICTJ-FormerYugoslavia-Justice-Facts-2009-English.pdf

Jay, S., Batruch, A., Jetten, J., McGarty, C. and Muldoon, O.T. (2019) Economic inequality and the rise of far-right populism: a social psychological analysis. *Journal of Community & Applied Social Psychology*, 29(5): 418–428.

Jetten, J., Haslam, C., Haslam, S.A., Dingle, G. and Jones, J.M. (2014) How groups affect our health and well-being: the path from theory to policy. *Social Issues and Policy Review*, 8(1): 103–130.

Jetten, J., Wang, Z., Steffens, N.K., Mols, F., Peters, K. and Verkuyten, M. (2017) A social identity analysis of responses to economic inequality. *Current Opinion in Psychology*, 18: 1–5.

Jovanović, R. and Bermúdez, Á. (2021) The next generation: nationalism and violence in the narratives of Serbian students on the break-up of Yugoslavia. *Studies in Ethnicity and Nationalism*, 21(1): 2–25.

Jovanović, V. (2016) Trust and subjective well-being: the case of Serbia. *Personality and Individual Differences*, 98: 284–288.

Kostovicova, D. (2006) Civil society and post-communist democratization: facing a double challenge in post-Milošević Serbia. *Journal of Civil Society*, 2(1): 21–37.

Lazarević, L., Knezevic, G., Purić, D., Teovanovic, P., Petrović, M., Ninković, M., et al (2023) Tracking variations in daily questionable health behaviors and their psychological roots: a preregistered experience sampling study. *Scientific Reports*, 13: 14058.

Lazarevik, V., Donev, D., Gudeva Nikovska, D. and Kasapinov, B. (2012) Three periods of health system reforms in the Republic of Macedonia (1991–2011). *Contributions of Macedonian Academy of Sciences & Arts*, 33(2): 175–189.

Lečić Toševski, D., Draganić, S. and Pejović Milovančević, M. (2010) Mental healthcare in Serbia. *International Psychiatry*, 7(1): 13–15.

Lečić Toševski, D., Pejušković, B., Miladinović, T., Tošković, O. and Priebe, S. (2013) Posttraumatic stress disorder in a Serbian community: seven years after trauma exposure. *Journal of Nervous & Mental Disease*, 201(12): 1040–1044.

Ledgerwood, D.M. and Milošević, A. (2015) Clinical and personality characteristics associated with post traumatic stress disorder in problem and pathological gamblers recruited from the community. *Journal of Gambling Studies*, 31(2): 501–512.

Marić, N.P., Lazarević, L.J.B., Priebe, S., Mihić, L.J., Pejović-Milovančević, M., Terzić-Šupić, Z., et al (2022) COVID-19-related stressors, mental disorders, depressive and anxiety symptoms: a cross-sectional, nationally-representative, face-to-face survey in Serbia. *Epidemiology and Psychiatric Sciences*, 31: e36.

Marshall, R.D., Olfson, M., Hellman, F., Blanco, C., Guardino, M. and Struening, E.L. (2001) Comorbidity, impairment, and suicidality in subthreshold PTSD. *American Journal of Psychiatry*, 158(9): 1467–1473.

McGregor, H.A., Lieberman, J.D., Greenberg, J., Solomon, S., Arndt, J., Simon, L., et al (1998) Terror management and aggression: evidence that mortality salience motivates aggression against worldview-threatening others. *Journal of Personality and Social Psychology*, 74(3): 590–605.

Milačić, F. (2022) Stateness and democratic backsliding in the former Yugoslavia: how political actors subvert democracy in the name of the nation. *Nations and Nationalism*, 28(4): 1474–1493.

Ninković, M. (2020) My ethnicity is older than yours! Delegitimizing other's ethnic identity as a correlate of inter-ethnic attitudes. In M. Videnović, I. Stepanović Ilić, N. Simić and M. Rajić (eds), *Proceedings of the XXVI Scientific Conference Empirical Studies in Psychology*. Institute of Psychology and Laboratory for Experimental Psychology, Belgrade. https://empirij skaistrazivanja.org/wp-content/uploads/2021/04/EIP2020_conf_proc eedings.pdf#page=132

Ninković, M., Damnjanović, K. and Ilić, S. (2024) Women's trust in the healthcare system in Serbia: Validation of the Women's Trust and Confidence in Healthcare System scale. *Women's Health, 20*, 17455057241249864.

Popadić, D., Pavlović, Z. and Mihailović, S. (2019) *Mladi u Srbiji 2018/2019* [*Youth in Serbia 2018/2019*]. Friedrich-Ebert-Stiftung, Belgrade

Priebe, S., Matanov, A., Janković Gavrilović, J., McCrone, P., Ljubotina, D., Knežević, G., et al (2009) Consequences of untreated posttraumatic stress disorder following war in former Yugoslavia: morbidity, subjective quality of life, and care costs. *Croatian Medical Journal*, 50(5): 465–475.

Priebe, S., Bogić, M., Ajduković, D., Frančišković, T., Galeazzi, G.M., Kucukalic, A., et al (2010) Mental disorders following war in the Balkans: a study in 5 countries. *Archives of General Psychiatry*, 67(5): 518–528.

Priebe, S., Janković Gavrilović, J., Bremner, S., Ajduković, D., Frančišković, T., Galeazzi, G.M., et al (2013) Psychological symptoms as long-term consequences of war experiences. *Psychopathology*, 46(1): 45–54.

Primary Health Care in Yugoslavia (1992) *European Journal of Public Health*, 2(3–4): 211.

Psychosocial Innovation Network (2022a) *Mental Health in Serbia: Assessment of Needs, Risk Factors, and Barriers to Receiving Professional Health*. Psychosocial Innovation Network. Available at: https://psychosocialinnovation.net/ wp-content/uploads/2022/11/Mental-Health-in-Serbia_Assessment-of-Needs-Risk-Factors-and-Barriers-to-Receiving-Professional-Help_2 022-study-results.pdf

Psychosocial Innovation Network (2022b) *Mental Health in Serbia: Availability of Psychosocial Support Services*. Available at: https://psychosocialinnovation. net/wp-content/uploads/2022/11/Mental-Health-in-Serbia_Availability-of-Psychosocial-Support-Services_2022-study-results.pdf

Purić, D., Petrović, M.B., Živanović, M., Lukić, P., Zupan, Z., Branković, M., et al (2023) Development of a novel instrument for assessing intentional non-adherence to official medical recommendations (iNAR-12): a sequential mixed-methods study in Serbia. *BMJ Open*, 13(6): e069978.

Pyszczynski, T., Abdollahi, A., Solomon, S., Greenberg, J., Cohen, F. and Weise, D. (2006) Mortality salience, martyrdom, and military might: the great satan versus the axis of evil. *Personality and Social Psychology Bulletin*, 32(4): 525–537.

Pyszczynski, T., Rothschild, Z. and Abdollahi, A. (2008) Terrorism, violence, and hope for peace: a terror management perspective. *Current Directions in Psychological Science*, 17(5): 318–322.

Savelli, M. (2018) 'Peace and happiness await us': psychotherapy in Yugoslavia, 1945–85. *History of the Human Sciences*, 31(4): 38–57.

Schermer, J.A., Branković, M., Oviedo-Trespalacios, O., Volkodav, T., Ha, T.T.K., Krammer, G., et al (2022) Humor styles are related to loneliness across 15 countries. *Europe's Journal of Psychology*, 18(4): 422–436.

Simon, G. (2003) Economic transition in Yugoslavia: a view from outside. *Medjunarodni Problemi*, 55(1): 104–128.

Solomon, S., Greenberg, J. and Pyszczynski, T. (2004) The cultural animal: twenty years of Terror Management Theory and research. In J. Greenberg, S. Koole and T. Pyszczynski (eds), *Handbook of Experimental Existential Psychology*. New York: The Guilford Press, pp 13–34.

Spinhoven, P., Penninx, B.W., Van Hemert, A.M., De Rooij, M. and Elzinga, B.M. (2014) Comorbidity of PTSD in anxiety and depressive disorders: prevalence and shared risk factors. *Child Abuse & Neglect*, 38(8): 1320–1330.

Subotić, J. (2019) The church, the nation, and the state: the Serbian Orthodox Church after communism. In S. Ramet (ed), *Orthodox Churches and Politics in Southeastern Europe*. Cham: Palgrave Macmillan, pp 85–110.

Tajfel, H. and Turner, J.C. (1986) The social identity theory of intergroup behavior. In S. Worchel and W.G. Austin (eds), *Psychology of Intergroup Relations*, Vol 2. Chicago: Nelson-Hall, pp 7–24.

Turjačanin, V. (2014) *Socijalna psihologija etničkog identiteta* [*Social Psychology of Ethnic Identity*]. Banja Luka: Filozofski fakultet.

Turjačanin, V., Žeželj, I., Maloku, E. and Branković, M. (2017) Taming conflicted identities: searching for new youth values in the western Balkans. In T.P. Trošt and D. Mandić (eds), *Changing Youth Values in Southeast Europe:Beyond Ethnicity*. Oxford; Routledge, pp 151–176.

United Nations Development Program (2022) *Nasilje u porodici – šta govore podaci.* [*Domestic Violence – What the Data Say*]. Available at: https://www.undp.org/sites/g/files/zskgke326/files/migration/rs/undp_rs_Nasilje_u_porodici_Sta_govore_podaci.pdf

Vejvoda, I. (2004) Zašto se dogodio rat? In M. Hadžić (ed), *Nasilno rasturanje Jugoslavije—Uzroci, dinamika, posledice* [*The Violent Dissolution of Yugoslavia – Causes, Dynamics, Consequences*]. Beograd: Centar za civilno-vojne odnose, pp 65–80.

World Health Organization (2010) *A Conceptual Framework for Action on the Social Determinants of Health.* Available at: https://www.who.int/publications/i/item/9789241500852

7

Psychosocial and educational perspectives from Ukraine: cultural identity and the nurturing of children

Bohdana Tymoskyshyn, Svitlana Semaniv,
Andrii Parkhoma and Gillian Bonner

Introduction

The war in Europe, following the invasion of Ukraine by the Russian army in February 2022, has resulted in many thousands of deaths in the Ukrainian civilian populations and Ukrainian and Russian soldiers, leading to *indirect* socioeconomic global impacts such as the rising cost of living, disruption of energy markets and the large-scale migration of one-third of the Ukrainian population. This chapter is written by a psychologist (SS), a psychotherapist (AP) and teacher (BT) who were displaced, with their children, from Ukraine to the UK. Their critical review of the changing attitudes and aspirations of Ukrainians from the Soviet era to the Orange Revolution to the Russian invasion, provide a context for reviewing the changing nurturing, education and cultural development of displaced children and children remaining in a country at war. Schemes such as Homes for Ukraine in the UK (see Chapter 12), have been most welcome. However, children's learning and cultural experiences, being significantly disrupted with the added challenge of needing to learn a new language, will have life-long consequences on health and wellbeing.

This chapter will consider the psychological and educational experiences of children and provide an insight into the optimal approaches to rehabilitation of families and their children as they prepare to return to their own country or resettle in a new country.

Svitlana Semaniv: My main online work with Ukrainians who have chosen to stay in their homeland is focused on alleviating heightened anxiety within the community. A significant portion of this population consists of internally displaced persons, grappling with the complexities of adapting to new environments and forging a path in a completely different way of life.

Figure 7.1: Svitlana Semaniv is a psychologist with a wide range of lecturing experience across public and private health care services. She has a diploma from Ivano-Frankivsk Medical College, Ukraine, graduated from Vasyl Stefanyk Precarpathian National University, and has a Family Consultant Certificate from the National Academy of Educational Sciences of Ukraine and a Certificate of a Basic Consultant in Positive Psychotherapy from the World Association of Positive and Transcultural Psychotherapy (WAPP). Currently she is employed by the London Borough of Sutton to support Ukrainians and continues to support families in Ukraine affected by the war in Ukraine.

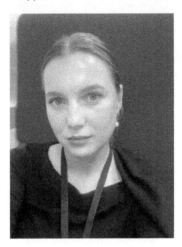

Moreover, families choose to remain in regions that may not be entirely secure, driven by an unwavering desire to stay close to their loved ones despite potential danger. However, the overarching reality for these individuals is the ongoing war, leading to the emergence of various psychological disorders triggered by traumatic events.

This spectrum of disorders includes not only expected anxiety but also more complex forms such as panic attacks, depressive tendencies, obsessive-compulsive behaviours and a variety of phobias. Additionally, the toll of the ongoing war is evident in the frequent and heart-wrenching experiences of losing family members. It is against this challenging backdrop that psychological support becomes crucial.

Addressing these multifaceted challenges requires a vigilant and nuanced approach. My efforts extend beyond acknowledging psychological struggles; I strive to provide tailored support and interventions to preserve overall wellbeing. Through counselling, psycho education and community engagement, I aim to facilitate a semblance of normalcy in the lives of these individuals, fostering resilience and empowering them to navigate the complexities of their present reality with strength and hope (Moskalets, 2019, 2017;

Maksymenko, 2020; McWillams, 2020; Shevchenko, 2022; 2023; Zhukova, 2022).

I previously worked at a rehabilitation center focused on addiction prevention, where I served as the founder and director. Currently, I work with Ukrainian refugees and maintain a private online practice with Ukrainians. (Figure 7.1)

Andrii Parkhoma: In Sutton, Svitlana and myself organise support groups for the Ukrainian community. These sessions focus on emotional wellbeing, offering activities like psychocorrection, warm support and education. Our main goal is to help individuals adapt to change and encourage self-realisation and independence.

During these sessions, participants can openly discuss their emotions, especially those related to family changes and challenges. We aim to create a supportive environment for people to navigate their feelings.

We also discuss adapting to a new environment, explaining parent–child relationships at different stages of development. This provides insights to help participants understand family dynamics during the adaptation process.

Beyond emotional support, we keep an eye out for potential psychological issues, prioritising participants' mental wellbeing. In urgent cases, we offer crisis psychological counselling to address and alleviate distress.

These support groups are a crucial community resource, fostering unity and understanding. By providing a space for shared experiences and collective growth, we contribute to the wellbeing of the Ukrainian community in Sutton, promoting resilience and a sense of belonging.

Figure 7.2: Andrii Parkhoma is a psychotherapist who studied at the Ukrainian Gestalt Institute (https://gestalt.org.ua/) National Association, completing two stages of the programme. Andrii specialises in 'Crisis and Trauma' and is currently furthering his education in the specialisation of 'Group Psychotherapy in the Gestalt Method'.

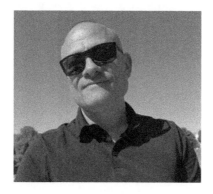

In summary, our approach addresses emotional, social, and psychological aspects, offering comprehensive support to those facing challenges in a new environment (Joyce and Sill, 2001; Ginger and Ginger, 2012; Heinz, 2013; Clarkin et al, 2015, Hinshelwood, 2016; McWilliams, 2020; Ivanova and Lebedeva, 2024)

Changing concepts of mental health and therapeutic support for children in Ukraine and the UK

Bodhana Tymoskyshyn

Soviet-era effects on children and parent–child relationships

The Ukrainian-Socialist Soviet Republic was born in 1922 and came to an end in 1991 when independence was declared. That political regime had a profound impact on children and parent–child relationships, shaping dynamics that persisted for decades. State-controlled ideologies heavily influenced family life, emphasising collectivism and loyalty to the communist regime. Parents often grappled with balancing political conformity and traditional parenting. Children growing up in this era were exposed to state-driven education and propaganda, fostering a sense of duty to the state over familial ties. The state's omnipresence extended to the home, with authorities encouraging children to report any anti-Soviet sentiments expressed by their parents. This created an atmosphere of surveillance, straining trust within families.

The Soviet emphasis on women's participation in the workforce altered traditional family roles. Mothers faced the dual challenge of fulfilling professional duties and maintaining domestic responsibilities, leading to strained parent–child relationships as time spent with children diminished.

Moreover, state-sponsored youth organisations like the Young Pioneers played a significant role in shaping children's ideologies. These organisations instilled communist values and loyalty to the state, often at the expense of strong familial bonds. Children were encouraged to prioritise their allegiance to the party, sometimes leading to generational divides and strained relationships between parents and their politically active offspring. The collapse of the Soviet Union in 1991 marked a seismic shift, but its echoes lingered in family dynamics. The abrupt socioeconomic changes brought uncertainty, impacting parents' ability to provide stability. As traditional values resurged, a tension between old and new ideologies emerged within families.

In conclusion, the Soviet era left an enduring imprint on children and parent–child relationships. The pervasive influence of state ideology, altered gender roles and the erosion of trust within families defined an era where political conformity often overshadowed familial bonds. Understanding this historical context is crucial for comprehending the complexities of contemporary family dynamics in post-Soviet societies.

Development of social and clinical psychology occurred from the Soviet to the post-Soviet era. The evolution of social and clinical psychology in Ukraine reflects a dynamic interplay of political, social and cultural forces. The emergence of modern psychology in this region is intricately tied to historical shifts and ideological transformations.

During the Soviet era, psychology in Ukraine, much like in the rest of the Soviet Union, was heavily influenced by Marxist–Leninist ideology. The state controlled the narrative, and psychology was expected to align with socialist principles. Psychologists often operated within strict ideological boundaries, with a focus on *collective wellbeing* over individual mental health. Clinical psychology, in particular, was subordinated to the needs of the state, emphasising rehabilitation over personalised care.

The concept of mental health was viewed through a societal lens, with dissent or deviance often pathologised. Dissidents were sometimes diagnosed with psychiatric disorders, leading to a conflation of political and clinical issues. Social psychology, too, served the state by studying collective behaviour and conformity, reinforcing the importance of socialist values.

The seeds of modern psychology in Ukraine were sown in the late Soviet period, as the system began to liberalise. With the dissolution of the Soviet Union in 1991, there was a significant shift. Academic freedom expanded, allowing psychologists to explore a broader range of theories and approaches. Western psychological ideas, previously restricted, became accessible, fostering a more diverse intellectual landscape. The early post-Soviet years were characterised by a surge in interest in Western psychological theories, research methodologies and therapeutic practices. Psychology departments in universities expanded their curricula to include a more diverse range of perspectives, contributing to the development of a distinct Ukrainian psychological identity.

In the post-Soviet era, social psychology underwent a notable transformation. The focus shifted from studying conformity to exploring the complexities of identity in a rapidly changing society. Researchers began to investigate issues such as nationalism, ethnic identity and the impact of historical traumas on collective memory. Social psychology became a tool for understanding the challenges of building a new national identity.

Clinical psychology also experienced significant changes. The emphasis on individual wellbeing and mental health gained prominence. Therapeutic approaches diversified, incorporating psychoanalytic, humanistic and cognitive-behavioural frameworks. The shift towards a more client-centred approach marked a departure from the previously state-centric model of mental health.

The transition was not without challenges. The sudden shift from a state-controlled system to a more open one brought both opportunities and difficulties. There was a need to establish ethical standards, professional organisations and a robust infrastructure for psychological research and practice.

Economic hardships in the post-Soviet period presented challenges for mental health services. Access to quality mental health care became an issue, and societal stigma around seeking psychological help persisted.

Today, the field of psychology in Ukraine continues to evolve. Research output has increased, and psychologists actively contribute to global discussions on various psychological phenomena. The integration of Ukrainian psychology into the broader international community has facilitated the exchange of ideas and methodologies.

The legacy of developments from the Soviet to the post-Soviet era on family relationships today reflects a complex interplay of historical, cultural and socioeconomic factors. The shifts in parent–child relationships during the post-Soviet era have left a lasting imprint on the dynamics within Ukrainian families, shaping how individuals navigate their roles and connections in contemporary society.

Individualism and autonomy: The emphasis on individualism instilled during the post-independence period continues to influence Ukrainian family relationships. Today, there is a recognition of *individual autonomy* and personal aspirations within families. Children are often encouraged to pursue diverse paths, and parents play a supportive role in helping them achieve their goals. This has fostered a sense of independence among the younger generation, impacting decision-making processes and life choices.

Cultural identity and national pride: The resurgence of Ukrainian cultural identity post-independence remains a potent force in family relationships. Families actively engage in preserving and transmitting cultural heritage, instilling a sense of national pride in their children. Cultural traditions, language and historical awareness are often cherished and passed down through generations, contributing to a strong sense of identity within Ukrainian families.

Communication and emotional wellbeing: The shift towards open communication and emotional expression has endured, promoting healthier family dynamics. Parents are more attuned to their children's emotional needs, fostering an environment where feelings are acknowledged and discussed. This has strengthened familial bonds, creating a space where individuals feel understood and supported within their family units.

Educational and career choices: The expanded freedom of educational and career choices continues to shape family relationships. Parents often play a role in guiding their children through diverse educational paths and supporting their career aspirations. The acceptance of varied professions and the pursuit of personal passions contribute to a more flexible and dynamic family structure, where individuals are encouraged to follow their interests.

Challenges of economic realities: The economic challenges faced during the post-Soviet transition have left a lasting impact on family relationships. Economic uncertainties, job instability and financial pressures continue to influence decision-making within families. Balancing economic realities with aspirations for personal and familial success remains an ongoing challenge, shaping how families navigate their financial and professional landscapes.

Globalisation and technological integration: The globalisation of information and technological influences persist in shaping family relationships. Families are interconnected with global trends and influences, impacting communication styles, entertainment choices and even family traditions. The integration of technology into daily life has both connected and, in some cases, challenged traditional family dynamics.

Generational dynamics: The legacy of the post-Soviet era is particularly evident in generational dynamics within Ukrainian families. Older generations, who experienced the Soviet era, may hold different perspectives on family roles and societal expectations than their younger counterparts. Negotiating these generational differences becomes an integral part of contemporary family relationships.

Effects of the war on children, for children left in Ukraine and for children who have come to the UK

The war in Ukraine has had profound effects on children, both for those who remain in the country and those who have sought refuge in the UK. The impact is multifaceted, encompassing negative consequences stemming from the trauma of conflict, displacement and loss, as well as positive aspects related to resilience, community support and opportunities for a new beginning.

Negative effects on children in Ukraine

Trauma and mental health: Children exposed to the horrors of war often experience trauma, leading to a range of mental health challenges such as anxiety, depression and post-traumatic stress disorder. The constant threat of violence, loss of loved ones and displacement contribute to the psychological burden carried by many Ukrainian children.

Displacement and loss: Families forced to flee conflict zones face the challenges of displacement, with children often losing their homes, schools and communities. This disruption can result in a sense of loss, instability and uncertainty about the future.

Educational disruption: The war has significantly disrupted the education system in affected areas, limiting children's access to quality education.

Displacement may lead to gaps in learning, hindering academic progress and future opportunities for these children.

Health and wellbeing: Humanitarian crises accompanying war can compromise children's health and wellbeing. Limited access to medical care, malnutrition and exposure to hazardous conditions pose serious risks to the physical health of Ukrainian children.

Positive aspects for children in Ukraine

Resilience: Despite facing immense challenges, many Ukrainian children exhibit remarkable resilience. The ability to cope with adversity, adapt to changing circumstances and maintain hope for a better future is a testament to the strength of the human spirit.

Community support: Tight-knit communities often come together in times of crisis, providing emotional and practical support to affected children. Community bonds can serve as a source of strength, fostering a sense of belonging and solidarity.

Educational innovation: While conflict disrupts traditional education, it can also spur innovation in learning methods. Non-governmental organisations and community initiatives may introduce creative approaches to ensure that children continue to receive education, even in challenging circumstances.

Negative effects on Ukrainian children in the UK

Acculturation stress: Children who have sought refuge in the UK may experience acculturation stress, grappling with the challenges of adapting to a new culture, language and educational system. This adjustment can be emotionally taxing, impacting mental health and wellbeing.

Separation and loss: Many refugee children have experienced the separation from their families and the loss of their homeland. The grief and trauma associated with these experiences can have long-lasting effects on their emotional and psychological development.

Educational disparities: Children arriving in the UK from conflict zones may face educational disparities, including language barriers and differences in curriculum. These challenges can hinder their academic progress and integration into the educational system.

Positive aspects for Ukrainian children in the UK

Safety and security: One of the most significant positive effects is the provision of safety and security for children who have sought refuge in the UK. The escape from the immediate dangers of conflict zones offers an opportunity for these children to rebuild their lives in a stable environment.

Figure 7.3: Bodhana Tymoskyshyn is a teacher of English. She worked and is still contracted to work in a primary school in Ukraine, but has been displaced to the UK. She trained at Vasyl Stefanyk Precarpathian National University, following studies at Kolomyia Organisation of The Red Cross Society. She maintains her academic studies on a yearly basis at IvanoFrankivsk Institute of Postgraduate Pedagogical Education.

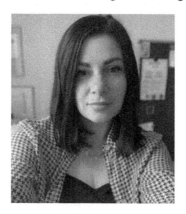

Educational opportunities: The UK, with its commitment to providing education for all, offers refugee children the chance to access quality schooling and pursue their academic goals. This can be a transformative experience, opening doors to future opportunities.

Community integration: Many communities in the UK actively support the integration of refugee children. Initiatives that promote inclusivity, cultural exchange and social engagement contribute to the positive adjustment of these children to their new surroundings.

Impact of the war on children's education in Ukraine and the UK

Before the war I had a calm life. I had a job, my husband had a job and my children were very happy. They were able to do all the things they liked, enjoyed school and playing football and had lots of friends.

People were talking about the possibility of war but didn't really believe it could happen and we were not prepared for it. When the invasion happened, I had to go to school that day and very quickly we organised online learning for all the children. However, because of all the alarms it was difficult for children to study because they had to keep going into hiding. Children began to lose much more learning even than they had lost during Covid.

Families started to move to other countries where some children continued with online learning because there were not enough places in schools for them. Many of the children who went abroad were still struggling even though they were safe, because they didn't know the language. This is very concerning for parents because the future of Ukraine depends on the education of each generation. A good education is viewed as being very important now in an independent Ukraine, because for many years very few people were able to have a good education during the Soviet era.

My parents did not have the possibility to study in the Soviet Union and their life was very hard so they were determined to give me a better life by making sure I had a good education but that was difficult for them. They had to work in factories for long hours but still didn't have much money, so they had to grow their own food in order to send me to a better school in the city. I had to walk to school, and it took me up to an hour to walk there. It was dark when I went and dark when I walked home. We didn't have many clothes and once my mother bought me some boots, but they were so cold that my legs were frozen all the time and even now I have problems with my toes, but my parents did their best.

My generation is determined to make things better for our children. The sacrifices my parents made meant that I could provide my children with things that I never had, because I was able to get a university education. Although my parents did get a basic education in the Soviet era it was very harsh, and children were not treated well at that time, there was very little nurturing. People had to work very long hours, so children were often left alone from a very young age. If a child behaved badly at school, the parents were told, and they would punish the child at home too. If a child was seen as being rebellious, this made the authorities suspicious of the parents who could be punished and even sent to prison or to Siberia. My mother is smart but was not given any opportunities.

The experiences that my parents and their parents had as children, still has an effect on families in Ukraine now. They were taught never to question authority and so it is hard for them to accept questioning attitudes from younger generations. It is also difficult for them to understand the relationship I have with my children because it is so different from how they see the parent-child roles.

It has taken time to change the education system and is only possible when a new generation of teachers, like myself, have studied Psychology which was part of my degree course in addition to English and History. These are subjects valued now in Ukraine in addition to Maths, specifically Ukrainian history so that children are well-informed about their country's struggles in the past. My generation has known freedom, but because my parents did not have this experience, they are still afraid of authority, and this can make difficulties in family relationships. Although Ukraine became a free country, that came at an economic cost and it was a poor country, still suffering from a system which contained corruption at every level and change was very slow. It was hard to fight against the old systems and it had to begin with education. Fortunately for me, I was able to access university for free in 2004 and that made possible a big change for my family.

When I first began teaching, I met with scepticism and misunderstanding from older teachers who were still using many of the methods from the previous generation. An example of this, that I was expected to continue, was that a measure of reading success was judged each week solely on the number of words that could be read by a child in one minute with no consideration given to understanding, and children were ranked according to their word count. However, over time, new methods and theories of education became adopted by schools and my children were having a good education by the time the war happened. Ukraine had made an economic recovery and was developing along lines in keeping with Western Europe although there were still generational differences of opinion and regional variations. (Bodhana Tymoskyshyn [see Figure 7.3]; based on https://osvita.ua/vnz/reports/culture/10251/; https://osvita.ua/school/method/22193/; https://osvita.ua/school/method/787/; https://vseosvita.ua/library/suchasna-systema-osvity-v-ukraini-ta-vyklyky-v-umov akh-viiny-634280.html)

Impact on children's education and wellbeing

Trauma: If there are students with trauma in the classroom, it is important for the teacher to be aware of the signs of this trauma. The teacher can work with students who are easily frightened, start to withdraw or show uncharacteristic reactions. Such behaviour can be observed in colleagues. Acute trauma is the result of exposure to a single extraordinary event, such as the death of a loved one. Students may 'relive' detailed memories and exhibit overreactions.

Chronic trauma results from prolonged exposure to traumatic situations, such as prolonged exposure to violence or bullying. Students may experience denial, anger and social withdrawal.

Complex trauma is the result of a single traumatic event that is devastating enough to have lasting effects. It can be war or displacement of refugees. Schoolchildren may experience depression, irritability and concentration problems (Yalom and Yalom, 1989; Tustin, 1990).

Signs and symptoms of a child's learning injury can take many forms. They can include problems with attention, information processing, concentration and performance of tasks, and language development. Other symptoms that affect a child's learning and social life may include: sadness/depression; physical symptoms, such as headaches; aggressive behaviour; bad relationships with peers; response to reminders or triggers.

Trauma-sensitive strategies in education: Effective work with students who have experienced trauma cannot be achieved by using one technique or checklist for all students. Instead, using trauma-informed strategies in the classroom is an effective approach to providing emotional and/or psychological support to all students.

These strategies can also be adapted to help students from displaced families develop resilience skills and prepare them for social and emotional learning (Yalom and Yalom, 1989; Tustin, 1990).

Strategy 1. Students feel safe. Deep feelings of insecurity and fear arising from trauma can manifest in many areas of people's lives, including play, interpersonal interactions and school. Teachers can make their classrooms physically, intellectually and emotionally safer by establishing certain norms and agreements. Effective rules include:

- respect the privacy of others; strive for improvement;
- respect others when they speak;
- speak from the heart; and
- allow time for improved health and personal development.

Strategy 2. Be consistent and predictable. Children of any age with a traumatic experience can be under constant stress. Teachers can make students feel safe and relaxed. Providing consistency and predictability through the teacher's mood, fairness, and the use of routines and schedules can help students feel at ease.

For example, a teacher can plan her lessons in the same way throughout the week: 10 minutes for a mini-lesson, 20 minutes for work and 10 minutes for reflection and summaries.

Strategy 3. Empathise with students. A teacher's ability to empathise with students is extremely important, especially if the teacher does not have direct experience. Teachers don't have to be injury detectives, but they can be proactive in learning about types of injuries.

Strategy 4. Create a team that has information about mental health damage. Successfully supporting displaced students requires everyone in the school to work together. This means that it is important for school administrators, principals, counselors, teachers, parents and organisations that support students to be aware of and work with trauma, and to support each other.

Strategy 5. Know your limits. When psychological trauma becomes extremely difficult for displaced students, families can be assisted in finding professional therapy for their child. It is important to remember that trauma-informed strategies are intended to help students cope and begin recovery but are not a substitute for professional trauma care. Helpful tips from experts on using trauma-sensitive strategies in the educational process:

- Accept children's reactions: this is how children learn from you that their reactions are normal, that there are no right and wrong ways to feel, and that showing their emotions is completely normal.
- Be honest with children: answer their questions as openly as possible, present information calmly and reasonably, in simple and understandable sentences.
- Adapt the details to the age of children, keeping in mind how much they are able to understand and perceive information.
- Talk about those who help during war: doctors, rescuers, volunteers, humanitarian aid, charities, local and global fundraisers, international organisations, and so on – this will help to shift the conversation about war away from the topic of death and destruction, and direct it in a positive direction.
- Involve students in positive activities: fundraising events at school, writing letters to the military, designing peace posters, and so on.
  (These tips are based on https://nushub.org.ua/lt/news/strategiyi-pidtry mky-uchniv-travmu/)

Conclusion

The journey of *social and clinical psychology* in Ukraine from the Soviet to the post-Soviet era reflects a complex interplay of historical, political and societal factors. The shift from a state-controlled ideological framework to a more diverse and open system has allowed for the growth and diversification of psychology in Ukraine, contributing to a richer understanding of human behaviour and mental health in the region.

The legacy of the sociopolitical *Soviet to the post-Soviet era* described in this chapter on Ukrainian family relationships today is a multifaceted tapestry, woven with threads of cultural revival, individual empowerment, economic challenges and global influences. Ukrainian families navigate a dynamic landscape, balancing the preservation of cultural identity with the embrace of modern values. The enduring legacy of the post-Soviet era continues to shape family relationships, contributing to the ongoing evolution of Ukrainian society in the 21st century.

The *effects of war on children* in Ukraine and those who seek refuge in the UK are far-reaching and complex.

An understanding of the appropriate education strategies for children still in Ukraine and displaced, informed by insights from clinical psychology, is important to provide to the best cultural and educational support for children affected by war.

While the negative consequences highlight the urgent need for humanitarian intervention and support, the positive aspects underscore the resilience of children and the potential for healing and growth, even in the face of adversity. Addressing the needs of these children requires a comprehensive and compassionate approach, encompassing mental health support, educational opportunities, and community engagement to ensure their wellbeing and successful integration into their new environments.

References

Clarkin, F., Yeomans, F.E. and Kernberg, O.F. (2015) *Transference-Focused Psychotherapy for Borderline Personality Disorder: A Clinical Guide*. New York: American Psychiatric Publishing. Available at: https://www.borderlinedisorders.com/book-TFP-for-Borderline-Personality-Disorder-A-Clinical-Guide.php

Ginger, S. and Ginger, A. (2012) *A Practical Guide for the Humanistic Psychotherapist*. Routledge, Online. Available at: https://www.karnacbooks.com/product/a-practical-guide-for-the-humanistic-psychotherapist/32307/

Heinz, K. (2013) *The Analysis of the Self: A Systematic Approach to the Psychoanalytic Treatment of Narcissistic Personality Disorders*. The University of Chicago Press, Online-Kindle.Available at: https://www.amazon.co.uk/Analysis-Self-Psychoanalytic-Narcissistic-Personality-ebook/dp/B00FXMPJKG

Hinshelwood, R. (2016) *Countertransference and Alive Moments: Help or Hindrance*. Process Press. Available at: https://www.amazon.co.uk/Countertransference-Alive-Moments-Help-Hindrance/dp/1899209174

Ivanova, E and Lebedeva, N. (2024) *Journey to Gestalt: Theory and Practice*. Gramatnica. Available at: https://kniga.lv/en/shop/puteshestvie-v-geshtalt-teorija-i-praktika/

Joyce, P. and Sill, C. (2001) *Skills in Gestalt Counselling & Psychotherapy*. New York: Sage.

Maksymenko, S. (2020) Systemic nature of human psyche and psychology of education. Available at: https://www.semanticscholar.org/paper/Systemic-Nature-of-Human-Psyche-and-Psychology-of-Maksymenko-Maksymenko/ece02f631c8a635e29017b04cdf1221948503695

McWilliams, N. (2020) *Psychoanalytic Diagnosis: Understanding Personality Structure in the Clinical Process*. New York: Guilford Press.

Moskalets, V. (2017) *Psychology of Personality*. Journal of Vasyl Stefanyk Precapathian National University, 4(2): 79–87.

Moskalets, V. (2019) *General Psychology (013 Primary Education): Theoretical Course*. Kyiv: Centre for Educational Literature. Available at: https://pedagogy.lnu.edu.ua/en/course/psychology-of-general-age-and-prdagogical-013-primary-education

Shevchenko, T. (2023) Health Psychology. Front Psychiatry 14 1134780 https://pubmed.ncbi.nlm.nih.gov/37575573/

Shevchenko, Y. (2022) Experimental psychology: open lab: a web application for running and sharing online experiments. *Behavior Research Methods*, 54(6): 3118–3125.

Tustin, F. (1990) *The Protective Shell in Children and Adults*. London: Karnac Books.

Yalom, I.D. and Yalom, M. (1989) *A Matter of Death and Life*. New York: McGraw-Hill.

Zhukova, A. (2022) Evidence-based psychotherapy practices for preschool child: a brief review for clinicians. *Clinical Psychology and Special Education*, 11(2): 22–42.

Indicative training materials (in Ukrainian) – Andrii Parkhoma

Белькина Ю. Этика и экология работы с травмой насилия и инцеста. Лекция. 12 March 2020. Available at: https://www.youtube.com/watch?v=C9vVErm-v4c

Голосова Н. «Травма. Посттравматическое расстройство. Особенности процессов и работы». Лекция. Available at: https://www.youtube.com/watch?v=qpOMd5G0xK8

Защиринская О.В., Винтер В.Л., Крутов С.Ю. Психическая травма как трансформационный ресурс личности. Круглый стол.// Вторая конференция медиажурнала «Психотерапия в России». Available at: https://www.youtube.com/watch?v=HxNCHTgDccA

Малинина О. Что не убивает нас – делает нас сильнее. Посттравматический рост. Вебинар. 5 March 2020. Available at: https://www.youtube.com/@NAGTU-MEDIA https://www.youtube.com/watch?v=G_7ooeAKQCo&list=PLThLg_RLEJfh2sz9SEm9H7QQz-j_VwFWo https://www.youtube.com/@agtuukraine4982 https://www.youtube.com/channel/UCo_NJx-EgJ3_2fAH6HVUACQ https://www.youtube.com/channel/UCnbOz8dyHzwW8Co-X0GStJQ https://www.youtube.com/@user-wr9ll1fd9o https://www.youtube.com/@kguorguaGESTALT https://www.youtube.com/@Beyoufully https://www.youtube.com/watch?v=NNvTjWKa5VQ

8

Mothering as a resource in countering adverse childhood experiences among Ukrainian refugee children

Rebecca Harrocks

Introduction

Writers featured in previous *Social Determinants of Health* volumes have documented how adverse childhood experiences (ACEs) can have far-reaching consequences for individuals, families and societies. ACEs are types of childhood trauma occurring before the age of 18 years that can impact the realms of physical and mental health (Bonner, 2017; Luscombe, 2017), with effects that can follow children into adulthood, redirecting them onto paths that can have consequences for the rest of their lives (Bonner and Luscombe, 2008). Related to this is the close relationship of health and education (Kerr, 2017), and the effects in either one of these areas can be long-term when inequalities are triggered or exacerbated by ACEs.

In the UK, regardless of whether they have experienced ACEs, children of the 2020s are facing additional challenges. Irrespective of regional variations, the constricting effects of austerity on the support services that local authorities are able to offer has been to the detriment of children and their families (Munro and Clements, 2020), though this has also necessitated development of a greater emphasis on collaboration across a range of agencies (Farrell et al, 2020). In addition, political and economic instability caused by Brexit is likely to increase the number of people living in poverty (Alston, 2018) while the effects of COVID-19 and its associated lockdowns on society's youngest are still emerging (Kunonga et al, 2022).

In the first volume of this series Munro considered the health and wellbeing of refugees and migrants, noting that 'in the case of those forced to flee conflict within the country of origin ... circumstances related to their original flight can have an impact on the physical and mental well-being of refugees for years following the original departure' (Munro, 2017: 304). While Munro's implicit focus was on adult refugees, closely related to her work is the increased risk for refugee children of experiencing ACEs due to potential exposure to armed conflict, physical trauma, death, sexual violence, loss of a parent or close family member, or displacement. Flight and displacement are in themselves also associated with the threat of physical or sexual violence and risk of trafficking.

Countering the long-term detriment of ACEs in refugee children is dependent on many factors, but is vital for reducing the heightened risk of long-term ill-health (Calam, 2017). This chapter will consider but one of these potential interventional factors, that is the role of the primary carer (often but not always the mother) whose significance is foundational in ACEs (Felitti et al, 1998) and attachment theory (Bowlby, 1969; 1973; 1988). In facing how to best support Ukrainian refugee children who have experienced ACEs since the Russian invasion on 24 February 2022, a challenge of immeasurable scale, this chapter argues that the primary carer of a child is a precious resource who must be appropriately supported and invested in for mitigating the long-term effects of ACEs on the child.

Ukrainian refugees

It is challenging to provide accurate, up-to-date figures of people displaced from Ukraine as the situation is continuously developing. At the time of writing, the war still goes on. Ukrainians continue to leave their homeland to escape the Russian invasion, but conversely, some of those who left in the earliest stages of the war have since returned. Others have been internally displaced within Ukraine, while yet more have been forcibly moved to Russia; these forced deportations are thought to include tens of thousands of children. The refugee picture is therefore complex, varied and ever-changing. It is also important to note that although Ukrainians displaced by the war are refugees by definition, in some host countries (such as in the countries of the UK) they do not usually have legal refugee status but instead can apply for visas for a set time period.

Despite these notes of caution, some observations can be made around the scale of displacement. Just prior to the 2022 Russian invasion (and it should be noted that many Ukrainians see the war as commencing with the annexation of Crimea in 2014), the population of Ukraine (including occupied Crimea) was 43.8 million (World Bank, 2023). As of the autumn of 2023, the United Nations High Commissioner for Refugees had recorded 5.8 million Ukrainian refugees across Europe, down from 7.9 million (or 18 per cent of its pre-war population) at the beginning of the year, with 5.2 million of these registered for temporary protection or similar national protection schemes across Europe (UNHCR, 2023); these are considered conservative estimates in the absence of official figures and they do not include the many tens of thousands of Ukrainians who have been granted refuge further afield such as in the United States, Canada or Australia. In addition, within Ukraine an estimated 5.1 million people had been internally displaced (or 11.6 per cent of its pre-war population) by May 2023, though a year prior this number had been calculated at an even higher 8 million people, a difference that reflects those who in the interim have either died, returned home within Ukraine, or left beyond its borders (IOM, 2022a; 2022b). In summary, by the end of 2022 a conservative estimate of almost *one-third* of Ukraine's pre-war population had been displaced, and by the autumn of 2023 (the time of writing) this remains at over a quarter (USA for UNHCR, 2023).

An additional 65,400 Ukrainians are believed to have been granted refugee or temporary asylum status in Russia out of an estimated 1.3 million refugees that were recorded in the country by the end of 2022 (UNHCR, 2023). There was a significant Russian minority in Ukraine; the most recent census in 2001 identified this group as comprising 17.3 per cent of Ukraine's total population, though this figure may well have fallen in the 20 years since, having already substantially decreased from 22 per cent since the preceding census in 1989 and Ukraine's independence from the Soviet Union in 1991 (Romaniuk and Gladun, 2015). Russia has also admitted to transporting civilians from conflict zones in Ukraine to Russia, often to its far east, and frames these as humanitarian evacuations. Ukraine has countered that these are forced relocations, and thus both a war crime and a crime against humanity under international law (HRW, 2022). Evidence from those affected certainly points towards the use of coercion at the very least.

The European countries with the highest figures of Ukrainians are Poland and Germany with 1.6 million and 1 million registered in their national protection schemes respectively, at the time of writing. Other high numbers of Ukrainian refugees (over 100,000) are also each recorded in the Czech Republic, Bulgaria, Slovakia, Romania, Austria, Italy, Spain and the UK (UNHCR, 2023). These figures are substantial and such sudden and sizeable population increases cannot fail to place huge pressure on governments, local authorities and services related to education, housing and healthcare. Beyond that are, of course, additional factors to address such as that those arriving from Ukraine usually have little more than the clothes they arrive in and no means to support themselves; that they often do not know the language of their host country, or do not know it well; and that many of these displaced people have encountered extreme trauma before, during and sometimes after their journeys.

Due to the restrictions on men aged 18 to 60 from leaving Ukraine, most of those who have crossed over into other countries are women and children, whilst as of June 2022, four months into the invasion, it was already estimated that two-thirds of Ukraine's children had been displaced both internally and outside of the country (UNICEF, 2022). The scope of this is staggering. The commentary that follows regarding ACEs is taken from and mostly transferable to different international contexts but it is important to note that with the exception of Case Study 8.1, it is written from a UK setting. The UK has thus far welcomed 169,000 displaced Ukrainians on its national protection scheme (Home Office, 2023) as well as providing extensive military support to Ukraine in 2022 (Prime Minister's Office et al, 2022). However, as with other countries that have opened their borders in response to this sudden great humanitarian need, the UK was ill-prepared to unexpectedly provide support services such as housing, education and healthcare to the tens of thousands of traumatised adults and children who have been forced to flee Ukraine.

Adverse childhood experiences among child refugee and asylum-seeking populations

Several studies have demonstrated that the greater the number of ACEs a child experiences, the more likely they are to face unfavourable behavioural, mental and physical outcomes throughout their lives (Bonner and Luscombe, 2008; Webster, 2022). Typically, ACEs can be caused by experiencing any form of abuse (that is, physical, emotional, sexual); living with someone who abuses alcohol or other drugs; exposure to domestic violence; living with someone who has serious mental health problems; living with someone who has gone to prison; or losing a close family member through death, divorce or abandonment. This list is far from exhaustive as trauma can come in many forms, for example, through war and conflict-induced displacement, to which we now turn.

Children who flee conflict are not immune from these 'typical' ACEs, but they are also at risk of further ones. Pre-migration, this might include heightened risk of abuse; witnessing, experiencing or committing violence; experiencing bombings or destruction of one's home; and death or abduction of loved ones. On the migration journey itself there is also an increased risk of abuse and vulnerability to traffickers; witnessing violence; risk to life; and severe deprivation of basic necessities. Post-migration upon arrival to a 'safe' location there remains increased vulnerability to abuse, living with and processing trauma, and the potential for ongoing separation from close family members. Other risk factors that may increase the harm caused by ACEs include being unaccompanied, poor family cohesion, discrimination and multiple relocations (Wood et al, 2020). There is also the shock and difficulty of arriving to a usually unfamiliar environment, possibly with an alien language, culture and systems to navigate, and often reduced to a state of poverty.

Unsurprisingly, many of the health consequences of experiencing ACEs – both due to and unrelated to conflict – are psychological. Both children and adults who have experienced ACEs are more likely to face poor mental health and mental illness including depression, anxiety, post-traumatic stress disorder, psychosis and personality disorders (Yen et al, 2002; Varese et al, 2012; Frewen et al, 2019; Sheffler et al, 2020. Associated with this are difficulties forming relationships, reduced academic achievement, and an increased risk of substance abuse, homelessness and criminal behaviour (Bellis et al, 2023). Both in association and in addition, effects on biological 'hardwiring' during the crucial development stages of infancy, childhood and adolescence can cause negative health outcomes over the life course (Bonner and Luscombe, 2008; Miller et al, 2011). Those who experience ACEs are at increased risk of illness and chronic medical conditions both in childhood and adulthood, and a recent study suggested that by the age of 49 years those who had experienced four or more ACEs were almost four times as likely to have been diagnosed with one or more chronic diseases than those with no ACEs (Ashton et al, 2016).

Apart from the moral imperative, there are obvious social and cost benefits to trying to minimise the long-term detriment that ACEs can cause in the form of reduced spending on healthcare, housing and the justice system. In supporting displaced people from Ukraine and elsewhere, the existing research around ACEs among child refugee and asylum-seeking populations can educate us on some of the key drivers of change in supporting those who have faced trauma in early life to mitigate its long-term effects. This includes existing research around language and integration, social support, finances, refugee/settled status and mental health.

Attachment theory and the centrality of the main caregiving parent

Bowlby's formulation of attachment theory in the 1960s and 1970s has sat as a basis for study into human relationships ever since (Bowlby, 1969; 1973). Its premise is that the hardwiring by which we form and maintain relationships as humans is developed in infancy through the nature of the relationship with our primary caregiver/s. Ideally, and for forging resilience and our ability to maintain healthy relationships throughout later life, the primary caregiver should act as a secure base and safe haven providing a 'circle of security' that supplies support, comfort and protection. There are defined desired attributes for the roles of both caregiver and child that maintain a sense of hierarchy and security.

Attachment theory and ACEs are intrinsically and inextricably connected. Though not limited to the person of primary caregiver, the 'classic' ACEs of abuse, losing a close family member, or living with someone who is violent, abusing substances or mentally unwell, all demonstrate the cruciality of these relationships. The presence and behaviour of the primary caregiver/s is paramount to whether a child experiences ACEs, and thus also their long-term prognosis (Wood et al, 2020). As such, appropriate support of parents and caregivers has direct correlation with outcomes for their children.

To effectively support displaced Ukrainian children, consideration of how to also assist their primary caregivers is therefore crucial. As already noted, among displaced Ukrainian families the primary caregiver is often the child's biological mother, but the following observations are applicable to the primary caregiver regardless of gender or biological relationship.

Key learning from previous research

Supporting both parent and child refugees for the mitigation of ACEs in a context of shared trauma and forced migration requires the straddling of several bodies of extensive research and as such it is only possible here to draw out some brief headlines of what might be useful. It is also important to recognise that much of these have already informed refugee responses.

Language

Trauma has been shown to impair adults' language-learning abilities not only due to the cognitive limitations caused by poor mental health but also the social isolation that it can cause (Finn, 2010). Yet knowledge of the host language is fundamental for mothers to be able to access services, education and employment, and ultimately for successful social integration. Access to these also contributes to their emotional and physical wellbeing, which also affects that of their children; as such, provision of trauma-informed language teaching is crucial for parents who are not fluent in the host language.

In addition, higher host language proficiency has been associated with lower levels of psychological distress among refugee minors (Müller et al, 2019). The impact of this on family life is that children's integration into the host society is often faster than that of their parents which can cause a shift in family dynamics when parents become dependent on their offspring to provide key information about the culture or systems of the new country (Osman et al, 2016). Therefore, authorities could best support refugee parents by providing information in their first language, ideally through a facilitator who is familiar with both the home and host cultures. To this end, there is already much native-language guidance on the UK government's website (Gov.uk et al, 2023).

Social support and integration

Social support is a key determinant of health and is vital for wellbeing and integration, yet by circumstance of their relocation, refugee families often face reduced social support. Social support can take different forms, being provided through formal systems such as governments or professional services, as well as through supportive personal relationships. It is a resource that can provide support to refugees for both pre-settlement trauma and the stress that resettlement challenges can bring about, with demonstrated psychological and health benefits such as decreased loneliness and increased sense of self-worth (Stewart et al, 2010).

As with language, social support is also a significant contributor to social integration, countering loneliness and isolation by supporting parents with access to information and services that can further assist them; this also leads to better health outcomes (Alegria et al, 2004). As well as being accessible by being available in refugees' native language/s, social support should also be culturally appropriate, particularly in the case of 'formal' support (Stewart et al, 2010). Informally, many community groups for Ukrainian refugees have been established, creating opportunities for mothers and primary caregivers to meet socially and access information and support. It is important that those in areas of lower Ukrainian population density, such as in rural locations, also have access to communities that can provide social support.

Finances

The detrimental effects of poverty on families are extensive and well-documented. While there is debate as to whether financial poverty should be considered an ACE in itself, what is more certain is that a lack of sufficient funds and material resources can act as a stressor on parents and family relationships, with the potential to trigger family breakdown as well as poor mental health or criminal behaviour in both adults and children alike (Bellis et al, 2023). Families' financial difficulties are significantly associated with higher levels of depression (Heptinstall et al, 2004), and financial pressures are a common additional stressor of refugee life, especially for parents.

Unfortunately, economic challenges tend to be the norm for many displaced persons who have usually fled homes, jobs, family support and material possessions, while low language proficiency is a barrier to employment. Many refugees want to work, not only for the economic benefits this brings, but also for the positive psychological effects of being an active member of the workforce. In the case of Ukrainian refugees many of these are – financially – effectively lone-parent families in their host countries, reliant on a sole income for those who are in employment, or even less for those who are not. For migrant and refugee mothers in employment, the absence of family support for childcare provision can lead to children being left unattended at home far more than may hitherto have been the case, resulting in increased child disobedience and prompting harsh parenting (Wood et al, 2020).

Refugee/settled status

It is again important to note that while this book considers European perspectives, this chapter is written from a UK position. The approach of the

British Home Office since the start of 2022 has been to not grant refugee or asylum seeker status to those arriving or extending stays from Ukraine, but instead it has created several schemes to issue Ukrainians with visas. A visa provides time-limited leave to remain but has the advantages (over asylum seeker status) that the beneficiary has the right to work and to claim government benefits. As of the time of writing in November 2023, the UK visa schemes for Ukrainian nationals grant permission for a three-year stay. Beyond this, the outcome of the war is of course unknown, and thus so is also what will be developed around legal status to remain.

For our purposes this approach also means that much of the research regarding experiences in asylum systems and the precarity of life when awaiting leave to remain is not immediately relevant. Regardless, it should be noted that there is a strong correlation between insecurity of legal status/right to remain in a country and elevated rates of post-traumatic stress disorder and depression (Heptinstall et al, 2004), and that the effect of such long-term legal precarity has been shown to have a significantly worse effect on women than men (Phillimore and Cheung, 2021). In addition, refugee status – even when not legally defined as such – can evoke feelings of powerlessness and damage a parent's vision of themselves as a source of protection for their child (Wood et al, 2020), again leading to disruptions in the parent–child relationship and poor mental health.

Mental health

As with ACEs in non-conflict/displacement contexts, the mental health of the main caregiving parent can significantly impact their offspring. In a context of forced migration it is inevitable that the risk of trauma and impact on mental health is magnified for adults, just as it is for children, and a growing body of work has demonstrated that caregiver mental health is particularly crucial in predicting long-term outcomes for children affected by conflict (for example, Betancourt and Khan, 2008; Sim et al, 2018).

The parenting and attachment behaviours of parents who have experienced trauma can change, such as if the parent withdraws, causing attachment insecurity for the child(ren) that can result in difficulties for their own emotional regulation (Dalgaard et al, 2016; Kaplan et al, 2016). Parents suffering from trauma, mental illness or exile-related stress may be more prone to adopting harsher parenting styles, which can result in increased child conduct problems (Bryant et al, 2018).

The mental health of refugee families can be affected not only by what happens before and during migration, but also by daily stressors at the host location such as inadequate housing or multiple relocations, economic hardship and family separation (Stewart et al, 2010). Therefore, it is crucial for refugee caregivers to receive emotional and mental health support that is ongoing and not only supports them in processing previous trauma, but also in navigating the ongoing adjustment to life in their host country.

Conclusion

The factors of language and integration, social support, finances, legal status and mental health are some of the key social determinants of health for both refugee adults and children, and these should be central considerations when designing approaches and services to best support displaced Ukrainians. In addition, the role of the main caregiver must be understood as crucial to the health and wellbeing of children under their care, with appropriate targeted support that addresses not only short-term but also long-term outcomes. However, this list is far from exhaustive, and each concern is complex with its own associated challenges and issues. As with other wicked problems, in the crisis of refugee displacement the interconnectedness of each of these factors, as viewed from a social determinants of health perspective, means that the implementation of support in any of these areas should have positive repercussions in some or all of the others.

In the face of complex and overwhelming challenges it is vital to provide any and whatever support is possible (even if resources dictate that this is not quite the optimal desired response) and, in many areas, this is already happening. Adequate long-term support does come at a cost, but this can be offset not only financially but also morally against its long-term benefits. The avoidance and mitigation of ACEs for Ukraine's children is crucial for their long-term health and wellbeing and thus – though a dramatic assertion – eventually also to the rebuilding of Ukraine and, hopefully, the re-establishment of a lasting peace in Europe. Recognising and acting upon the primacy of the main caregiver's role in this is key to effectively embracing mothering as a resource in countering ACEs among Ukrainian refugee children.

Case Study 8.1: Ukrainians being supported in Norway
Emilie Søyseth and Therese Trygg Hannevik

Events, conversations and observations that are described in this case study are based on experiences from our work in the Children's Department and Department for Special Needs at The Salvation Army's refugee centre in Kongsberg, Norway.

The refugee centre in Kongsberg has the capacity to receive 700 refugees. Of these places, 550 are intended for Ukrainian refugees who are waiting for placements in various municipalities all over Norway. The average length of stay in an emergency refugee centre before resettlement is three months.

Ukrainian refugees in Norway

As in the UK, there is a special legal pathway in Norway for refugees coming from Ukraine, who are, because of the war, under *collective protection*, a form of protection given to people in a mass evacuation situation. The asylum-seeking proceedings in such cases are simplified and beneficiaries receive a temporary residence permit valid for one year, with the possibility of extension.

'The introduction programme'

Immigrants are obliged to participate in an introduction programme with the aim of preparing people who have been granted asylum and/or a residence permit for a life in Norway, and to support them in becoming financially independent. They are taught basic skills in Norwegian, a good understanding of Norwegian society, and are prepared for Norwegian working life (IMDi, 2021). The length of the programme varies and is tailored to the needs, goals and experiences of each individual. In addition, those who have children will receive guidance around what it is like to be a parent in Norway, as well as what their rights and duties are. Their children are also supported into the Norwegian education system.

Experiences from working with Ukrainian families with children at The Salvation Army's refugee centre in Kongsberg

In a previously published article, Emilie described an experience with a recently arrived family at the refugee centre:

> Now there is a mother standing in front of me with her two children. The only luggage I see the family has with them is a small bag with room for ID cards and passports ... I welcome the little family and say we have saved some dinner for her and the children that's ready in the kitchen.

> The mother has bags under her eyes. She smiles at me and says thank you. The little brother clings on to his teddy bear as he assesses me with his eyes, unsure if he should give me a little smile or start crying. I look over to the older brother. He gives me a big grin that's missing two front teeth. I tell the mother that she has two beautiful boys. She doesn't understand English very well, but I point with two fingers towards her boys while making a heart in the air. She looks at me and holds up three fingers. I see her eyes well up with tears. She has three sons. Or had. (Søyseth, 2022)

This mother has lost a son in the war. And she will continue to be the mother of two young children. Children who constantly need an embrace to seek comfort in, a hand to hold when the world is to be explored, and a warm gaze to seek security in when the world feels unsafe.

This mother has a gaze that often turns away. That turns away when the tears come, in an attempt to hide her sadness from her children. A gaze that searches the mobile screen for information and messages from remaining family and friends in Ukraine. A gaze that turns towards home. Home, where life used to mean security.

The Circle of Security

Everything now feels unfamiliar and unsafe for the mother who is supposed to be a 'safe haven' for her children, as described in the theory of the Circle of Security. This considers how parents respond to signals children send out concerning comfort, exploration or just contact in general. The wish is for the children to be met where they are.

Sometimes children simply seek eye contact, and it will then be enough for the parents to meet their gaze. However, if the parents are in a stressful life situation, this can be reflected in how they interact with their own children and their ability to read and respond to the signals their children send out (Powell et al, 2018).

Experiences from the 'activities table'

Just outside our office, we have set up an activities table. Various activities for the children are laid out here. The wall between our office and this activities table is made of glass. We can look straight out at the children sitting there, and the children can look straight into our office. It gives us the opportunity to be present during several interactions with the children and their families.

One day, I looked up from my desk in the office. Through the glass I meet the eyes of the little boy, a big smile, and a Lego figure he has built entirely himself. He holds it up, before running into my office and giving me a high-five. His mother is sitting on the sofa across the room. She looks down at the mobile screen. The boy runs back to the table to start a new project. The mother looks up, just a little too late to catch her son's feat.

The boy sitting at the activities table expresses a need for confirmation and recognition in what he perceives as an important moment. I was present in this moment. The boy was seen, and his needs attended to. Such moments constantly appear in children's lives, and sharing these moments with them helps to strengthen both the child and the relationship. It is therefore also important that the mother can get the opportunity to gather enough strength to be present in the next moment when it arises.

This is not a unique story. Our activities table has become a place where we get the opportunity to share several of these moments with the children and the families who live here.

The families are only at the centre for a short period of time. The staff's supportive gaze can to some extent compensate for the mothers not being fully present in their caregiving role. It is nevertheless the mothers who will continue to be the children's safe haven, even when they move away from here.

We employees therefore try as much as possible to add something to the role of a caregiver, without taking over the mother's role. We're there to add new gazes the children can look to for support, not replace those of their mothers.

Other measures

There are several other ways we try to help and facilitate the mothers in their role. They often express that motherhood is experienced differently in Norway. Here, the language, parenting methods and the social structures are vastly different. We therefore have a focus on resident participation, to strengthen the mothers' sense of identity and control in a new and unfamiliar everyday life.

For example, the centre accommodates residents who wish to contribute as volunteers. This can be, for example, as hairdressers, yoga instructors, dance instructors, contributing during organised children's activities, or by serving food in our canteen. This helps to create the feeling of doing something meaningful both for oneself and for others and can also give an experience of a greater sense of control in one's everyday life.

Another important part of our work towards strengthening the role of mothers is to ensure access to information. The mothers approach us with various questions on a regular basis. Repeated questions are usually about how the Norwegian school system works, how Norwegians raise their children or about various rumours they have heard about Norwegian society on social media. We regularly hold both mandatory and voluntary parent meetings where we can provide information and families can ask us questions. Many of the parents' concerns are reduced when we provide new and accurate information.

Other measures that contribute to creating space for the mothers to breathe, and in addition can be a positive input in the children's everyday lives, are different activities arranged at the centre. These can be weekly organised children's activities, shorter and longer hikes, family outings, games nights, and various arts and crafts activities. These also contribute to creating new relationships and wider networks for both adults and children.

Summary/conclusion

The families we work with only live at the reception for a short period of time. Nevertheless, we consider this time to be an important first introduction to Norwegian society. Our role is largely about assisting in various ways and helping to strengthen the refugees' own experiences of control and mastery of their own everyday lives.

The way forward for the families who live with us is uncertain. Our wish is therefore that, together with the families, we can create the strength to keep walking and keep carrying – even when the road leads to the unknown.

References

Alegria, M., Takeuchi, D., Canino, G., Duan, N., Shrout, P., Meng, X., et al (2004) Considering context, place and culture: the national Latino and Asian American study. *International Journal of Methods in Psychiatric Research*, 13: 208–220.

Alston, P. (2018) *Statement on Visit to the United Kingdom*. Available at: https://www.ohchr.org/sites/default/files/Documents/Issues/Poverty/EOM_GB_16Nov2018.pdf

Ashton, K., Bellis, M., Davies, A., Hardcastle, K. and Hughes, K. (2016) *Adverse Childhood Experiences and their Association with Chronic Disease and Health Service Use in the Welsh Adult Population*. Cardiff: Public Health Wales.

Bellis, M.A., Wood, S., Hughes, K., Quigg, Z. and Butler, N. (2023) *Tackling Adverse Childhood Experiences (ACEs): State of the Art and Options for Action*. Available at: https://www.ljmu.ac.uk/-/media/phi-reports/pdf/2023-01-state-of-the-art-report-eng.pdf

Betancourt, T. and Khan, K. (2008) The mental health of children affected by armed conflict: protective processes and pathways to resilience. *International Review of Psychiatry*, 20: 317–328.

Bonner, A. (2017) The individual: growing into society. In A. Bonner (ed), *Social Determinants of Health: An Interdisciplinary Approach to Social Inequality and Wellbeing*. Bristol: Policy Press, pp 3–16.

Bonner, A. and Luscombe, C. (2008) *Seeds of Exclusion*. London: The Salvation Army.

Bowlby, J. (1969) *Attachment and Loss, Vol. 1: Attachment*. New York: Basic Books.

Bowlby, J. (1973) *Attachment and Loss: Vol. 2. Separation, Anxiety, and Anger*. New York: Basic Books.

Bowlby, J. (1988) *A Secure Base: Parent-Child Attachment and Healthy Human Development*. London: Basic Books.

Bryant, R., Edwards, B., Creamer, M., O'Donnell, M., Forbes, D., Felmingham, K., et al (2018) The effect of post-traumatic stress disorder on refugees' parenting and their children's mental health: a cohort study. *The Lancet: Public Health*, 3(5): 249–258.

Calam, R. (2017) Public health implications and risks for children and families resettled after exposure to armed conflict and displacement. *Scandinavian Journal of Public Health*, 45(3): 209–211.

Dalgaard, N., Todd, B., Daniel, S. and Montgomery, E. (2016) The transmission of trauma in refugee families: associations between intra-family trauma communication style, children's attachment security and psychosocial adjustment. *Attachment and Human Development*, 18(1): 69–89.

Farrell, C., Law, J. and Thomas, S. (2020) Public health and local government in Wales: every policy a health policy – a collaborative agenda. In A. Bonner (ed), *Local Authorities and the Social Determinants of Health*. Bristol: Policy Press, pp 385–400.

Felitti, V., Anda, R., Nordenberg, D., Williamson, D., Spitz, A., Edwards, V., et al (1998) Relationship of childhood abuse and household dysfunction to many of the leading causes of death in adults: the adverse childhood experiences (ACE) study. *American Journal of Preventive Medicine*, 14(4): 245–258.

Finn, H. (2010) Overcoming barriers: adult refugee trauma survivors in a learning community. *TESOL Quarterly*, 44(3): 586–596.

Frewen, P., Zhu, J. and Lanius, R. (2019) Lifetime traumatic stressors and adverse childhood experiences uniquely predict concurrent PTSD, complex PTSD, and dissociative subtype of PTSD symptoms whereas recent adult non-traumatic stressors do not: results from an online survey study. *European Journal of Psychotraumatology*, 10(1): 1606625.

Gov.uk, Ministry for Housing, Communities and Local Government and Department for Levelling Up, Housing and Communities (2023) *Homes for Ukraine: Guidance for Guests*. 3 April. Available at: https://www.gov.uk/government/collections/homes-for-ukraine-guidance-for-guests

Heptinstall, E., Sethna, V. and Taylor, E. (2004) PTSD and depression in refugee children. *European Child & Adolescent Psychiatry*, 13: 373–380.

Home Office (2023) Statistics on Ukrainians in the UK, updated 4 September 2023. Available at: https://www.gov.uk/government/statistics/immigration-system-statistics-year-ending-march-2023/statistics-on-ukrainians-in-the-uk

HRW (Human Rights Watch) (2022) 'We had no choice': 'filtration' and the crime of forcibly transferring Ukrainian civilians to Russia. Available at: https://www.hrw.org/report/2022/09/01/we-had-no-choice/filtration-and-crime-forcibly-transferring-ukrainian-civilians

IMDi (2021) Welcome to the introduction programme! Available at: https://www.imdi.no/globalassets/dokumenter/velkommet-til-introduksjonsprogrammet-20211/imdi_introduksjonsbrosjyre_engelsk.pdf

IOM (International Organization for Migration) (2022a) Ukraine internal displacement report: general population survey round 4, 29 April to 3 May 2022. Available at: https://displacement.iom.int/repo rts/ukraine-internal-displacement-report-general-population-sur vey-round-4-29-april-3-may-2022

IOM (International Organization for Migration) (2022b) Ukraine internal displacement report: general population survey round 13, June 2023. Available at: https://dtm.iom.int/reports/ukraine-internal-displacement-report-general-population-survey-round-13-11-may-14-june-2023

Kaplan, I., Stolk, Y., Valibhoy, M., Tucker, A. and Baker, J. (2016) Cognitive assessment of refugee children: effects of trauma and new language acquisition. *Transcultural Psychiatry*, 53(1): 81–109.

Kerr, K. (2017) Addressing inequalities in education: parallels with health. In A. Bonner (ed), *Social Determinants of Health: An Interdisciplinary Approach to Social Inequality and Wellbeing*. Bristol: Policy Press, pp 17–28.

Kunonga, E., Cooling, V., Chireka, B. and Chawatama, T. (2022) Giving children the best start in life? In A. Bonner (ed), *COVID-19 and Social Determinants of Health, Wicked Issues and Relationalism*. Bristol: Policy Press, pp 70–82.

Luscombe, C. (2017) Mental health, severe and multiple deprivation. In A. Bonner (ed), *Social Determinants of Health: An Interdisciplinary Approach to Social Inequality and Wellbeing*. Bristol: Policy Press, pp 241–254.

Miller, G.E., Chen, E. and Parker, K.J. (2011) Psychological stress in childhood and susceptibility to the chronic diseases of aging: moving toward a model of behavioral and biological mechanisms. *Psychological Bulletin*, 137(6): 959–997.

Müller, L., Büter, K., Rosner, R. and Unterhitzenberger, J. (2019) Mental health and associated stress factors in accompanied and unaccompanied refugee minors resettled in Germany: a cross-sectional study. *Child and Adolescent Psychiatry and Mental Health*, 13(8): 1–13.

Munro, G. (2017) Health and wellbeing of refugees and migrants within a politically-contested environment. In A. Bonner (ed), *Social Determinants of Health: An Interdisciplinary Approach to Social Inequality and Wellbeing*. Bristol: Policy Press, pp 299–310.

Munro, G. and Clements, K. (2020) The challenges facing local authorities in supporting children and families. In A. Bonner (ed), *Local Authorities and the Social Determinants of Health*. Bristol: Policy Press, pp 215–228.

Osman, F., Klingberg-Allvin, M., Flacking, R. and Schön, U. (2016) Parenthood in transition: Somali-born parents' experiences of and needs for parenting support programmes. *BMC International Health and Human Rights*, 16(7): 1–11.

Phillimore, J. and Cheung, S. (2021) The violence of uncertainty: empirical evidence on how asylum waiting time undermines refugee health. *Social Science & Medicine*, 282: 114154.

Powell, B., Cooper, G., Hoffman, K. and Marvin, B. (2018) *Trygghetssirkelen – en tilknytningsbasert intervensjon*. Oslo: Gyldendal Norsk forlag AS.

Prime Minister's Office, 10 Downing Street and the Rt Hon Liz Truss (2022) UK will match record Ukraine support in 2023, 20 September 2022 press release. Available at: https://www.gov.uk/government/news/uk-will-match-record-ukraine-support-in-2023#:~:text=The%20UK%20is%20already%20the,%C2%A32.3bn%20in%202022

Romaniuk, A. and Gladun, O (2015) Demographic trends in Ukraine: past, present, and future. *Population and Development Review*, 41(2): 315–337.

Sheffler, J., Stanley, I. and Sachs-Ericsson, N. (2020) ACEs and mental health outcomes. In G. Asmundson and T. Afifi (eds), *Adverse Childhood Experiences: Using Evidence to Advance Research, Practice, Policy, and Prevention*. San Diego: Academic Press, pp 47–69.

Sim, A., Bowes, L. and Gardner, F. (2018) Modeling the effects of war exposure and daily stressors on maternal mental health, parenting, and child psychosocial adjustment: a cross-sectional study with Syrian refugees in Lebanon. *Global Mental Health*, 5: 40–52.

Søyseth, E. (2022) Å Være Medmenneske I Det Umenneskelige. *Norges Kristne Råd*, 12 November. Trans. E. Søyseth. Available at: https://norgeskristnerad.no/2022/11/12/219190/

Stewart, M., Makwarimba, E., Beiser, M., Neufeld, A., Simich, L. and Spitzer, D. (2010) Social support and health: immigrants' and refugees' perspectives. *Diversity and Equality in Health and Care*, 7(2): 91–103.

UNHCR (2023) Operational data portal, Ukraine refugee situation. Available at: https://data.unhcr.org/en/situations/ukraine

UNICEF (2022) Briefing note on the situation of children in Ukraine. 14 June. Available at: https://www.unicef.org/press-releases/unicef-briefing-note-situation-children-ukraine#:~:text=Nearly%20two%2Dthirds%20of%20Ukraine's,facing%20uncertainty%20about%20the%20future

USA for UNHCR (2023) Ukraine emergency. Available at: https://www.unrefugees.org/emergencies/ukraine/#:~:text=Emergencies&text=There%20are%20nearly%205.1%20million,(as%20of%20May%202023).&text=More%20than%206.2%20million%20refugees,(as%20of%20July%202023)

Varese, F., Smeets, F., Drukker, M., Lieverse, R., Lataster, T., Viechtbauer, W., et al (2012) Childhood adversities increase the risk of psychosis: a meta-analysis of patient-control, prospective and cross-sectional cohort studies. *Schizophrenia Bulletin*, 38(4): 661–671.

Webster, E. (2022) The impact of adverse childhood experiences on health and development in young children. *Global Pediatric Health*, 9: 2333794.

Wood, S., Ford, K., Hardcastle, K., Hopkins, J., Hughes, K. and Bellis, M. (2020) *Adverse Childhood Experiences in Child Refugee and Asylum Seeking Populations*. Wrexham: Public Health Wales.

World Bank (2023) Population, total – Ukraine. Available at: https://data.worldbank.org/indicator/SP.POP.TOTL?locations=UA

Yen, S., Shea, M., Battle, C., Johnson, D., Zlotnick, C., Dolan-Sewell, R., et al (2002) Traumatic exposure and posttraumatic stress disorder in borderline, schizotypal, avoidant, and obsessive compulsive personality disorders: findings from the collaborative longitudinal personality disorders study. *Nervous and Mental Disease*, 190(8): 510–518.

9

Living in fear: the ongoing crisis of domestic violence and abuse

Amy Quinn-Graham

Introduction

In 2023, we find ourselves living in a time of multiple crises. In the UK, we are experiencing a cost of living crisis preceded by over a decade of austerity. We are still feeling the effects of the COVID-19 pandemic and since February 2022 we have been living with the direct and indirect consequences of Russia's invasion of Ukraine. The Cambridge Dictionary (2023) describes a 'crisis' as 'a time of great disagreement, confusion, or suffering'. It is a turning point when decisions must be made quickly (Oxford English Dictionary, 2023) and life becomes more unstable and insecure, especially for those already marginalised and vulnerable. However, a crisis isn't just a single moment of catastrophe, albeit with long-lasting and often devastating effects. A crisis can be something consistent that society has just accepted as part of its everyday reality, such as domestic violence and abuse (DVA) (Krishnadas and Taha, 2020). The World Health Organization (WHO)'s 2013 Director-General, Dr Margaret Chan, stated that violence against women and girls, which encompasses DVA, 'is a global public health problem of epidemic proportions' (World Health Organization, 2013). DVA is a human rights issue with severe impacts on both individuals and communities, as well as economic consequences. DVA cost England and Wales GBP£66 billion from 2016 to 2017 (Oliver et al, 2019).

DVA is described by the UK government as abusive behaviour committed by someone 'personally connected' to you (an intimate (ex)partner, parent, child or relative), with 'abusive behaviour' described as consisting of 'physical or sexual abuse … violent or threatening behaviour … controlling or coercive behaviour … economic abuse … psychological, emotional or other abuse' (Home Office, 2022c: 21). The year ending March 2022 saw a 7.7 per cent increase in domestic abuse-related crimes in England and Wales from the previous year, taking the figure over 900,000. This was a 14.1 per cent increase from the year ending March 2020, but only represents around two-fifths of instances of DVA that occur across the two countries. The Crime Survey for England and Wales estimates that 6.9 per cent of women (1.7 million) and 3 per cent of men (699,000) aged over 16 years across England and Wales experienced DVA in the year ending March 2022 (ONS, 2022), totalling approximately 2.4 million. This is hardly surprising given that 'more than one in ten of all offences recorded by the police are domestic abuse related' (Home Office, 2022c) and the police in England and Wales receive over 100 calls relating to DVA every hour (HMIC, 2015).

For women, DVA is the most common form of violence they face (Heise, 2011). In fact, on average, one woman is killed in the UK every three days by a man intimately known to them (Femicide Census, 2020). By committing the new Domestic Abuse Bill into law in 2021, the government promised to raise awareness of DVA and its impact, improve the effectiveness of the justice system in both providing protection to victims and prosecuting perpetrators, and equip statutory agencies to better support victims (Home Office, 2022a). However, there are questions around the government's ability to meet these objectives given cuts throughout the last decade to police and the criminal justice system (McRobie, 2013), which have been shown to negatively impact convictions related to violence against women offences (Femicide Census, 2020), and the exclusion of a gendered analysis of DVA accounting for the broader inequalities women face, a gap which will only hinder attempts to enact long-lasting change (Aldridge, 2021).

Therefore, this chapter begins by briefly outlining how DVA is conceptualised in research and practice, with a focus on violence and abuse directed at a partner or ex-partner, including how the social determinants of health (SDH) framework can help us to recognise the linkages between the socioeconomic political context and the structural determinants influencing vulnerability to DVA. This chapter then goes on to explore how the crises of austerity, COVID-19 and the Russian war in Ukraine have shifted elements of the socioeconomic political context outlined in the framework, changing the face of DVA and increasing vulnerabilities. It is widely recognised that DVA increases during times of crisis, including wars, recessions, virus outbreaks and natural disasters (McRobie, 2013; Lyons and Brewer, 2022; Kourti et al., 2023), and this chapter will explore how these crises intersect, exacerbating each other and illuminating DVA in a new way.

Defining domestic violence and abuse

The WHO uses the language of 'intimate partner violence' when talking about DVA as it recognises that in many parts of the world, 'domestic violence' and/or 'domestic abuse' encompass violence and abuse against children and other family members outside of the intimate partner relationship. This chapter focuses on what the WHO refers to as intimate partner violence, however it uses the language of DVA as 'domestic violence and abuse' is more familiar in the UK setting. The impacts of DVA are severe and long-lasting, ranging from physical injury, depression and anxiety, self-harm, and suicidal thoughts to sexual and reproductive health consequences, miscarriage, and even death (World Health Organization, 2012). The WHO recognises that DVA is disproportionately committed against women.

Prior to 2015, there was a perception shared among DVA practitioners and researchers in England and Wales that the existing criminal justice response was too narrow in its focus on discrete incidences and therefore ill-equipped to pick up patterns of coercion and control that were appearing in many women's personal testimonies of DVA, as well as in a growing body of research (Stark and Hester, 2019). When conceptualising the different types of DVA in the early to mid-1990s, Johnson (1995: 284) outlined how the control demonstrated by men within 'intimate terrorism' (the most severe form of DVA and the one most often perpetrated by men against women) was based on patriarchal traditions of a man's right to control 'his' woman, and relied not only on the systematic use of violence but also on 'economic subordination, threats, isolation, and other control tactics'. Consequently, in 2015 and in order to 'supplement current legal responses to partner assaults by enhancing the probability that the subset of chronic abusive partners would be identified and charged with a broad range of their offenses' (Stark and Hester, 2019: 86), England and Wales expanded its definition of 'domestic abuse' to include coercive control, defined as 'a pattern of behaviour, often encompassing a range of abusive behaviours such as physical, sexual and economic abuse' (Home Office, 2022b: 4).

Historically, sociological frameworks to explain the causes and prevalence of DVA have sat within two wider – often opposing – theories: family violence/conflict theory and feminist theory. In 1998, Lori Heise brought these together in an integrated ecological model, arguing that 'male dominance is the foundation for any realistic theory of violence, but experience suggests that as a single factor explanation, it is inadequate' (Heise, 1998: 263). The model (updated in 2011, in line with an improved evidence base) recognises the need for theories of DVA to include risk factors that *contribute* to the perpetration of DVA (rather than cause it) while maintaining gender as a category of analysis at the centre of the different ecological levels. Heise's model is helpful for identifying specific points for intervention at the individual (both victim and perpetrator), relationship, community and macrosocial levels to challenge and prevent DVA, however the *Conceptual Framework for Action on the Social Determinants of Health* (see Figure I.1, Introduction, this volume) is perhaps more useful in the context of crises covered in this chapter, as it draws our attention to possibilities for change in the socioeconomic political domain.

Social determinants of health framework

In the ever-changing context of crises, we can use the social determinants of health (SDH) framework to more deeply interrogate the role social determinants such as income, social networks, education and working conditions – to name a few – have on someone's vulnerability to DVA. It draws our attention to how changes in someone's socioeconomic position and the structures shaping their environment can increase or decrease their exposure to the social determinants that would otherwise serve as protective factors against DVA. The SDH is relatively unique to other models by highlighting the linkage between the socioeconomic political context and the structural determinants of health inequities, suggesting that purposive action in the socioeconomic political realm could address the [negative] effects of the structural determinants on individuals' health and wellbeing (World Health Organization, 2010).

Figure 9.1 utilises the SDH model for DVA specifically, focusing in on the socioeconomic political context of the crises outlined in this chapter and their interplay with both structural and intermediary determinants. These are not the only structural or intermediary determinants that act as risk factors to DVA, but they help us to see how the crises discussed in this chapter create an environment where these factors work together to increase vulnerability to DVA.

We know that gender is a structural determinant of DVA, so we can begin by situating the issue there, acknowledging that being a woman (or indeed identifying as non-male) makes one more vulnerable to DVA. However, we can then begin to see how other structural determinants can influence someone's experience of DVA and how they are shaped – and subsequently shape – the wider socioeconomic political context. For example, as explored in the following section, the wider political context of austerity and the decimation of the welfare state in the UK has led to public sector job losses that have disproportionately affected women, negatively changing their socioeconomic status as they've struggled to find alternative employment. Occupation and income are recognised in the SDH model as key structural determinants of health inequities, so we can see how negative changes to these elements could make someone more vulnerable to DVA and other health-related issues. In the case of DVA, this intersects with gender to increase this vulnerability.

Now we turn to a handful of the crises that have impacted, shaped and changed the socioeconomic political context of the UK and therefore exacerbated women's vulnerabilities to DVA.

Figure 9.1: Social determinants of domestic violence and abuse

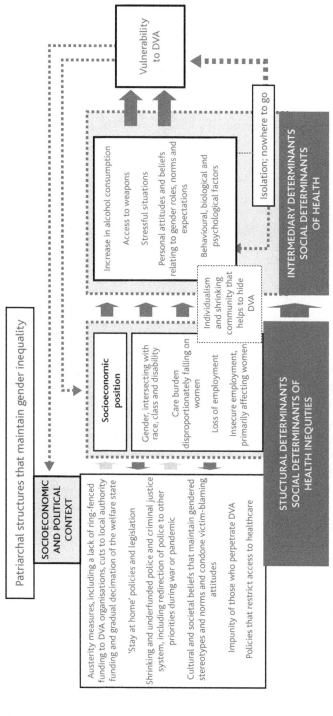

Source: Adapted from *A Conceptual Framework for Action on the Social Determinants of Health* (World Health Organization, 2010: 6) overlaid with author's own additions relevant to DVA

A decade of crises

Austerity

The UK has experienced an unprecedented number of crises at an alarming speed in the last decade. Burton (2023: 366) tells us that economists commonly refer to the years 2010–2020 as 'the lost decade', recognising it as one of the 'most volatile in modern British history' where many of the UK's poorest ended up worse off than they were ten years previously. The austerity measures proposed and enacted by the Conservative government in 2010 have contributed considerably to this volatility and led us into the cost of living crisis engulfing the UK at the time of writing (Parvez, 2022). It is widely argued that the dismantling of the welfare state has negatively impacted women's equality and safety (Sands, 2012; McRobie, 2013), and is very likely to have led to increasing levels of violence against women and girls (Sanders-McDonagh et al, 2016), including DVA.

There are the obvious manifestations of this austerity agenda on DVA services, through a lack of ring-fenced funding for DVA services at a national level, and primarily through significant cuts to local authority funding. This is typically the funding used to support non-statutory services such as DVA charities and organisations (Wakefield, 2019). Sands (2012: 19) tells us that due to funding cuts resulting in a lack of refuge spaces, on a typical day in 2011, Women's Aid had to turn away 230 women, almost 9 per cent of those seeking refuge. This led 'to support workers being forced to suggest places for women to sleep outside, such as the Occupy camps, A&E departments or night buses'. Refuge's CEO, Sandra Horley, reported in 2020 that austerity measures had led to 'Refuge seeing more than 80 per cent of its services experiencing cuts in real terms' despite the Domestic Abuse Bill legally mandating the government to provide refuge spaces for victims of DVA (Horley, 2020).

DVA provision is most often delivered by smaller organisations who are better equipped to meet the specific needs of those women who face increased vulnerabilities due to other aspects of their identity, such as LGBTQIA+ women, Black and minority ethnic women, and women without recourse to public funds. These smaller organisations have been hit the hardest by local authority cuts, with those receiving less than GBP£20,000 of local authority funding experiencing cuts of up to 70 per cent compared to those organisations receiving over GBP£100,000, who experienced much smaller cuts of up to 29 per cent (Sands, 2012). Sanders-McDonagh et al (2016: 1) refer to this decimation of the welfare state as 'structural violence', highlighting how it further violates and abuses those experiencing DVA.

Less obviously, there are other impacts of austerity that have disproportionately affected women and increased their vulnerability to DVA. Cuts to local authority funding has resulted in a high number of job losses across public services; jobs which are disproportionately held by women. Changes in housing benefit in 2013 made it harder for women, especially those under 25, to find secure housing, and the Fawcett Society and Institute for Fiscal Studies have recognised single mothers as the demographic hit hardest by benefit cuts (McRobie, 2013). These factors are just some of the wider impacts of austerity that have increased women's vulnerability to DVA and, as highlighted by Fahmy and Williamson (2018), whose work outlines poverty as a key intermediary determinant of DVA, increased the likelihood of women becoming trapped in violent relationships which they don't have the means to escape.

COVID-19

This increased vulnerability to becoming 'trapped' in relationships with a violent and abusive partner is something that the subsequent crisis of COVID-19 highlighted. Kourti et al (2023) describe how the mandate to 'stay at home', put in place to try to prevent the spread of the virus, forced victims into isolation with their perpetrators, and this led to an increase in violence and a decrease in reports of DVA. Compared to the last week in February, the first week of lockdown in the UK saw a 25 per cent rise in phone calls to the National Domestic Abuse Helpline alongside a 150 per cent rise in visits to their website (Chipakupaku, 2020).

While this correlation should not be used to conclude that COVID-19 was the *cause* of DVA, we can see how COVID-19 exacerbated certain triggers that led to more frequent and more intensely violent behaviour, such as isolation, anger, stress and boredom (Williamson et al, 2020). We know from previous epidemics, such as the Ebola and Zika viruses, that 'public health emergencies have often illuminated the hidden everyday crisis of domestic violence' (Krishnadas and Taha, 2020: 48), intensifying the violence and abuse women are already experiencing through restrictions on movement and a fear of infection (UN Women et al, 2020).

Despite the UK government updating its guidance during the first lockdown to reflect that home may not be safe for certain people, such as victims of DVA, and creating an exemption for these people to leave their homes, isolation was still a significant issue facing victims. When analysing 48 posts on the popular social media site Reddit, written by victims of DVA during the COVID-19 lockdowns, Lyons and Brewer (2022) found that not only were victims isolated with their perpetrators, which increased suicidal thoughts in some of the victims, they became even further isolated because they didn't want to visit their usual support networks of friends and family for fear of infecting them with the virus. Additionally, they were reluctant to try to access refuge or shelter spaces because of their communal nature and therefore the subsequent fear of being infected (Moreira and Pinto Da

Costa, 2020). This fear of becoming infected, or passing infection onto children, friends or family, was also used by perpetrators to keep victims at home (Kourti et al, 2023). Isolation is a common tactic used by abusers in 'everyday' situations of DVA, to increase their victims' vulnerability and reliance on them. COVID-19 exacerbated this, providing perpetrators with a 'legitimate' reason to further isolate their partners (Gupta, 2020).

Moreira and Pinto Da Costa's (2020) literature review highlighted other factors exacerbated by COVID-19 that contributed to the perpetration of DVA, particularly in relationships where DVA was already present. A change in economic circumstances, with one or both partners losing their jobs, was seen as increasing stress, which in turn often intensified the DVA, increased instances of economic abuse and/or removed the victim's financial means to leave. It was noted that this was likely further exacerbated when men lost their jobs and women didn't, because of the pressure gendered norms put on men to be the 'provider'. Support services, helplines and healthcare provision changed and reduced their provision during lockdowns, making it harder for victims to access support and advice, especially where everything moved online and victims had no freedom within the house to make a phone call or send an email. Additionally, police provision usually dedicated to responding to DVA was redirected to policing lockdown adherence (Lyons and Brewer, 2022).

The war in Ukraine

This loss of dedicated police provision for DVA is mirrored in the crisis of war, when police efforts get diverted to catching war criminals and saboteurs (Semeryn, 2022), as has been the case in the Russian war in Ukraine. It is widely reported and evidenced that the perpetration of gender-based violence, particularly sexual violence, against women and girls increases during war and conflict (Arango et al, 2021). However, this is most commonly referring to the violence committed against women and girls by enemy forces; in the case of the Russian war against Ukraine, much of the reporting on gender-based violence has been focused on Russian soldiers committing sexual violence against Ukrainian women and girls.

Nevertheless, running alongside this violence, and less reported on, is a rise in cases of DVA committed by Ukrainian men against their Ukrainian wives or female partners. Analysing previously unreleased national police data, Reuters reported that while 'registered cases of domestic violence in Ukraine initially fell after Russia invaded in February 2022, as millions of people fled the fighting ... as families have returned to their old homes or re-settled in new ones, cases have soared' (Foroudi, 2023). Multiple women have reported having 'perfect' relationships before the war, and then finding that as their husbands have returned from conflict, they've become violent towards them (Williams, 2023). Officials, including the country's commissioner for gender policy and experts working in DVA, claim that 'rising stress, economic hardship, unemployment and trauma related to the conflict' are to blame for this increase in DVA (Foroudi, 2023). This has been seen previously, when in 2016, during a time of conflict in eastern Ukraine, 'over 30 per cent of the women whose partner returned from the front suffered physical or sexual violence', according to the United Nations (Semeryn, 2022).

However, the fact that DVA was a significant problem in Ukraine before the war should not be overlooked, with Barbara Araujo, International Rescue Committee's Women's Protection and Empowerment Manager, claiming that two out of three women in Ukraine had experienced gender-based violence before the Russian war (International Rescue Committee, 2022). DVA was only criminalised in Ukraine in 2019, meaning that even before the war, shelters for victims and survivors were few and far between and social services support was stretched to its limit (Williams, 2023). A study carried out in 2023 by USAID, which asked Ukrainian citizens about their perceptions of sexual violence against women during the Russian war found that the majority of respondents identified and supported biased attitudes towards survivors of sexual violence and DVA, which discouraged survivors from coming forward and seeking help. These included victim-blaming beliefs such as the view that if a woman had been drinking alcohol then she automatically consented to sexual activity (USAID, 2023). Attitudes like these condone and therefore hide the real rates of DVA and sexual violence. War simply helps to further hide DVA as police attention is diverted, funding is redirected to the war effort and shelters become filled with internally displaced people rather than staying open and reserved for victims and survivors of DVA (Semeryn, 2022).

Additionally, it should not be assumed that women fleeing Ukraine are automatically safe from DVA. In fact, research undertaken by the World Bank and supported by the UK's Foreign, Commonwealth and Development Office (FCDO) concluded that 'women who were forcibly displaced are more likely to experience intimate partner violence' (Arango et al, 2021: 3). Women are particularly vulnerable entering a new place where they don't speak the language and are forced to rely solely on existing family members who already live outside of Ukraine, either due to work or study (Semeryn, 2022). Men remaining in Ukraine may still be able to control their wife or partner's movements, finances and support network if they also have access to the family outside Ukraine.

Discussion: the role of the social determinants of health framework

Exploring the examples of austerity measures, COVID-19 and the war in Ukraine has revealed various ways in which the hidden, everyday reality of

DVA is illuminated and exacerbated during times of crisis. However, these crises do not occur in a vacuum, and we can see ways that these crises have built on each other to further complicate and frustrate the issue of DVA. In fact, Krishnadas and Taha (2020: 53) describe the disruption that came with COVID-19 as hitting the UK when we'd 'already been in a state of crisis for some time'.

This is where the SDH framework can be helpful in highlighting the relationship between aspects of the socioeconomic political context and structural determinants. For example, the policy decisions made around the COVID-19 pandemic, such as closing schools and initiating 'stay-at-home' orders, intersected with 'gender' as a structural determinant to increase the care burden facing women specifically (due to prevailing and institutionalised gender stereotypes, roles and expectations). This led to many women becoming 'shock absorbers of poverty, sacrificing their careers and security by leaving work to take on unpaid care' (Women's Budget Group, 2022), which, in turn, has made them more vulnerable in our current cost of living crisis, another element of the socioeconomic political context that has been shown to increase vulnerability to DVA.

Consequently, the SDH framework points to places where interventions could be made at the socioeconomic political level that interrupt this downward spiral of interconnectedness, particularly in the realm of what we may perceive as unrelated social policy (Gill and Thériault, 2005). In this example, where COVID-19 policies have exacerbated structural gender inequalities and deepened the negative impact of austerity measures and the cost of living crisis for women specifically, these could be policies that better protect women's jobs and job opportunities when they take on an increased care burden, reverse austerity measures that have decimated the welfare state, increase accessible childcare provision, or commit to providing education initiatives that challenge gender stereotypes about who is responsible for the care burden. This focus on policies at the state level is integral to gaining a fuller understanding of DVA as an issue of health inequity and is an aspect of SDH often neglected by analysts, as the quality of social determinants is 'shaped by the policies that guide how societies (re)distribute material resources among their members' (World Health Organization, 2010: 25).

The SDH framework is also therefore a helpful tool in recognising the intersectionality involved in DVA vulnerability. For example, while Heise's (2011) ecological model on preventing DVA places gender at the centre, the SDH framework also draws attention to the role of race and class. We see this play out in the crises explored in this chapter through the identification of the particular vulnerabilities facing refugee women fleeing the war in Ukraine. As well as severely decimating generalised DVA services and resources, McRobie (2013) tells us that austerity measures have 'dried up access points' for refugee and ethnic minority women experiencing abuse, alongside general cuts to services created to support refugees and other particularly marginalised groups.

Finally, using the SDH framework to outline how each of these crises have shaped – and continue to shape – the DVA landscape, prompts us to challenge our assumptions about what influences DVA vulnerability and prevalence and think more creatively about where we may be missing data on these connections. In their discussion paper exploring the connections between social determinants of health and women abuse, Gill and Thériault (2005) start by asking, 'what determines health?' to generate a list of determinants that they then use to explore linkages with domestic violence and abuse against women. They conclude that due to the complexity of the issue, 'looking at woman abuse through a focused discussion on the social determinants of health can therefore be one of many possible avenues to contribute to the understanding of this issue' (Gill and Thériault, 2005: 9).

Conclusion

Unfortunately, even as we emerge from the COVID-19 pandemic, we are still faced with a series of ongoing crises, including the previously discussed cost of living crisis and the war in Ukraine. Climate change, economic instability and global conflict continue to contribute to increases in violence against women and girls, including DVA, both globally and within the UK (Women's Budget Group, 2022). Therefore, action is required to respond to the growing crisis of DVA and mitigate against its further exacerbation.

One of the first recommendations, which COVID-19 helped to shed a light on, is the need to shift public opinion from seeing DVA as a private matter to something which has significance in the public sphere (Krishnadas and Tada, 2020; Moreira and Pinto Da Costa, 2020). For Krishnadas and Tada (2020) this needs to be a collective, community effort; one in which people feel empowered to identify the signs of DVA and support victims to report it. This would also help to challenge traditional ideas, systems and structures that relegate women to the private sphere more generally, making them more vulnerable. Be that soaring childcare costs that push women out of employment and back into the home, or the devaluing of public sector jobs typically undertaken by women. This should also include ensuring that healthcare workers are equipped to ask the right questions, in a non-judgemental, non-directive way, that encourage a DVA victim to disclose their experience, and not to 'write off' psychological symptoms such as anxiety as simply a result of the current crisis, as happened during the COVID-19 lockdowns (Moreira and Pinto Da Costa, 2020).

Second, while it is unlikely that during a crisis legislation related to DVA would change, efforts must be made to ensure that access to support, legal and health services, and the police and the criminal justice system are not compromised (Moreira and Pinto Da Costa, 2020). DVA must be seen as a continued priority, not something that resources can just be diverted from and reinstated once 'normal life' has resumed. This could include building strong multi-agency partnerships and pathways that don't collapse under the pressure of a new crisis.

Third, given the UK context of austerity, DVA services must be protected from local authority cuts (Sands, 2012). Once local authority funding has been 'restored to a level which enables councils to meet their statutory obligations' (Wakefield, 2019: 12), funding for specialist services must be ring-fenced and DVA services must be granted the same level of funding as other public services, with a focus on supporting preventative, non-statutory services (Sands, 2012; Wakefield, 2019). Sands (2012) and Wakefield (2019) also detail various other economic recommendations designed to remove the burden of austerity from women's shoulders and reduce their vulnerability to dependence on a potentially abusive partner.

Lastly, whether in a time of crisis or 'everyday' life, the focus must be on preventing DVA from happening in the first place. As clearly stated by the WHO in the SDH framework, 'interventions and policies to reduce health inequities must not limit themselves to intermediary determinants, but must include policies specifically crafted to tackle the social mechanisms that systematically produce an inequitable distribution of the determinants of health among population groups' (World Health Organization, 2010: 7). In other words, alongside recommendations specific to times of crisis, and as alluded to in some of those recommendations mentioned earlier, resources must be allocated to cutting off DVA at its root.

DVA prevention efforts are wide-ranging and must work towards change across the individual, interpersonal, community and societal levels (Michau et al, 2015) as well as recognise the impact of policies and state intervention in the socioeconomic political context. Evidence points towards the need to shift 'norms, attitudes and beliefs related to gender' (Heise, 2011: viii), such as male authority and female obedience. At an individual level, this is often done through small, participatory, age-appropriate workshops with adults or children, focused on identifying DVA, defining healthy relationships, challenging gender stereotypes, roles and expectations, and promoting gender equality. At a societal and systemic level, 'transformation of the long standing political structures, deeply entrenched socially accepted practices, and normative behaviours that maintain women's and girls' inequality and tolerance of violence against women and girls' is necessary (Michau et al, 2015: 1674).

Ultimately, DVA must be recognised as a crisis in and of itself; one with devastating consequences that continues to be exacerbated by every new crisis that emerges. We must not forget about DVA as we scramble to deal with each new crisis and must not forget how many people – predominantly women and children – are *already* living in fear.

References

Aldridge, J. (2021) 'Not an either/or situation': the minimization of violence against women in United Kingdom 'domestic abuse' policy. *Violence Against Women*, 27(11): 1823–1839.

Arango, D.J., Kelly, J., Klugman, J. and Ortiz, E. (2021) *Forced Displacement and Violence against Women: A Policy Brief*, Washington, DC: World Bank Group.

Burton, M. (2023) The impact of 'the lost decade' on developing a relational culture in public-private partnering. In A. Bonner (ed), *COVID-19 and Social Determinants of Health: Wicked Issues and Relationalism*. Bristol: Policy Press, pp 366–375.

Cambridge Dictionary (2023) Crisis. *Cambridge Dictionary*. Available at: https://dictionary.cambridge.org/dictionary/english/crisis

Chipakupaku, D. (2020) Coronavirus: calls to national domestic abuse helpline rise by 25% in lockdown. *Sky News*. Available at: https://news.sky.com/story/coronavirus-calls-to-national-domestic-abuse-helpline-rise-by-25-in-lockdown-11969184

Fahmy, E. and Williamson, E. (2018) Poverty and domestic violence and abuse (DVA) in the UK. *Journal of Gender-Based Violence*, 2(3): 481–501.

Femicide Census (2020) *Femicide Census 2020*. Available at: https://www.femicidecensus.org/wp-content/uploads/2022/02/010998-2020-Femicide-Report_V2.pdf

Foroudi, L. (2023) Rising domestic violence is a hidden front in Ukraine's war. *Reuters*. Available at: https://www.reuters.com/world/europe/rising-domestic-violence-is-hidden-front-ukraines-war-2023-08-03/

Gill, C. and Thériault, L. (2005) Connecting social determinants of health and woman abuse: a discussion paper. *Finding Common Ground: Creating a Healthier and Safer Atlantic Canada*, 23–26 August 2005, Charlottetown pp 1–20.

Gupta, J. (2020) What does coronavirus mean for violence against women? *Women's Media Center*. Available at: https://womensmediacenter.com/news-features/what-does-coronavirus-mean-for-violence-against-women

Heise, L.L. (1998) Violence against women: an integrated, ecological framework. *Violence Against Women*, 4(3): 262–290.

Heise, L.L. (2011) *What Works to Prevent Partner Violence? An Evidence Overview*. London: STRIVE Research Consortium.

HMIC (2015) *Increasingly Everyone's Business: A Progress Report on the Police Response to Domestic Abuse*. HMIC. Available at: https://assets-hmicfrs.justiceinspectorates.gov.uk/uploads/increasingly-everyones-business-domestic-abuse-progress-report.pdf

Home Office (2022a) *Domestic Abuse Act 2021: Overarching Factsheet*. Home Office. Available at: https://www.gov.uk/government/publications/domestic-abuse-bill-2020-factsheets/domestic-abuse-bill-2020-overarching-factsheet#when-will-the-measures-in-the-act-come-into-force

Home Office (2022b) *Controlling or Coercive Behaviour: Statutory Guidance Framework*. Home Office. Available at: https://assets.publishing.service.gov.uk/government/uploads/system/uploads/attachment_data/file/1072673/MASTER_ENGLISH_-Draft_Controlling_or_Coercive_Behaviour_Statutory_Guidance.pdf

Home Office (2022c) *Domestic Abuse: Statutory Guidance*. Home Office. Available at: https://assets.publishing.service.gov.uk/government/uploads/system/uploads/attachment_data/file/1089015/Domestic_Abuse_Act_2021_Statutory_Guidance.pdf

Horley, S. (2020) Refuge responds to the Spring Budget. *Refuge*. Available at: https://refuge.org.uk/refuge-responds-to-the-spring-budget/

International Rescue Committee (2022) Women continue to pay the highest price for the war in Ukraine, warns IRC. *Relief Web*. Available at: https://reliefweb.int/report/ukraine/women-continue-pay-highest-price-war-ukraine-warns-irc

Johnson, M.P. (1995) Patriarchal terrorism and common couple violence: two forms of violence against women. *Journal of Marriage and the Family*, 57(2): 283–294.

Kourti, A., Stavridou, A., Panagouli, E., Psaltopoulou, T., Spiliopoulou, C., Tsolia, M., et al (2023) Domestic violence during the COVID-19 pandemic: a systematic review. *Trauma, Violence, & Abuse*, 24(2): 719–745.

Krishnadas, J. and Taha, S.H. (2020) Domestic violence through the window of the COVID-19 lockdown: a public crisis embodied/exposed in the private/domestic sphere. *Journal of Global Faultlines*, 7(1): 46–58.

Lyons, M. and Brewer, G. (2022) Experiences of intimate partner violence during lockdown and the COVID-19 pandemic. *Journal of Family Violence*, 37(6): 969–977.

McRobie, H. (2013) Austerity and domestic violence: mapping the damage. *50:50*. Available at: https://www.opendemocracy.net/en/5050/austerity-and-domestic-violence-mapping-damage/

Michau, L., Horn, J., Bank, A., Dutt, M. and Zimmerman, C. (2015) Prevention of violence against women and girls: lessons from practice. *Lancet*, 385: 1672–1684.

Moreira, D.N. and Pinto Da Costa, M. (2020) The impact of the COVID-19 pandemic in the precipitation of intimate partner violence. *International Journal of Law and Psychiatry*, 71(101606): 1–6.

Oliver, R., Alexander, B., Roe, S. and Wlasny, M. (2019) *The Economic and Social Costs of Domestic Abuse*. London: Home Office. Available at: https://assets.publishing.service.gov.uk/media/5f637b8f8fa8f5106d15642a/horr107.pdf

ONS (2022) Domestic abuse in England and Wales overview: November 2022. Office for National Statistics. Available at: https://www.ons.gov.uk/peoplepopulationandcommunity/crimeandjustice/bulletins/domesticabuseinenglandandwalesoverview/november2022

Oxford English Dictionary (2023) Crisis. *Oxford English Dictionary*. Available at: https://www.oed.com/search/dictionary/?scope=Entries&q=crisis

Parvez, A. (2022) Governments' economic policies are a form of gender-based violence. *Oxfam GB*. Available at: https://www.oxfam.org.uk/oxfam-in-action/oxfam-blog/governments-economic-policies-are-a-form-of-gender-based-violence/

Sanders-McDonagh, E., Neville, L. and Nolas, S.-M. (2016) From pillar to post: understanding the victimisation of women and children who experience domestic violence in an age of austerity. *Feminist Review*, 112(1): 60–76.

Sands, D. (2012) *The Impact of Austerity on Women*. London: Fawcett Society.

Semeryn, K. (2022) Russian invasion overshadows domestic violence in Ukraine. Available at: https://iwpr.net/global-voices/russian-invasion-overshadows-domestic-violence-ukraine

Stark, E. and Hester, M. (2019) Coercive control: update and review. *Violence Against Women*, 25(1): 81–104.

UN Women, IDLO, UNDP, UNODC, World Bank and The Pathfinders (2020) *Justice for Women Amidst COVID-19*. New York: UN Women, IDLO, UNDP, UNODC, World Bank and The Pathfinders. Available at: https://www.undp.org/publications/justice-women-amidst-covid-19

USAID (2023) Society's attitudes towards sexual violence during the Russian-Ukrainian war. Available at: https://s3.documentcloud.org/documents/23923383/society_crsv_en.pdf

Wakefield, H. (2019) *Triple Whammy: The Impact of Local Government Cuts on Women*. London: UK Women's Budget Group.

Williams, J. (2023) 'This war made him a monster': Ukrainian women fear the return of their partners from war. *Time*. Available at: https://time.com/6261977/ukraine-women-domestic-violence/

Williamson, E., Lombard, N. and Brooks-Hay, O. (2020) Domestic violence and abuse, coronavirus, and the media narrative. *Journal of Gender-Based Violence*, 4(2): 289–294.

Women's Budget Group (2022) Austerity is gender-based violence. *Women's Budget Group*. Available at: https://wbg.org.uk/blog/austerity-is-gender-based-violence/

World Health Organization (2010) *A Conceptual Framework for Action on the Social Determinants of Health*. Geneva: World Health Organization. Available at: https://apps.who.int/iris/rest/bitstreams/52952/retrieve

World Health Organization (2012) *Intimate Partner Violence*. New York: World Health Organization. Available at: https://iris.who.int/bitstream/handle/10665/77432/WHO_RHR_12.36_eng.pdf

World Health Organization (2013) Violence against women: a 'global health problem of epidemic proportions'. *World Health Organization.* Available at: https://www.who.int/news/item/20-06-2013-violence-agai nst-women-a-global-health-problem-of-epidemic-proportions-#:~:text= 20%20June%202013%20%7C%20Geneva%20%2D%20Physical,South%20 African%20Medical%20Research%20Council

A life course approach to human development and ageing: impact of war and other contemporary crises

Catherine Hagan Hennessy and Elaine Douglas

Introduction

The context of prevailing social, economic and physical conditions in society is recognised as fundamental to health and wellbeing throughout the life course. The interaction and impact of these social determinants on human development and health across successive life stages has been an established area of interdisciplinary science since the 1980s. This chapter uses the perspective of life course health development (LCHD) (Halfon and Forrest, 2018) emerging from this work to consider the potential impact of current global and regional challenges on lifetime health trajectories and outcomes. The LCHD approach employed here is aligned with the World Health Organization (WHO) conceptual framework on social determinants of health on which other chapters in this volume are based, explicitly addressing these *structural* and *intermediary* health determinants over the human lifespan.

A principal focus of the chapter are inequalities in ageing associated with factors operating across the whole of the life course. This focus is informed by a critical perspective on the concept of 'healthy ageing' defined by the WHO as 'the process of developing and maintaining the functional capacity that enables well-being in older age' (2015: 28) which dominates public health policy discourse. A variety of concepts reflecting an optimal trajectory of the ageing process – for example, 'successful ageing', 'active ageing' and 'healthy ageing' are commonly used in gerontological research, policy and practice (Menassa et al, 2023). Adaptations to these concepts have been made over time in response to critical consideration of their shortcomings. Notably, Geronimus' (2023) critique of the notion of 'healthy ageing' reflects her view that social structural factors continue to be systematically ignored in efforts to explain and address inequities in ageing processes and outcomes. The use of the term healthy ageing in this chapter, therefore, is in line with critical perspectives on the concept and the corresponding emphasis on social determinants of health in the LCHD framework. Prospects for realising healthy ageing are interrogated in relation to three contemporary and interacting societal issues and events: the Ukrainian conflict, the COVID-19 pandemic and the cost of living crisis. Each of these issues is examined in regard to evidence of the risks they pose to development and health at various life stages and cumulatively across the life course.

The demographic ageing of world populations is highlighted by the United Nations as 'one of the most significant social transformations of the twenty-first century with implications for nearly all sectors of society' (United Nations, 2022). In view of the impact of 'greying' populations on societies and economies globally, international goals for maximising healthy ageing are increasingly informed by a LCHD perspective aimed at reducing health inequalities at all ages (World Health Organization, 2016). This perspective highlights the physical and social exposures that contribute to building an individual's 'health capital' and ultimately determining their chances of healthy ageing that are known to influence health and adaptive capacity from the earliest stages of life. This chapter addresses the three focal issues identified earlier through a synthesis of relevant evidence on the lifetime impact of social determinants of health on healthy ageing.

The LCHD framework has its origins in studies demonstrating the relationship of growth in early life stages to the subsequent development of chronic disease in midlife and older age (Barker, 1990). The research that has emerged over the past three decades out of this developmental perspective highlights the multifactorial and dynamic interaction of behavioural, social and environmental influences on genetic expression and the regulation of physiologic and behavioural functions that are intrinsic to health (Halfon and Forrest, 2018). The relationship of a range of prenatal, childhood and adult exposures and impacts to disease conditions such as cardiovascular disease, Type 2 diabetes (Forouhi et al, 2004), respiratory disease and cancer (Kuh and Ben-Shlomo, 2004), among others, has been demonstrated through a life course perspective on chronic disease epidemiology. More recently (Hatch et al, 2007), an explicitly life course approach to health and wellbeing outcomes in later life has been employed to examine influences on physical capability, cognitive functioning, and psychological and social wellbeing in later life (Kuh et al, 2014). For example, in the landmark HALCyon project that used data from a set of longitudinal British birth cohort studies, childhood socioeconomic position was found to be related to all indicators of physical capability in older age. Findings from HALCyon and a growing body of evidence from other studies highlight the role of social determinants of health across the life course in patterning ageing outcomes (Marengoni and Calderon-Larranaga, 2020).

This chapter therefore considers the importance of resources and (dis) advantages accrued across successive life stages – for example, education, income, social networks and other protective factors – and their implications for later life health and wellbeing from a LCHD perspective. In addition to the developmental effects of adverse conditions and exposures on health outcomes in older age, the particular vulnerabilities of older people in current circumstances of societal economic downturn, conflict emergencies and a global pandemic are highlighted. The chapter concludes with a discussion of the significance and role of public policies and programmes internationally that address health inequalities and ensure social inclusion of persons at all ages as supports for the physical, cognitive and social aspects of healthy ageing.

The life course impact of war on ageing outcomes

The direct and indirect longer-term consequences of war on lifetime health and wellbeing have been investigated for several decades, particularly since the Second World War (Garfield, 2008). In addition to the mortality and morbidity experienced at the time of military conflict and its immediate consequences, epidemiologists have tracked the life course impact of exposure to war among combatant and civilian populations (Levy and Sidel, 2009). Findings from longitudinal cohort studies, for example, demonstrate the significance of prenatal factors such as maternal nutrition (Roseboom et al, 2011) and exposure to chronic stresses of conflict during pregnancy to ageing outcomes of their offspring.

A classic example are studies of the long-term effects of the so-called Dutch 'Hunger Winter' of 1944 when the German occupying force severely limited rations in areas of the Netherlands, affecting the entire population including pregnant women. In addition to food shortages, among the war-related stresses and trauma prevalent at this time were violence, infrastructure breakdown and extreme seasonal cold (Lumey et al, 2011). From detailed maternity hospital patient records, researchers have been able to link information about maternal health and gestational age during the famine with later life health outcomes of those who were in utero during the famine. Findings from these studies showed that maternal undernutrition during pregnancy had a range of adverse health outcomes across the life course of their offspring, including, for example, addiction (Franzek et al, 2008), obesity (Ravelli et al, 1976), hypertension (Stein et al, 2006) and coronary heart disease (Roseboom et al, 2000) as well as evidence of possible accelerated cognitive ageing (de Rooij et al, 2010). Further studies using linked registry data for Dutch cohorts who were children during the famine period and those born in the immediate post-famine years have demonstrated the additional effects of these war exposures beyond their lifetime impact on health. Ramirez and Haas (2022), for example, have shown decreased overall odds of subsequent educational and income attainment in these cohorts, especially for males. This research indicates that some of the fundamental supports for life course health and wellbeing were compromised by exposures to war in early life, decreasing the prospects for healthy ageing.

The lifetime effects of childhood exposure to war have also been examined, for example, using data from SHARELIFE, a retrospective survey conducted as part of the European Survey of Health, Aging and Retirement in Europe (SHARE) (Kesternich et al, 2014). Data were collected from over 20,000 individuals in 13 European countries on childhood events experienced during and after the Second World War. Using measures of war exposure including experience of dispossession, persecution, proximity to combat and periods of hunger, subjection to these conditions was found to increase the probability of developing diabetes, depression and heart disease, and to significantly lower self-rated health as adults. As in the Dutch Hunger Winter research, experiencing war in childhood was also found to be associated with circumstances and supports known to affect ageing outcomes, in this case less education, lower life satisfaction and a decreased probability of ever being married for women.

The long-term sequelae of exposure to wartime stresses in young adulthood have been examined for a number of armed conflicts, including notably the Vietnam War. Data from the 2018 Vietnam Health and Aging Study (VHAS) conducted with 2,447 older adults aged 60 and over in northern Vietnam has been used to investigate the association between war traumas and a range of later life health outcomes. Zimmer et al (2021) established the association between early adult exposure to three types of war experiences (death and injury, stressful living conditions, and fearing death and/or injury) and several health outcomes including increased number of diagnosed health conditions, greater mental distress and somatic symptoms, poorer physical functioning, higher prevalence of post-traumatic stress symptoms and chronic pain. Further studies using the VHAS cohort data have demonstrated the negative impact of wartime stress exposure on later life mental health outcomes (Kovnick et al, 2021), cardiovascular health (Korinek et al, 2020) and frailty (Zimmer et al, 2022).

Older people are recognised as one of the most vulnerable groups in populations affected by war, both in terms of its immediate and long-term consequences (Kar, 2022). Older individuals are often among the last to leave conflict areas, and once displaced are at risk due to problems with mobility and chronic health conditions and related needs for care. Previous research in other conflict areas has indicated the particular vulnerability of older people in respect to mental health outcomes. A study by Kimhi et al (2012), for example, examined coping among different age groups of adults one year after the Second Lebanon War in 2006. Compared to adults aged 20–45 and 46–64, older adults aged 65 years and over reported significantly higher levels of stress symptoms and lower levels post-traumatic recovery.

There is a growing body of evidence on the impacts of the current Ukrainian conflict relevant to the life course perspective on healthy ageing and the range of negative outcomes associated with wartime stresses. A report by UNICEF (2022) estimated that within one month of the onset of the war, some 4.3 million children, or more than half of Ukraine's child population, had been displaced. Of these, some 1.8 million had left the country as refugees and an additional 2.5 million were internally displaced. The impact of war-related stresses on Ukrainian children is highlighted by Martsenkovskyi et al's (2023) study of the prevalence of war-related negative mental health outcomes in the children of a national opportunistic sample of Ukrainian parents. Using a parent-reported screen, post-traumatic stress disorder (PTSD) was found in 17.5 per cent of preschoolers and 12.6 per cent of school age children. Delay in developmental milestones, having a parent attached to the emergency services or army, parental PTSD status and changes in parental anxiety were some of the strongest predictors of increased risk of PTSD in children.

The multiplicity of war-related stresses and trauma on young Ukrainians and their psychological impact has been highlighted by Chaaya et al (2022). Although not directly physically affected by the war in Ukraine, studies of adolescents and young adults in neighbouring Central European countries have demonstrated the impact of proximity to the conflict on psychological wellbeing. For example, studies of university students in the Czech Republic (Riad et al, 2022) and in Poland (Skwirczynska et al, 2022) have shown elevated levels of anxiety and depression in young people associated with increased concerns about the conflict.

The mental health impact of the Ukrainian conflict on the wider adult population is evidenced by findings from a study of adults aged 18 to 65 six months after the Russian invasion (Kurapov et al, 2023). The experience of a range of war-related exposures and trauma was shown to result in heightened levels of anxiety, depression and conditions including PTSD, with those between ages 28 and 45, women and those who had left the country most affected. The psychological effects of the conflict on adults was similarly established among a representative adult population sample (Khan and Altalbe, 2023) with levels of mental distress significantly associated with vulnerabilities such as residing in areas occupied by Russian forces and having older people and children living in the household.

Insight into the potential effects of the current Ukrainian war specifically on older persons is provided by findings of a survey in 2016 of persons aged 60 and over in conflict-affected areas of eastern Ukraine during earlier hostilities with Russia that began in 2014 (Summers et al, 2019). High prevalences of serious psychological distress were found among individuals with moderate or severe dependency due to disability, those having a chronic disease, and among women. The situation of older people (aged 60+) early in the current conflict is delineated in findings from a survey conducted by HelpAge International (2022). Among the risks to health and wellbeing reported by this population group – the vast majority of whom did not want to relocate from their homes – were high levels of need for assistance with obtaining basic provisions due to mobility limitations and living alone, lack of access to clean drinking water, exposure to cold resulting from electricity cuts, and urgent demand for medications for chronic disease and basic supplies for personal hygiene.

Seen from a LCHD perspective, the Ukrainian conflict presents serious threats to health and wellbeing across all age groups and life stages of the population. Damage to the building blocks and structural supports for life course health and healthy ageing in Ukraine is further suggested by findings from a large household survey undertaken during the earlier conflict in eastern Ukraine (Osiichuk and Shepotylo, 2020). Having enough money to cover living costs or buy food significantly decreased as a result of the conflict, as did people's expectations of their future financial situation. At the same time, the proportion of the Ukrainian population self-reporting having a chronic disease increased from 44 per cent in 2012 to 50 per cent in 2016. Thus prospects for optimal ageing outcomes are being systematically undermined as armed conflict in the region continues.

COVID-19

Another major contemporaneous threat to life course health outcomes is the global COVID-19 pandemic which began in early 2020. Although the preponderance of the burden of morbidity and mortality has been among older adults, the longer-term population health and social impacts of the disease cannot yet be determined. However, the value of examining the consequences of the COVID-19 pandemic from a life course perspective has been argued by Settersten et al (2020: 3): 'Infection cases that do not result in death can nonetheless have long-term consequences for the health and wellbeing of individuals and populations of all ages. In addition, infection and post-infection risks are not equally distributed across the population and are likely to exacerbate existing social inequalities in health.'

Using a life course framework, Benner and Mistry (2020) have considered the potential negative effects of the COVID-19 pandemic on the developmental outcomes of children and adolescents. They point to risks in younger individuals' life contexts associated with the pandemic, including family disruption due to illness or death, financial precarity resulting from job loss, and interruption of education with school closures and the move to alternative modes of education. The introduction of social distancing guidelines is also identified as posing potential hazards to physical and social development of children and adolescents with the curtailment of normal physical activities and social interactions. National data for England, for example, has demonstrated post-pandemic developmental delays in reaching milestones for key language, cognitive and social skills among children aged two to two-and-a-half years (Adams, 2024). The value of a life course perspective that foregrounds social determinants of health to assessing the impact of COVID-19 on child development and maternal wellbeing is emphasised by Witt et al (2023). They argue that identifying the direct and indirect impacts of COVID-19 must be considered within an understanding of the structural and socioeconomic issues that affect population groups and condition their prospects for lifelong health.

The developmental risks to children and adolescents of COVID-19 restriction measures have similarly been elaborated on by Arantes de Araujo et al (2020) through a systematic literature review of the impacts of epidemics and social restrictions on the health and wellbeing of younger persons. The study findings underlined the significant potential effects of these events and associated risk mitigation measures on the mental and emotional health of younger individuals including acute stress disorder, post-traumatic stress, anxiety disorders and depression. The researchers note that a variety of the epidemic-related conditions and circumstances affecting children and youth can be related to the evidence on the consequences of adverse childhood experiences (see Chapters 7 and 8, this volume). Factors such as parental loss and exposure to toxic home environments including domestic violence and substance abuse exacerbated by disruptions in family circumstances and social isolation are known predictors of diminished health and wellbeing in later life. The negative impacts of adverse childhood experiences on ageing trajectories are supported by an increasing body of longitudinal research globally (for example, Cheval et al, 2019), and the potential life course repercussions of the COVID-19 pandemic merit examination in light of this growing evidence.

The impact of the COVID-19 pandemic on the health behaviours and mental and social health of younger and working age adults has been investigated in a number of studies from different global settings. Findings from a longitudinal study with persons aged 18 to 34 in several metropolitan areas across the United States (Romm et al, 2021), for example, showed negative impacts on physical activity (almost half of participants) and sedentary behaviour (three-quarters of participants). About 40 per cent of participants also reported increased alcohol use and a third indicated eating less healthily during the pandemic. More than half reported increases in indicators of mental health impact, with women and sexual minorities at greater risk for depression. Turnic et al's study (2022) of working age adults (aged 20 to 49 years) in central Serbia likewise examined physical activity, nutritional habits, and mental and social health in individuals with recent COVID-19 infection. Negative impacts in this group were found on levels of exercise, on social and educational activities, and quality of life. Thus existing evidence points to a variety of risks to building 'health capital' in younger and middle-aged adults that have resulted from the pandemic.

The effects of the COVID-19 pandemic and associated safeguarding measures on older adults (aged 60 and over) have been synthesised in a review of the published literature by Lebrasseur et al (2021). The included studies reported heightened prevalence of psychological symptoms, increases in experiences of ageism and decline in physical health among the study populations. Decreased socialising and in-person social contact were associated in some studies with worsened quality of life and increased depression. Other challenges related to maintaining health and wellbeing in later life identified in this research included decreased levels of physical activity, problems with sleep and difficulties accessing needed services.

Other subsequent studies examining the impact of the pandemic on older adults are notable for employing longitudinal cohorts to assess changes in health and wellbeing. For example, using nationally representative data from the Canadian Longitudinal Study on Aging, Raina et al (2021) demonstrated a doubling of the odds of experiencing depressive symptoms during the period of the pandemic. A number of factors were found to produce vulnerability to the deterioration of depressive symptoms during the pandemic, among them poorer health, lower/loss of income, loneliness, and challenges in accessing usual provisions and needed healthcare and medications.

Reviewing the evidence of how COVID-19 has affected health and wellbeing across different life stages and age groups highlights the utility of understanding how risks to healthy ageing are patterned and influenced by diverse individual and societal factors.

Cost of living crisis

The disruptive effects of both the Russian invasion of Ukraine and the COVID-19 pandemic on supply chains of basic goods with ensuing increases in inflation rates are major drivers in the current global escalation of the cost of living (The Lancet Regional Health – Europe, 2023). According to a recent Eurobarometer survey (European Parliament, 2023), the rising cost of living is the most urgent worry for 93 per cent of Europeans, followed by the threat of poverty and social exclusion, mentioned by 82 per cent. Increases in the prices of food, fuel and energy characterise the 'cost of living crisis' that is accompanied by a chain of risks to population health as depicted in Figure 10.1.

The various pathways by which material conditions and the psychosocial repercussions of the cost of living crisis affect health are proposed by Broadbent et al (2023). The financial impact on households of rising costs produces downstream effects such as food insecurity, the inability

Figure 10.1: Increases in cost of living crisis that is accompanied by a chain of risks to population health

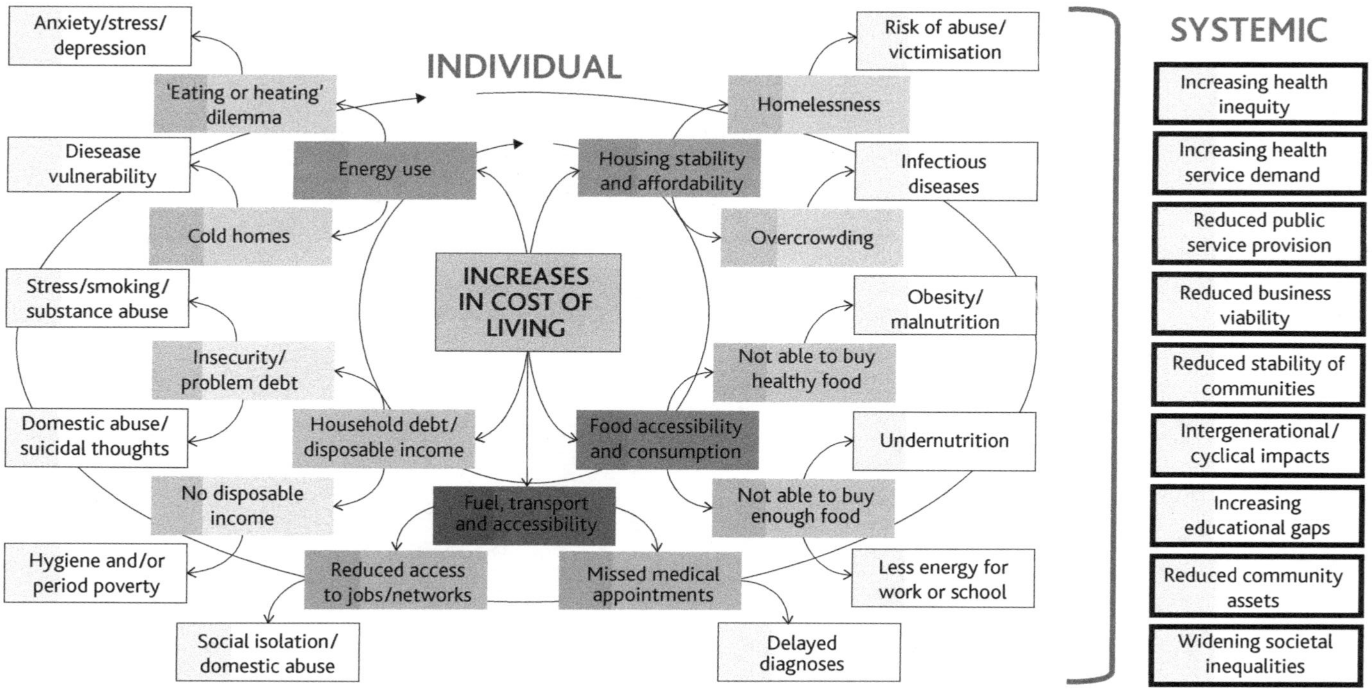

Source: Public Health Wales (2022)

to adequately heat homes or to actively participate in wider social and educational opportunities. Moreover, the impact on mental wellbeing of reduced or precarious financial circumstances is itself a gateway to poorer mental and physical health outcomes over time. As highlighted in Figure 10.1, the direct and indirect consequences of the cost of living emergency includes immediate and longer-term impacts on a host of social determinants of life course health and ageing.

Abundant evidence on low family income in childhood has demonstrated its negative causal effects on multiple aspects of childhood development. A systematic review of 54 studies on the impact of child poverty (Cooper and Stewart, 2021), for example, showed its adverse consequences on a range of children's cognitive, health and social-behavioural outcomes. In view of this evidence, conditions such as the reported prevalence of food insecurity in the past month in a recent household survey in the UK (The Food Foundation, 2022) offer significant cause for concern. According to the survey, one in four households with children (25.8 per cent) in the UK had experienced food insecurity during that timeframe, affecting an estimated four million children.

While the health and wellbeing effects of the current cost of living crisis are still to be determined, a variety of studies from other recent economic downturns – such as the 2007 to 2009 'Great Recession' – provide an indication of the types of potential impacts of the present crisis (England et al, 2023). The physical and mental health repercussions of this major macroeconomic event were summarised in a review of research conducted in developed countries (Margerison–Zilko et al, 2016). Impacts were evident for a range of outcomes across stages of the life course. Findings from this body of research offer evidence, for example, of various adverse effects on birth outcomes (for example, birth weight) and on indicators of child health. Detrimental impacts on adult health, in particular mental health, were reported across these studies. Self-rated health – a sentinel measure of health status and predictor of health outcomes – was found to have declined for those experiencing job loss, financial stresses and difficulties with housing. Overall, men and racial/ethnic minorities were identified as being at elevated risk of negative outcomes associated with this economic disruption.

Although evidence on the impact of the present cost of living crisis continues to emerge, findings from a robust literature on the multiple repercussions of recent major economic crises demonstrate the effects on key indicators and life course supports for optimal human development and healthy ageing.

Conclusion

It is well documented that social determinants of health influence physical, mental and emotional outcomes for people across the life course. They determine the number of years lived and the proportion of those that are lived well. They can negatively impact the trajectory of people's health from the womb, during childhood and adolescence, into adulthood and through to older ages. This chapter has explored three contemporary and interacting societal issues and events: the Ukrainian conflict, the COVID-19 pandemic and the cost of living crisis using a life course approach to human development and ageing. It is evident that each of the societal events has the capacity to derail and devastate the lives of individuals as they age, even when those events occurred at the beginning of their lives. Adverse childhood experiences not only impact childhood and adolescence but can alter the likelihood of healthy, longer lives by impeding physical, emotional and psychological development from the outset. However, older adults without such poor beginnings can also find themselves vulnerable to the impact of such events. The increased likelihood of chronic health conditions and cognitive decline can mean some older adults have fewer options to escape or take recourse from negative social events, and hence may be slower, or refuse, to take these up. Older adults are, of course, not homogeneous, and the negative impacts may be disproportionate, as in Ukraine, where women, those aged 70 and over, and those with disabilities were especially vulnerable (HelpAge International, 2023).

Internationally, there are a range of public policies, programmes and laws that seek to address health inequalities but not all explicitly advocate for older people per se. For example, the International Covenant on Economic, Social and Cultural Rights includes the rights to an adequate standard of living, to work, to social security and to the highest attainable standard of physical and mental health. The Convention on the Elimination of all Forms of Discrimination against Women includes human rights protection and prohibits discrimination against women, including older women. While the Convention on the Rights of Persons with Disabilities offers protections for older people with disabilities, including access to poverty programmes. These international laws, despite being signed up to by many countries across the globe, are limited in terms of making real change.

The United Nations, in conjunction with the WHO, declared the 2020s as the Decade of Healthy Ageing and highlights four key action areas including Combatting Ageism as part of the Global Campaign to Combat Ageism. The latest progress report (November 2023) cites advances in terms of developing legislation and national policies on health and social care needs assessments and establishing national programmes in some member states. However, less than a third of the countries involved currently have adequate support or resources to act upon its objectives. While work is ongoing to engage stakeholders, time will tell on the outcomes of this important initiative.

Challenging societal issues and events can adversely affect people across the life course, yet people can display great resilience in the face of adversity.

Legislation to address inequalities needs to be supported by a variety of stakeholders to effect change at the individual, community and societal level. International programmes may be able to support these endeavours and bring about longer-term change.

References

Adams, R. (2024) Rapid help needed for Covid babies who fell behind, says former Ofsted chief. *The Guardian*, 5 January.

Arantes de Araújo, L., Veloso, C.F., de Campos Souza, M., de Azevedo, J.M. and Tarro, G. (2020) The potential impact of the COVID-19 pandemic on child growth and development: a systematic review. *Jornal de Pediatria*, 97: 369–377.

Barker, D.J. (1990) The fetal and infant origins of adult disease. *British Medical Journal*, 301(6761): 1111.

Benner, A.D. and Mistry, R.S. (2020) Child development during the COVID-19 pandemic through a life course theory lens. *Child Development Perspectives*, 14(4): 236–243.

Broadbent, P., Thomson, R., Kopasker, D., McCartney, G., Meier, P., Richiardi, M., et al (2023) The public health implications of the cost-of-living crisis: outlining mechanisms and modelling consequences. *The Lancet Regional Health Europe*, 27: 100585.

Chaaya, C., Chambi, V.D., Sabuncu, Ö., Abedi, R., Osman, A., Osman, A., et al (2022) Ukraine – Russia crisis and its impacts on the mental health of Ukrainian young people during the COVID-19 pandemic. *Annals of Medicine & Surgery*, 79: 104033.

Cheval, B., Chabal, C., Sieber, S., Orsholits, D., Cooper, R., Guessous, I., et al (2019) Association between diverse childhood experiences and muscle strength in older age. *Gerontology*, 65(5): 474–484.

Cooper, K. and Stewart, K. (2021) Does household income affect children's outcomes? A systematic review of the evidence. *Child Indicators Research*, 14: 981–1005.

De Rooij, S.R., Wouters, H., Yonker, J.E., Painter, R.C. and Roseboom, T.J. (2010) Prenatal undernutrition and cognitive function in late adulthood. *Proceedings of the National Academy of Sciences of the United States of America*, 107(39): 16881–16886.

England, C., Jarrom, D., Washington, J., Hasler, E., Batten, L., Lewis, R., et al (2023) Measuring mental health in a cost-of-living crisis: a rapid review. Health Technology Wales.

European Parliament (2023) Europeans concerned by cost of living crisis and expect additional EU measures. Press release. Available at: https://www.europarl.europa.eu/news/en/press-room/20230109IPR65918/europeans-concerned-by-cost-of-living-crisis-and-expect-additional-eu-measures

The Food Foundation (2022) New data show 4 million children in households affected by food insecurity. The Food Foundation. Available at: https://foodfoundation.org.uk/publication/new-data-show-4-million-children-households-affected-food-insecurity

Forouhi, N., Hall, E. and McKeigue, P. (2004) A life course approach to diabetes. In D. Kuh, Y. Ben Shlomo and E. Susser (eds), *A Life Course Approach to Chronic Disease Epidemiology*, 2nd edn. Oxford: Oxford University Press, pp 165–188.

Franzek, E.J., Sprangers, N., Janssens, A.C.J.W., Van Duijn, C.M. and Van De Wetting, B.J.M. (2008) Prenatal exposure to the 1944–45 Dutch 'hunger winter' and addiction later in life. *Addiction*, 103(3): 433–448.

Garfield, R. (2008) The epidemiology of war. In B.S. Levy and V.W. Sidel (eds), *War and Public Health*, 2nd edn. New York: Oxford University Press, pp 23–36.

Geronimus, A.T. (2023) *Weathering: The Extraordinary Stress of Ordinary Life on the Body in an Unjust Society*. London: Virago.

Halfon, N. and Forrest, C.B. (2018) The emerging theoretical framework of lifecourse health development. In N. Halfon, C.B. Forrest, R.M. Lerner and E.M. Faustman (eds), *Handbook for Life Course Health Development*. Cham: Springer, pp 19–43.

Hatch, S., Huppert, F. A., Abbott, R., Croudace, T., Ploubidis, G., Wadsworth, M., Richards, M., and Kuh, D. (2007) 'A life course approach to well-being', in J. Haworth and G. Hart (eds) *Well-Being: Individual, Community and Social Perspectives*, London: Palgrave Macmillan, pp 187–205.

HelpAge International (2022) Ukraine: Older people face abandonment and isolation as conflict with Russia intensifies. HelpAge International. Available at: https://www.helpage.org/news/ukraine-older-people-face-abandonment-and-isolation-as-conflict-with-russia-intensifies/

HelpAge International (2023) *'I've lost the life I knew': Older People's Experiences of the Ukraine War and their Inclusion in the Humanitarian Response*. London: HelpAge International.

Kar, N. (2022) War and older adults: consequences and challenges. *Journal of Geriatric Care and Research*, 9(1): 1–3.

Kesternich, I., Siflinger, B., Smith, J.P. and Winter, J.K. (2014) The effects of World War II on economic and health outcomes across Europe. *The Review of Economics and Statistics*, 96(1): 103–118.

Khan, A.R. and Altalbe, A. (2023) Potential impacts of Russo-Ukraine conflict and its psychological consequences among Ukrainian adults: the post-COVID-19 era. *Public Health*, 11: 1280423.

Kimhi, S., Hantman, S., Goroshit, M., Eshel, Y. and Zysberg, L. (2012) Elderly people coping with the aftermath of war: resilience versus vulnerability. *American Journal of Geriatric Psychiatry*, 20(5): 391–401.

Korinek, K., Young, Y., Teerawichitchainan, B., Chuc, N.T.K., Kovnick, M. and Zimmer, Z. (2020) Is war hard on the heart? Gender, wartime stress and late life cardiovascular conditions in a population of Vietnamese older adults. *Social Science & Medicine*, 265: 113380.

Kovnick, M.O., Young, Y., Tran, N., Teerawichitchainan, B., Tran, T.K. and Korinek, K. (2021) The impact of early life war exposure on mental health among older adults in northern and central Vietnam. *Journal of Health and Social Behavior*, 62(4): 526–544.

Kuh, D. and Ben-Shlomo, Y. (2004) A life course approach to chronic disease epidemiology. In D. Kuh, Y. Ben Shlomo and E. Susser (eds), *A Life Course Approach to Chronic Disease Epidemiology*, 2nd edn. Oxford: Oxford University Press, pp 240–259.

Kuh, D., Karunananthan, S., Bergman, H. and Cooper, R. (2014) A life-course approach to healthy ageing: maintaining physical capability. *Proceedings of the Nutrition Society*, 73(2): 237–248.

Kurapov, A., Kalaitzaki, A., Keller, V., Danyliuk, I. and Kowatsch, T. (2023) The mental health impact of the ongoing Russian-Ukrainian war 6 months after the Russian invasion of Ukraine. *Frontiers in Psychiatry*, 14: 1134780.

The Lancet Regional Health – Europe (2023) Editorial: the cost-of-living crisis is also a health crisis. *The Lancet*, 27: 100632.

Lebrasseur, A., Fortin-Bédard, N., Lettre, J., Raymond, E., Bussières, E., Lapierre, N., et al (2021) Impact of the COVID-19 pandemic on older adults: rapid review. *JMIR Aging*, 4(2): e26474.

Levy, B.S. and Sidel, V.W. (2009) Health effects of combat: a life-course perspective. *Annual Review of Public Health*, 30(1): 123–136.

Lumey, L.H., Stein, A.D. and Susser, E. (2011) Prenatal famine and adult health. *Annual Review of Public Health*, 32: 237–262.

Marengoni, A. and Calderon-Larranaga, A. (2020) Health inequalities in ageing: towards a multidimensional lifecourse approach. *The Lancet Public Health*, 5(7): E364–E365.

Margerison-Zilko, C., Goldman-Mellor, S., Falconi, A. and Downing, J. (2016) Health impacts of the Great Recession: a critical review. *Current Epidemiology Reports*, 3(1): 81–91.

Martsenkovskyi, D., Karatzias, T., Hyland, P., Shevlin, M., Ben-Ezra, M., McElroy, E., et al (2023) Parent-reported posttraumatic stress reactions in children and adolescents: findings from the Mental Health of Parents and Children in Ukraine Study. *Psychological Trauma: Theory, Research, Practice, and Policy*. https://dx.doi.org/10.1037/tra0001583

Menassa, M., Stronks, K., Khatami, F., Diaz, Z.M.R., Espinola, O.P., Gamba, M., et al (2023) Concepts and definitions of healthy aging: a systematic review and synthesis of theoretical models. *eClinical Medicine*, 51: 101821.

Osiichuk, M. and Shepotylo, O. (2020) Conflict and well-being of civilians: the case of the Russian-Ukrainian hybrid war. *Economic Systems*, 44(1): 100736.

Public Health Wales (2022) *Cost of Living Crisis in Wales: A Public Health Lens*. Report.

Raina, P., Wolfson, C., Griffith, L., et al (2021) A longitudinal analysis of the impact of the COVID-19 pandemic on the mental health of middle-aged and older adults from the Canadian Longitudinal Study on Aging. *Nature Aging*, 1: 1137–1147.

Ramirez, D. and Haas, S.A. (2022) Windows of vulnerability: consequences of exposure timing during the Dutch Hunger Winter. *Population and Development Review*, 48(4): 959–989.

Ravelli, G.P., Stein, Z.A. and Susser, M.W. (1976) Obesity in young men after famine exposure in utero and early infancy. *New England Journal of Medicine*, 295: 349–353.

Riad, A., Drobov, A., Krobot, M., Antalová, N., Alkasaby, M.A., Peřina, A., et al (2022) Mental health burden of the Russian–Ukrainian War 2022 (RUW-22): anxiety and depression levels among young adults in Central Europe. *International Journal of Environmental Research and Public Health*, 19: 8418.

Romm, K.F., Patterson, B., Wysota, C.N., Wang, Y. and Berg, C.J. (2022) Predictors of negative psychosocial and health behavior impact of COVID-19 among young adults. *Health Education Research*, 36(4): 385–397.

Roseboom, T.J., van der Meulen, J.H.P., Osmond, C., et al (2000) Coronary heart disease after prenatal exposure to the Dutch famine 1944–45. *Heart*, 84(6): 595–598.

Roseboom, T.J., Painter, R.C., van Abeelen, A.F.M., Marjolein, V.E., Veenendaal, S. and de Rooij, R. (2011) Hungry in the womb: what are the consequences? lessons from the Dutch famine. *Maturitas*, 70(2): 141–145.

Settersten, R.A., Bernardi, L., Härkönen, J., Antonucci, T.C., Dykstra, P.A., Heckhausen, J., et al (2020) Understanding the effects of COVID-19 through a life course lens. *Advances in Life Course Research*, 45: 100360.

Skwirczynska, E., Kozłowski, M., Nowak, K., Wróblewski, O., Sompolska-Rzechuła, A., Kwiatkowski, S. et al (2022) Anxiety assessment in Polish students during the Russian–Ukrainian war. *International Journal of Environmental Research and Public Health*, 19: 13284.

Stein, A.D., Zybert, P.A., van der Pal-de Bruin, K. and Lumey, L.H. (2006) Exposure to famine during gestation, size at birth, and blood pressure at age 59 year: evidence from the Dutch famine. *European Journal of Epidemiology*, 21: 759–765.

Summers, A., Leidman, E., Pereira Figueira Periquito, I.M. and Bilukha, O.O. (2019) Serious psychological distress and disability among older persons living in conflict affected areas in eastern Ukraine: a cluster-randomized cross-sectional household survey. *Conflict and Health*, 13: 10.

Turnic, N., Vasiljevic, T.I., Stanic, M., Jakovljevic, B., Mikerova, M., Ekkert, N., et al (2022) Post-COVID-19 status and its physical, nutritional, psychological, and social effects in working-age adults: a prospective questionnaire study. *Journal of Clinical Medicine*, 11(22): 6668.

UNICEF (2022) More than half of Ukraine's children displaced after one month of war.

United Nations (2022) Global issues: ageing. Available at: https:/www.un.org/en/global-issues/ageing

Witt, W.P., Harlaar, N. and Palmer, A. (2023) The impact of COVID-19 on pregnant women and children: recommendations for health promotion. *American Journal of Health Promotion*, 37(2): 282–288.

World Health Organization (2015) *World Report on Ageing and Health*. Geneva: World Health Organization.

World Health Organization (2016) *Multisectoral Action for a Life Course Approach to Healthy Ageing: Draft Global Strategy and Plan of Action on Ageing and Health*. Sixty-ninth World Health Assembly. Geneva: World Health Organization.

Zimmer, Z., Fraser, K., Korinek, K., Akbulut-Yuksel, M., Young, Y.M. and Khanh Toan, T. (2021) War across the life course: examining the impact of exposure to conflict on a comprehensive inventory of health measures in an aging Vietnamese population. *International Journal of Epidemiology*, 50(3): 866–879.

Zimmer, Z., Korinek, K., Young, Y., Teerawichitchainan, B. and Toan, T.K. (2022) Early-life war exposure and later-life frailty among older adults in Vietnam: does war hasten aging? *The Journals of Gerontology: Series B*, 77(9): 1674–1685.

Relationalism, local and national authority governance: responding to the Ukrainian refugee crisis

Introduction to Part III

Richard Smith

When it comes to the importance of *relationalism*, the case can clearly be made, in the context of partnering, when one sees the dire consequences of war in Europe and the Middle East and its impact on the cost of living (Burton, this volume). Part III addresses a number of the issues affecting a fundamental breakdown of relationships between organisations and people across UK and Europe. It addresses some of the complex governance issues that arise when public, commercial and community interests are engaged.

At the heart of *relationalism* reviewed in the previous volume of this series (Bonner, 2023)and in this part of the book is a recognition of the need for a change in behaviour. A change in the manner that organisations and sectoral interests relate to each other in response to the external environment. The chapters in this section examine the strategic and financial complexities that arise through the expertise of the contributors including a number of case studies related to Finland (Chapter 11), Sutton Homes for Ukraine (Chapter 12) and Norway, including a section relating to The Salvation Army (Chapter 14). Comparisons are drawn between UK and Europe.

The perspectives in this section serve to illustrate the value of *relationalism*. There were four issues attributed to enabling relational partnering to be more effective in terms of its outcomes. These were identified as: the *functional roles* [and relationships of the partners]the *financial arrangements* [including attention to risk factors]; the *social consequences* of the partnership in terms of what it delivered to the community and involving the third sector. It is also, most importantly, the reaction of the partners and beneficiaries to the relationship in terms of recognising the change in behaviour that comes from a culture of equal partners (that is, less adherence to contractor/client requirements which are generally governed through application of procurement rules and interpretation of contract terms).

Significantly, the bringing together of a number of disparate people and organisations with differing backgrounds and experience began to crystallise the considerable value that can be gained from effective relational partnering. The 'conversations' (via Zoom and Teams) that occurred through the COVID-19 period began to focus on these four factors and while the discussions were focused mainly on the UK (and in particular local government), the same principles are equally relevant to international governance.

When it comes to *internationalism* the functional aspects of international partnering are particularly self-evident when one talks about nation-states. The current wars are a direct result of territorial ambitions, both proactive and reactive, coupled with the impact of historical legacy. It is clear from the following chapters that relational continuity will be impacted through social instability, particularly, as in Chapter 11 the issue of homelessness is considered. A second issue identified in Chapter 12 is the positive value that can be generated through partnerships between a (local) governmental organisation, the third sector and the community. This is clear when functionality in the form of good governance works. Internationally, *relational partnerships* are important when the crises such as the Russian–Ukraine war and in the Middle East result in the displacement of populations and the need for support from receiving countries.

Of course, in an international context when it comes to war or a diminution of social values (see Chapter 5) there is a considerable human and financial cost. However, through working in a *relational* manner and within a *relational culture*, the positives of human experience can be seen ahead of its tragedies. A powerful *relational dividend* that has been identified through work within the UK has been a re-focus on the value of a legal framework (which, in the context of internationalism, includes international law) that needs to be both flexible and innovative enough to accommodate new initiatives. Such a regime demands *mutual trust* and respect between parties. It demands a more positive attempt at delivering new outcomes which are mutually beneficial with less emphasis upon the nature of the legal relationship and the process leading up to it. These same principles are applicable when one examines different legal regimes across different nation-states.

Relationalism demands a re-education of individuals and organisations, including a change to culture and behaviour, ensuring that the right people occupy the right place in the right time frame. This has much to do with the nature of the governance and the legal framework within which they operate. Some form of 'accreditation' is urged, the need for which is made through the examples detailed in this part of the book. An *accreditation model* (see Smith,2023, Introduction to Part V in the previous volume,) facilitated by universities and other higher education bodies will necessarily focus on building trust between the individuals and organisations as a prerequisite to forming contract agreements to undertake services. This contrasts with today's partnering in which relationships between contracting parties largely emerges after financial agreements and placement of the contract.

When it comes to internationalism and accreditation, it is clear from the experiences detailed in the case studies in this section that this opportunity to build *relationalism* is much more difficult. The case studies described in part the consequences of the war in Ukraine, where precipitative military action was taken by one party and the opportunity to change any relationship or culture was lost. The question therefore remains for the future – what kind of re-education/accreditation process is possible between nation–states recognising the role that the United Nations and International Court of Justice would have to play. With regard to any role that the United Nations might play in the context of accrediting relationalism, it is interesting to note its charter (see Appendix A) with its focus upon 'Peace, dignity and equality on a healthy planet'. These principles of course lie at the heart of relationalism. It can be seen that the

> United Nations can take action on a wide variety of issues due to its unique international character and the powers vested in its charter which is considered an international treaty. The UN charter codifies the major principles of international relations from sovereign equality of States to the prohibition of the use of force in international relations. (United Nations, 1945)

As the accreditation process evolves for *relationalism* in the UK, it will be interesting to note the future roles the UN, with reference to its charter, and the International Court of Justice might play. It is especially important that the right international legal framework is created embodying the principles of *relational contracting*.

The chapters and case studies that follow recognise the value of the *relational dividends* in a number of different ways. In the case of the Finnish housing and homelessness strategy (Chapter 11), *relational activities* were carried out despite political discontinuity. This would have been a recognition of the various partners' functionality and the different types of relationship that impacted on homelessness. It is noted there have been various *relational instruments* ranging from agreements that reflect individual clients and those between the state and the largest cities.

In the case of the London Borough Sutton Council (Chapter 12), the strong relationship that exists between the Borough of Sutton and the community (Chapter 13) or third sector has underpinned 'The Sutton Plan'. The *emotional consequence* of this plan is to make Sutton a place where everyone feels welcome and works with refugees, migrants and asylum seekers. It was also clear from the Sutton experience that building up community and peer support networks for refugees, therefore evolving strong *relational support* for these groups, was beneficial and led to a successful community sponsorship policy, involving a funded voluntary sector organisation (Case Study 12.1) and hosts in the community (see Chapters 7 and 12). It is also interesting to note the mechanisms through which the support network was developed, including video calls which helped to reduce the state of fear, uncertainty and inability to create long-term planning.

When it comes to the Norwegian case study (8.1 in Chapter 8) and support for refugees in other chapters, there was a recognition of the *emotional dividend* factors coupled with social consequences that arose with the increasing number of migrants/refugees. It emphasised the need to carry out 'our social mission in a correct and considerate manner with great awareness that there are people who are strongly affected by the work we do'.

It is also clear from the chapters and case studies described in this part of the book that the work of The Salvation Army was based upon good relationships with a clear focus (mission) on helping to resolve problems of capacity and places for refugees and asylum seekers to live. The role of education and accreditation, and recognition, by government departments in the long-standing and highly respected work of The Salvation Army was important when it came to ensuring that the right people were placed in the right jobs within the refugee centres.

As is discussed in Chapter 14, the theological foundations of The Salvation Army also emphasises the value of *relationalism*. In this respect, the term *relationalism* has exactly the same meaning as the Latin term 'con venire', which is the coming together of individuals or parties to make a bond (or contract). It is also noted in Chapter 14 that there is a mutual interest in establishing a relationship which is 'non-hierarchical and equal in the sense that although there is order and process, everyone has an equal space around the table'.

Relationalism can mean many things to many people. There has long been a need for a coordinated response to the development of the idea of *relationalism*. In today's society, there is too little attention paid to the need to build *mutual trust* between people. A trust that enables partners, whether socially or commercially, to share a working relationship on an equal footing. The 'tick box culture' negates the opportunity to take time and have the benefit, for example, of face-to-face discussions in order to build such a relationship. *Relationalism* will result in more effective organisational relationships when their function and purpose in partnering is recognised. Through a more flexible legal framework it is possible to mitigate risks and improve financial returns. From the case studies in this book it is easy to see the social benefits to communities and the third sector that can be obtained, alongside the emotional consequences that are generally positive, even though they have arisen from great adversity.

It is apparent that when there is a fundamental breakdown of relationships, as we have observed between Russia and Ukraine and more recently between Israel and Hamas, the most difficult side of human experience is to be witnessed. Perhaps though, through having to witness and in many cases experience war with its consequences domestically and internationally, we can at least draw lessons of value for development of our future relationships. This section aims to capture these experiences. This *Social Determinants of Health* publication begins the journey.

References

Bonner, A. (ed) (2023) *COVID-19 and Social Determinants of Health: Wicked Issues and Relationalism.* Bristol: Policy Press.

Smith, R. (2023) Introduction to Part V: The case for relationalism. In A. Bonner (ed) *COVID-19 and Social Determinants of Health: Wicked Issues and Relationalism.* Bristol: Policy Press.

United Nations (1945) United Nations Charter. https://www.un.org/en/about-us/un-charter

11

Relational continuity despite instability: distributed local and national governance towards the eradication of homelessness in Finland

Annalisa Sannino and Yrjö Engeström

Introduction

The effects of socioeconomic factors on health and on health inequalities across groups are generally presented as firmly supported by research in numerous fields (Marmot and Wilkinson, 2005). Social determinants of health refer to 'factors apart from medical care that can be influenced by social policies and shape health in powerful ways' (Braveman and Gottlieb, 2014: 19). Homelessness as a socioeconomic condition definitely represents in a major way such factors.

Homelessness is a major wicked challenge faced by all countries, including the most affluent ones. Ever since 2007 Finland has pursued an exceptionally coherent and successful policy of homelessness reduction. Differently from top-down policies, this has been created with the involvement of multiple layers of governance of civil society coming together around the generative principle of Housing First.

This chapter gives a brief overview of a series of participatory studies conducted in Finland to support a multi-level effort towards the eradication of homelessness. A common denominator among these studies is that they were carried out during a period from 2018 to 2023 in which the local challenges with homelessness in Finland coincided with the impact of a series of global upheavals, ranging from the refugee crisis, to COVID-19 and the war in Ukraine. The chapter is a proposition on distributed governance by showing how the Finnish Housing First (FHF) homelessness strategy could continue to develop despite political discontinuity and large-scale instabilities.

The chapter starts by introducing FHF, its history and current circumstances. A section follows with an account of continuing developments of the strategy despite unprecedented obstacles. The chapter ends with a reflection on the role distributed local and national governance can play in the face of discontinuity risks threatening the unprecedented advances and realistic prospects of definite solutions to homelessness in Finland.

Finnish Housing First, its history and the current circumstances

The homelessness strategy in Finland is a valuable example of an alternative to top-down policies, having been created by multiple layers of governance of civil society coming together around the generative principle of Housing First (Pleace et al, 2016). A dense texture of relational instruments has been established over the past 15 years, ranging from agreements and commitments with individual clients to agreements and commitments between the state and cities. This chapter illuminates how, despite instability, distributed and national governance could be maintained and even strengthened by a deliberate longitudinal effort at elevating relational ties to a qualitatively new level which goes by the name of FHF 2.0.

Homelessness is a phenomenon of great complexity and a widespread humanitarian crisis globally. Its proliferation is fuelled by pervasive stigma profoundly rooted in capitalist structures and in the *homo economicus*. It is an acute societal challenge filled with tensions, due to the economic resources and extensive transformation it demands. Overcoming homelessness requires homes as well as dealing with a wide range of vulnerabilities including sustained exposure to violence, growing up in childcare institutions, involvement in crimes, mental and physical health issues, debts, and substance abuse. As such, homelessness requires determined collaborative coalitions which cross sectors and hierarchical levels and expand into learning ecosystems with strong roots in civil engagement.

Coalitions of that kind are in place in the field of homelessness in Finland thanks to the FHF approach initiated by four activists in 2007 and pursued by means of three interconnected national programmes from 2008 to 2019 (Pleace et al, 2016). With FHF people with a history of homelessness or at risk of becoming homeless are offered affordable housing and tailored services to face social and healthcare needs (Y-Foundation, 2017; 2022). FHF's guiding principle is that living in one's own apartment is a precondition for a person to make the most of services towards functional independent living. The processes and results of FHF since the first national programme represent a vivid example of the effectiveness of multi-layered relational ties afforded by the welfare society.

Finland has distinguished itself as the only nation in Europe that has been able to significantly reduce homelessness since 2008 (Abbé Pierre Foundation and FEANTSA, 2018). Yet in recent years a number of factors have emerged which threaten the possibility for this country to continue in this direction and eventually eradicate homelessness. In 2018–2019, when the third national programme was coming to an end, there was no clear continuation commitment on the part of Juha Sipilä's government. This was also a period in the history of homelessness work in Finland filled with uncertainties due to a major generation change among administrators and practitioners, evidence of new emerging needs among clients whose conditions require services from multiple sectors and complex solutions, and identification of a particularly challenging group of clients whose housing solutions repeatedly failed. In 2019–2023, Sanna Marin's government programme supported homelessness work but the turmoil caused by the pandemic and then by Russia's attack of Ukraine obstructed a timely and focused approach. Currently, with Petteri Orpo's strongly market ideology-based government, the planned extensive cuts in public funding from 2024 onward may significantly damage the progress made in homelessness work for 15 years.

In other words, at a point when eradicating homelessness has become a realistic perspective in Finland, the past five years have cast new shadows on this prospect. The portion of people living in rental homes has grown steadily, the portion of market-based rental homes has rapidly increased, the number of evictions rose by 13 per cent in 2022, and mortality risks among young homeless has been found to be tenfold compared to the population average.

Continuity against all odds: developments of the Finnish Housing First homelessness strategy from 2018 to 2023

The following is a chronological account of a series of participatory studies of our team with homelessness practitioners from 2018 to 2023. The studies focused on change efforts taking place locally at the level of a supported housing unit for young people, at the city level with two municipalities in Finland, and at the national level, with a collective comprising the coordinator of the national programme for the prevention of homelessness at the Ministry of Environment, four prominent non-governmental organisations, six cities, nine regions and the largest national non-profit landlord for affordable rental housing in the country.

2018–2020

The first study was conducted in 2018–2020, despite unsuccessful attempts at gathering external research funding. It consisted of three interconnected Change Laboratories (CLs; Engeström et al, 1996) in which the researchers and practitioners collectively analysed current circumstances and change prospects locally at the level of a supported housing unit, at the city level with one of the largest municipalities in Finland, and at the national level, with the collective described earlier (Sannino, 2020; 2022). The sectors of the organisations and actors represented in the CLs ranged from housing, criminal justice and healthcare to psychiatric and addiction care, psychosocial services and social work.

Despite some of these actors having never sat around the same table before, they joined a total of 18 CL sessions over a period of ten months, to analyse the history and current developments of homelessness work within and across their respective organisations and to explore reasons behind possible gaps between them. Throughout this process, they also reconceptualised priorities in their joint work and designed models meant to support collaborative future initiatives to be undertaken towards eradicating homelessness.

The CLs at the municipal and national level strongly benefited from the impulses stemming from the CL at the ground level of the housing unit. At each level the participants built on jointly produced analyses to elaborate action plans for keeping up the momentum of homelessness work in the 2020s. In particular the CL at the national level defined a vision for FHF 2.0 to be brought to the attention of political forces and decision-makers.

From 2012 to 2018 the housing unit in which the local-level CL took place was in the limelight as one of the most challenging units in the country, with serious incidents, complaints from neighbours, frequent police visits and ambulance calls. There was great turmoil as the staff included practitioners who were afraid of the residents. At the same time, however, possibilities for a new beginning emerged with a unit manager leading the staff to experiment with novel ways of working, discovering new capabilities they had ignored before in themselves as well as in the residents (Sannino, 2020).

The numerous references to changes underway in this housing unit in the sessions of the other two CLs indicate that the changes in frontline work of this housing unit started to become a real source of inspiration and transformative envisioning across the organisations, sectors and hierarchical levels. The studies provide evidence of systematic cross-fertilisation across the three CLs that helped building momentum within and between the processes at the local, city and national levels. The housing unit is today serving as a model for other units nationally, with projects stemming from the analyses and design realised during the CL.

In the large city where the second CL was conducted, the numbers of homeless started to increase in 2018, especially among the youth, after more than a decade of sustained decrease. What appeared as particularly challenging for this city was to shift from the criterion of sobriety and no intoxicants to the FHF ethos. Attempts to overcome this challenge were made along the CL process, with strong signs of resistance caused by fear and structural obstacles. Due to the awareness of the financial constraints in the city, the participants in the city-level CL started exploring alternative intermediate remedies which could be realistically established with existing resources.

At the end of both the city-level and the national-level CL, proposals for action plans written by the participants were presented in public events and were used in interactions with decision-makers. The document produced at the national level was titled *Housing First 2.0: Let Us Make Together a Possibility for Everyone.*

2020–2022

The three CLs generated a partnership between the research team and key homelessness actors which led to a second study in 2020–2022. The COVID-19 pandemic made it difficult to work in supported housing units and low-threshold meeting places. The numbers of homeless young people who use substances had started to increase. It became clear that new operating models are needed for homelessness work, especially to help clients who have difficulties to settle and who need many support services. With this new study, the CL participatory approach was adapted online to bring together practitioners from different locations in Finland with a combination of synchronous interactions by means of online workshops and asynchronous interactions by means of a video library and web forums for discussion (Sannino et al, 2021). This study involved a total number of 276 homelessness practitioners who took part in ten workshops and made use of the video library and the ten web forums. The practitioners were geographically distributed across 15 Finnish municipalities.

This study focused on the development of newly identified ways of working among frontline homelessness practitioners. Also, this study followed up on the implementation of a number of innovations designed during the three CLs of the previous study, and supported the consolidation of partnerships between the researchers and the actors in the field. This study, as the previous one, was deliberately initiated by the research team to support the critical transition phase in the history of FHF.

The three CLs in the first study produced models that gave meaning and direction to the involved collectives and helped identifying alternatives to no longer viable perspectives in homelessness work. Also, steps were undertaken to implement spearhead projects designed on the basis of these models within and across the levels (Sannino, 2020; 2022). One of such spearheads was the approach of mobile multi-professional service teams named Deerfoot, envisioned in the CL at the city-level in the first study. The word chosen by the practitioners for this spearhead is borrowed from the Deerfoot books by Edward S. Ellis. In the context of homelessness work, the word *Deerfoot* refers to a new type of agile and flexible service.

The clients of homelessness work today have to increasingly move between different housing solutions and different services to meet very diverse acute needs. The FHF solutions implemented during the decade after the first national programme in 2008 and based on permanent supported housing for dealing with substance abuse are no longer sufficient. These solutions must be complemented with mobile multi-professional teams aimed at preventing that these vulnerable people fall into cracks of relatively fragmented services.

As this second study progressed, the Deerfoot perspective and name was appropriated by a midsize city which had not participated in any of the CLs in the first study. The two cities applied for and received funding from the state for their respective Deerfoot projects, based on the same principles but also adapted to the specific needs of the two cities. The funding made possible the implementation of these projects in the two cities since the beginning of 2021. In one of the online workshops of the second study, representatives of the two cities decided to intensify their exchanges to further develop the envisioned solutions. In the third study, our team followed and supported with our CL formative intervention tools the progress of this initiative (Sannino et al, 2023). Building on the experiences in this midsize city, a fast-reacting, expert mobile multi-professional team was found to be effective in supporting hard-to-reach homelessness work clients with diverse problems.

Models of such mobile services have been developed in Europe and in the United States, especially to support mental health patients. The most well-known are the ACT (Assertive Community Treatment) models and the FACT and RACT models stemming from them. The midsize city's experimentation with the Deerfoot model is, however, displaying two distinctive promising functions of multi-professional mobile homelessness work: first, supporting each client so that s/he does not fall outside the services; second, mending gaps and ruptures in the service system together with different actors.

While the American ACT model emphasises very long-term care and requires for example that each team has a psychiatrist, the Deerfoot model created and implemented in this midsize city aims at serving the entire population of potential clients, with shorter client relationships and reorganisation of the collaboration and coordination between already existing services. The basic idea is that this is a team that opens doors and gets different professionals actively involved as needed by specific clients. The multi-professional mobile homelessness team in this midsize city is now being consolidated to serve clients at the level of the entire county. Preliminary calculations in this city also reveal that this type of work can lead to significant savings when it succeeds to eliminate gaps and ruptures in the service system, in other words, to prevent clients from falling outside the services.

Multi-professional mobile support in homelessness work is not new. So far, however, it has been implemented on the basis of practical experience and in addition to the practitioners' other tasks, often without carefully tested models, specific competences and resources. The experiences gained in the city mentioned earlier indicate that multi-professional mobile homelessness work requires a new work orientation and new kinds of competences to be systematically cultivated by means of education and peer learning.

There are signs now in Finland of awareness that multi-professional mobile homelessness work, such as Deerfoot, should be lifted up to a national strategic principle that is properly modelled and supported (Kaakinen, 2023).

2022–2023

As Finland was recovering from the turmoil of the COVID-19 pandemic, new unprecedented circumstances emerged with the war in Ukraine which further slowed down the prospects of eradicating homelessness highlighted in the Marin government programme. At the same time, the country was finalising a long reform process which led to the establishment of wellbeing services counties. These new administrative entities strive to adopt the most promising new services and working models from the municipalities that constitute them. This presents to homelessness practitioners a significant challenge and at the same time an opportunity to foster the potential of multi-professional mobile support. For this, a fourth study was designed with CL-type formative intervention research, this time by initiative of the Housing First Network Developers for homelessness work at the Y-Foundation, in collaboration with our research team.

The aim of this project was to form over a period of ten months a network where the representatives of the wellbeing services counties interested in the development of multi-professional mobile support would produce a comprehensive description of alternative operating models of this type of work, by discussing and comparing together their experiences. Representatives of nine wellbeing services counties participated in this process. The final report, co-written with management-level and other practitioners participating in the workshops, was published in December 2023. The report presents key principles of multi-professional mobile support for local, regional and national use in homelessness work. The report was presented in a public seminar attended by policy makers and authorities from wellbeing services counties, along with frontline practitioners.

A perspective on distributed local and national governance towards the eradication of homelessness in Finland

The chronological account of the four successive studies presented in this chapter offers a useful empirical basis to reflect on the role of distributed local and national governance. The role this type of governance can play is particularly important in the face of discontinuity risks of approaches such as FHF which have been proven successful and which represent significant resources for the common good.

In the literature on social determinants of health, it is understood that upstream determinants such as financial and educational resources are central in modelling downstream behavioural determinants. As the latter are prioritised in typical linear interventions, the CL participatory approach mobilised in our series of studies indicates that non-linear interventions aimed at inter-organisational and cross-sectoral learning may be able to counteract financial and political upstream constraints. The literature points also at the fact that, as long as the various relevant research fields and areas of practice remain poorly integrated, if not altogether separate, it will not be possible to impactfully address such upstream socioeconomic determinants of health, homelessness included.

Critical perspectives (for example, Braveman et al, 2011; Preda and Voigt, 2015) on this vast body of knowledge emphasise the need of finding ways to translate local knowledge into action prospects which can direct public policies (Ruger, 2004a; Marmot et al, 2008). Lack of political will is often referred to as the key barrier to this end, and alternative types of interventions are also considered as a possible way forward (Ruger, 2004b).

Conclusion

This chapter offers an empirically grounded perspective on the importance of addressing homelessness on multiple fronts, in multiple domains of research, policy and practice, and in an integrated manner. It presents sustained experiences to integrate practice, research and policy into a process led by a plurality of very diverse yet highly complementary actors and institutions. Cohesion among these actors and institutions built since 2007 needs to be supported, strengthened and expanded for homelessness to be eradicated. This perspective contributes to recent discussions on reparative science (Breilh, 2023) and responsibility (Navarro, 2009) in response to the risk of not pursuing policy solutions already available even when they are urgently needed.

> Commercial sector wealth and power increase, whereas the countervailing forces having to meet these costs (notably individuals, governments, and civil society organisations) become correspondingly impoverished and disempowered or captured by commercial interests. This power imbalance leads to policy inertia; although many policy solutions are available, they are not being implemented. (Gilmore et al, 2023: 1194)

The perspective adopted in this article is much in line with Friel et al (2023: 1229):

> Evidence shows that progressive economic models, international frameworks, government regulation, compliance mechanisms for commercial entities, regenerative business types and models that incorporate health, social, and environmental goals, and strategic

civil society mobilization together offer possibilities of systemic, transformative change, reduce those harms arising from commercial forces, and foster human and planetary wellbeing. In our view, the most basic public health question is not whether the world has the resources or will to take such actions, but whether humanity can survive if society fails to make this effort.

The call for action in the social determinants of health literature is interpreted here also as a call to everyone concerned with or able to influence work on homelessness. Aligning with a critical bioethics perspective, we concur that the focus must be on

> the voices of the affected communities, of scientists or independent experts and public managers involved and linked to a real project of justice and the full ethics of life. That enunciation must be intercultural and meta-critical: it can only be worked on from a transdisciplinary platform, with open doors and structured within the framework of a participatory public–social programme. (Breilh, 2023: 16)

Participatory intervention efforts such as the ones presented here are also actions in themselves. Aimed at joint analyses of strengths and shortcomings of existing institutional arrangements in homelessness work and at exploring grey areas of possibilities on this basis, such actions may be relevant especially in times of great turmoil and uncertainly as the field of homelessness work in Finland is currently demonstrating.

Acknowledgements

The empirical studies discussed in this received no external funding, with the exception of the second study funded by the Finnish Work Environment Fund (2019–2021). We are very grateful to all experts and practitioners in these studies for their collaboration, inspiration, time and trust.

References

Abbé Pierre Foundation and FEANTSA (2018) *Third Overview of Housing Exclusion in Europe*. Available at: https://www.feantsa.org/download/full-report-en1029873431323901915.pdf

Braveman, P. and Gottlieb, L. (2014) The social determinants of health: it's time to consider the causes of the causes. *Public Health Reports*, 129(1/2): 19–31.

Braveman, P., Egerter, S. and Williams, D.R. (2011) The social determinants of health: coming of age. *Annual Review of Public Health*, 32: 381–398.

Breilh, J. (2023) The social determination of health and the transformation of rights and ethics: a meta-critical methodology for responsible and reparative science. *Global Public Health*, 18(1): 2193830.

Friel, S., Collin, J., Daube, M., et al (2023) Commercial determinants of health: future directions. *Lancet*, 401: 1229–1240.

Gilmore, A.B., Fabbri, A., Baum, F., et al (2023) Defining and conceptualising the commercial determinants of health. *Lancet*, 401: 1194–1213.

Kaakinen, J. (2023) *Kotiin: Selvitysraportti tarvittavista toimenpiteistä asunnottomuuden poistamiseksi vuoteen 2027 mennessä [Home: Report on the Measures Needed to End Homelessness by 2027]*. Helsinki: Ministry of the Environment.

Marmot, M. and Wilkinson, R. (eds) (2005) *Social Determinants of Health*. Oxford: Oxford University Press.

Navarro, V. (2009) What we mean by social determinants of health. *International Journal of Health Services*, 39(3): 423–441.

Pleace, N., Knutagård, M., Granfelt, R. and Culhane, D. (2016) The strategic response to homelessness in Finland. In N. Nichols and C. Doberstein (eds), *Exploring Effective Systems Responses to Homelessness*. Toronto: The Homeless Hub Press, pp 425–441.

Preda, A. and Voigt, K. (2015) The social determinants of health: why should we care? *The American Journal of Bioethics*, 15(3): 25–36.

Ruger, J.P. (2004a) Ethics of the social determinants of health. *Lancet*, 364: 1092–1097.

Ruger, J.P. (2004b) Health and social justice. *Lancet*, 364(9439): 1075–1080.

Sannino, A. (2020) Enacting the utopia of eradicating homelessness: toward a new generation of activity–theoretical studies of learning. *Studies in Continuing Education*, 42(2): 163–179.

Sannino, A. (2022) Transformative agency as warping: how collectives accomplish change amid uncertainty. *Pedagogy, Culture & Society*, 30(1): 9–33.

Sannino, A. (2023) Toward a power–sensitive conceptualization of transformative agency. In N. Hopwood and A. Sannino (eds), *Agency and Transformation: Motives, Mediation, and Motion*. Cambridge: Cambridge University Press.

Sannino, A. (2023) Problem identification in change laboratories: workplace learning to eradicate homelessness. In H. Bound, A. Edwards, K. Evans and A. Chia (eds), *Workplace Learning for Changing Social and Economic Circumstances*. London: Routledge, pp 201–218.

Sannino, A., Engeström, Y. and Kärki, E. (2023) *Multiprofessional Mobile Support for Overcoming Homelessness: A Study of Nopsajalka Work in Jyväskylä*. Tampere: Tampere University.

Y-Foundation (2017) *A Home of Your Own: Housing First and Ending Homelessness in Finland*. Keuruu: Otava.

Y-Foundation (2022) *Housing First in Finland*. Available at: https://ysaatio.fi/en/housing-first-finland

12

The power of partnerships: working with the third sector to build community support networks for displaced people

Fern Barber

Introduction

The London Borough of Sutton has a long and proud history of partnership working, including strong relationships with the voluntary and community or 'third' sector (VCS). The Council's approach to partnership working is underpinned by a set of shared principles set out in 'The Sutton Plan'. Within the Council's corporate plan, *Ambitious for Sutton*, there is a specific focus on making Sutton a place where everyone feels welcome, including a commitment to work with the local VCS to support refugees, migrants and asylum seekers.

The local response to the COVID-19 pandemic further strengthened relationships with VCS organisations, including improved communication through widespread use of video conferencing to have more frequent meetings between the Council, VCS leads, and other partners to relay vital public health messages and support with things like access to personal protective equipment. The COVID-19 pandemic also reminded local public sector leaders of the key role that the third sector plays in supporting our communities. Sutton's VCS organisations were instrumental in both the vaccination roll-out, through the recruitment and deployment of volunteers, and the shielding programme, through sourcing and delivering food parcels to vulnerable persons.

Over the past decade the population of Sutton has become increasingly diverse. According to the 2021 census 43 per cent of the population were from Asian, Black, Mixed/Multiple and White non-British ethnic backgrounds, up from 29 per cent in the 2011 census. Seventeen per cent of households in Sutton have members who do not speak English as their first language and over 80 languages are spoken as a first language in Sutton (Sutton Strategic Needs Assessment, 2023). More recently, Sutton has welcomed people that have been displaced from across the world, including refugees from Syria, Afghanistan and Ukraine, as well as over 3,000 migrants from Hong Kong who relocated to the UK under the British National Overseas or 'BN(O)' Visa Scheme after the Chinese parliament approved a new national security law for Hong Kong in 2020. Third sector organisations in Sutton have been closely involved in welcoming refugees and migrants into the borough for decades, and more recent schemes, such as the 2016–2020 Syrian Resettlement Scheme, allowed a number of local groups to play a more proactive role as part of a community sponsorship approach.

However, the numerous refugee and migrant resettlement schemes that the UK government has introduced in recent years have provided challenges for local authorities. The roles and responsibilities of local councils have varied widely across the different schemes, as have the levels of funding received to support communities and perform these difficult for local government officers to navigate, constantly having to keep abreast of the latest guidance, as well as councils facing legitimate criticism from local migrant communities of unequal treatment as a result of some schemes attracting higher levels of funding than others.

Homes for Ukraine scheme: the initial response

Although Sutton Council and local third sector organisations had supported a small number of families from Syria and Afghanistan to resettle in the borough between 2019 and 2021, the scale, nature and pace of the Homes for Ukraine scheme in spring 2022 was unprecedented. The scheme, launched on 14 March 2022 by the UK government, was an individual sponsorship model whereby Ukrainians (and their immediate family members) with no family ties to the UK could be sponsored as 'guests' by individuals or organisations offering a room in their home or a self-contained property. The response from the UK public was significant, within days of launching, more than 130,000 British people had signed up. At time of writing 274 groups (318 adults and 115 children) had arrived in Sutton via the Homes for Ukraine scheme and there were 112 live sponsorships, also known as 'host' families or individuals accommodating Ukrainians.

However, the pace at which the scheme was initially rolled out across the UK presented a significant number of risks and challenges for local authorities to manage; foremost of which was the need to ensure vulnerable women, children and older people were effectively safeguarded from potential harm and to quickly identify and reduce risks of homelessness due to inadequate accommodation or sponsorship breakdowns. In March 2022 a number of charities wrote an open letter to the Secretary of State for Levelling Up, Housing & Communities about how the scheme was open to exploitation from human traffickers, for example, with matching between sponsors and guests taking place via unregulated social media sites. In addition to these risks, there were also significant concerns across local government that while the scheme was well intentioned in its aims, many sponsors would be ill-equipped to live in close proximity with people who had recently experienced trauma, which could lead to the relationships breaking down and Ukrainian families becoming homeless soon after arriving in the UK.

Early on we recognised that after our safeguarding duties, preventing sponsorship breakdowns, wherever possible, was our second key objective in delivering the scheme locally. Research indicated that building up community and peer support networks for refugees, as well as their sponsors, was one of the best preventative measures we could take to support as many sponsorships as possible to flourish. For example, a report from the Bartlett Development and Planning Unit, University College London (2018) suggests that social support from the host community is one of the key benefits of a community sponsorship policy when compared with other refugee resettlement models. This was something we were keen to replicate locally to ensure that refugees and their sponsors had access to a wider community support network. However, we were also mindful that, as council officers, we had a more formal role to play in delivering the scheme; including completing safeguarding checks on sponsors and inspecting accommodation. We were therefore not the right people to offer peer support and advice to sponsors and guests. In light of this, council officers looked to play a more facilitative role in developing a local plan of action and reached out to a number of local VCS organisations, including Community Action Sutton, Volunteer Centre Sutton, Citizens Advice Sutton, Sutton Salvation Army, Sutton Deanery Refugee Support Group, Sutton Community Works and Refugee and Migrant Network Sutton.

It was clear in our first planning meeting with key leads from the different VCS groups in Sutton that there was a strong will among everyone involved to support sponsors and their Ukrainian guests and provide them with a warm welcome to our borough, although the 'what, when and how' were still to be determined together. Fortunately, two local organisations had been involved in community sponsorship before, helping Syrian families resettle in Sutton, and it was hoped that through this experience they would be able to offer common-sense advice and guidance to local sponsors and guests.

One of the first actions we took was for the Council's VCS infrastructure partner, Community Action Sutton (see Case Study 12.3), to host a Zoom webinar for sponsors where they could ask questions of a variety of partners and hear from those who had been involved in community sponsorship about their experiences; sharing advice on things like sharing their communal space and supporting children to settle into school. This virtual event was well attended by sponsors and although not all the questions could be answered we used the feedback to create a local frequently asked questions document which was regularly updated, translated and shared with sponsors and guests. A number of similar webinars were held following this, and as more Ukrainian guests arrived in the UK these webinars were replaced with in-person advice and information sessions for sponsors and Ukrainians hosted at The Salvation Army in Sutton with representatives from a variety of organisations including the Council, the NHSSutton College, and key third sector organisations such as Citizens Advice Sutton and Refugee and Migrant Network Sutton. In addition to these events, a WhatsApp group was set up for sponsors where they could share information and advice, and Facebook and other social media platforms were also used by community groups to share information.

Measures to build and sustain community support networks

As more and more Ukrainian families began to arrive in Sutton, the Council continued to hold regular video calls with local VCS representatives to plan activity and identify solutions to problems together. Through this work, community support activity developed iteratively and in response to the needs of Ukrainians and their sponsors. For example, a weekly drop in was hosted at the local Salvation Army, in Sutton, which allowed Ukrainians and sponsors to speak to peers and develop connections and friendships. This helped to create a wider social support network for guests and hosts akin to that of the community sponsorship model. This served to reduce isolation and enable Ukrainians to access support beyond their immediate host family. In addition to this, Ukrainian guests were able to access community-based English language classes through Refugee and Migrant Network Sutton and a variety of support from Citizens Advice Sutton, for example, to apply for financial assistance or register their children for a local school.

It was humbling to see that in the initial response phase, most VCS organisations delivered support activities through the goodwill and generosity of volunteers, without seeking funding from the Council. A number of Ukrainian nationals who had moved to the UK some time before the Russian invasion of Ukraine became active volunteers and community organisers; giving up their time to help with translation and support new arrivals to adjust to life in the UK. A case study from one of these individuals, Natalya, is included in this chapter (see Case Study 12.2) and they played a pivotal role in establishing local community support networks in Sutton. However, as the numbers grew and funding was provided to the local authority from central government, we were mindful of the need to sustain this good work and scale up some of the projects over the medium term by providing funding to VCS groups. In order to deliver funding to VCS groups in a responsive way, we worked with our VCS infrastructure partner, Community Action Sutton, to set up a small grants programme (see Case Study 12.3) whereby groups could bid for funding for support activities and projects for Ukrainian refugees and their sponsors.

One project that was supported via this grants programme was a summer school for Ukrainian children in 2022 which arose out of connections made through the weekly drop-ins and feedback from Ukrainians who had been attending them. Not only did this project provide benefits to the children, helping them to make friends, retain native language skills and celebrate their identity through art and performance, it also provided opportunities for some of the mothers who had been teachers back in Ukraine to gain the necessary voluntary experience and safeguarding checks to help them apply for jobs in the UK. Due to the positive outcomes from this project, and in response to feedback from the Ukrainian community, additional funding was provided to sustain momentum and the summer school was scaled up into a weekly Saturday school supporting between 50 and 100 children, delivered by one of the larger VCS organisations in the borough, Volunteer Centre Sutton, and a local church. Other VCS projects that were granted included fitness classes, football coaching and mentoring sessions for young people.

Reflections on supporting Ukrainian families in Sutton

Sutton's experience with the Homes for Ukraine programme has illustrated the importance of actively identifying and engaging VCS partners at the outset of any programme to resettle displaced persons. We were fortunate to be able to draw upon the skills, knowledge and experiences of members of the community who had been involved in community sponsorship of refugees in the past, as well as professionals from the Council and partner agencies who had experience of working with migrants, including unaccompanied and asylum-seeking children. In addition to this, the early involvement of Ukrainian nationals already living in the borough, like Natalya (see Case Study 12.1), was vital in fostering a wider sense of community for Ukrainian families who arrived in Sutton and in scaling up activities and projects that were successful in light of feedback from the community. However, there were also lessons learned, for example, around the need to set clear expectations about access to housing, which is an acute issue for many councils, especially London Boroughs, where demand for social housing far exceeds the available stock, making waiting lists extremely long.

However, one cannot underestimate how hard it has been for those families who came to the UK from Ukraine, and we can only hope that through our efforts as a partnership they felt welcome and supported in the face of an uncertain future. Many Ukrainians we worked with spoke about the difficulty of living in a perpetual state of fear and uncertainty, feeling unable to make long-term plans about their families' future as the conflict rumbles on. A number of Ukrainians who came to Sutton as part of the

Homes for Ukraine scheme have returned home, others have resettled in other countries, and some have chosen to build a life for themselves and their children in the UK. Whatever path they have chosen, it has not been an easy decision and this best illustrated through the reflections of Yanina (with her young daughter; see Case Study 12.2), who arrived in Sutton in May 2022. This resulting in her putting her PhD research, at Odessa State University, on hold.

A more detailed insight into the link between the public sector (the London Borough of Sutton) and the voluntary sector (Volunteer Centre Sutton) is provided in Case Study 12.3.

Case Study 12.1: Natalya Semchyshyn: Ukrainian community organiser and volunteer based in Sutton

I came to London in 2010 with my boyfriend who is now my husband. We came because there was a financial crisis in Ukraine and I worked in a bank. Many banks were closing down so work was difficult. My best friend lived in London at that time and she suggested to me that I should come and work here because of the unstable financial situation in Ukraine. We thought that if we came to the UK we would be able to find work, save money and then return to Ukraine. My friend explained to me that even if my qualifications were not accepted in the UK, I would easily find work such as cleaning or being a housekeeper and there was lots of work for men in the building trade.

When we arrived, we rented a room in a house and my husband quickly found work in the construction industry. I obtained a job as a housekeeper. Our life continued like this for about six years and at the end of that time the financial situation in Ukraine had improved. We then had to make a decision about where we would live, because we were hoping to start our family. It was good to see that things were improving in Ukraine, but the attitudes and behaviours in the UK were better for us, so we made the decision to stay. I felt that here my children would have a better experience in school than that experienced by myself. I liked the fact that London was a multicultural city and found that people are welcoming to those who come from another country, not every country is so accepting. This was important to me.

I remember the morning that Russia invaded Ukraine, as my sister called me just as I was getting my children ready to go to school. I couldn't believe her and started to check the news on my phone. Like all Ukrainians at that time, I started to cry and panicked. I called my husband and my family, and we started to call everyone we knew in Ukraine, to check that they were alive. Many of my family left to go to different countries, especially Poland, because that is close to Ukraine, and they felt it would be easy to return home. People arranged to go and stay with friends and family, especially mothers and children, as men 18 years and older were not allowed to leave. They left with a few possessions, anything that they could carry. I thought that I could help family members because I had lived in the UK for so long. Our house is very small but many of our family members came and stayed with us until they could find somewhere else to live. We had only moved to Sutton a couple of weeks before the war began. It was the first house that we had been able to buy, and it was a difficult time for me because I did not have friends nearby and it was hard to find a school place for my eldest child. Once he was in school, I met a Chinese lady and when she realised that I was Ukrainian, she got me involved in a project to raise money for Ukrainian refugees, at the school. I realised then that even simple things can help, and decided to do whatever I could.

After moving to Sutton, I wanted to improve my English, but because I have a young child at home, I couldn't afford to pay for a course at college. I heard about ESOL (English for Speakers of Other Languages) lessons at a local church, provided by volunteers from the Refugee Migrant Network Sutton (RMNS) and through going there I made a link with the London Borough of Sutton, who were about to welcome Ukrainian refugees. I realised that I would be able to help Ukrainians when they arrived because I understand how to apply for school places and how to find work, and so on. I appreciated that everyone who arrived would be feeling very scared especially if they could not speak English. I created a Facebook page to connect with people and became involved with the drop-in information mornings at The Salvation Army in Sutton. As the people arrived from Ukraine they were signposted to the drop-in and I was able to act as a translator, to answer many of their questions or direct them to people who could help. I found working with volunteers to be inspiring and began to see that voluntary organisations are vital to support people in the local community.

As I met these newly arrived Ukrainians, I felt proud to see how Ukraine had changed for the younger generation. Many of them could speak some English, and their resilience inspired me. The worst thing imaginable had already happened, but you have to keep going. The women had found some inner strength that made them brave enough to make very difficult decisions. I began to realise how empowering it was to work together as volunteers. The development of organised volunteering has only been evolving in Ukraine in recent years. During the school holidays in 2022 I worked with other volunteers to provide a five-week project based at The Salvation Army, Sutton, where children came to classes in English, Ukrainian, art and music as well as having fun together. This project was funded by the London Borough of Sutton Ukraine Response Team, and was so successful that many of the parents asked if this could continue. This led me to establish a Saturday school at another local church hall, based at Christ Church. It became clear that a funding stream was needed to support this venture in order to provide resources and employ teachers. The project manager from the Ukrainian drop-in at Sutton

Salvation Army Church (GB see Chapter 6) and the Churchwarden (CI) of Christ Church, supported a bidding process which resulted in funding being released to the Volunteer Centre Sutton with myself being employed as the Ukrainian Project Coordinator. (15 October 2023)

Case Study 12.2: Yanina Pushkar: PhD student displaced from Ukraine

The night of 24 February changed the life of my family, the life of the whole country and not only. Before the Russian invasion, I lived in the south of Ukraine in the port and historical city of Odesa. I had a happy life, a loving family, doing what I loved and planning a happy future.

I finished my master's degree at Odesa State Agrarian University and decided to study further and get a PhD. After submitting documents to Odesa State Agrarian University, I successfully passed the exams and was enrolled in the Faculty of Veterinary Medicine and Biotechnology, Department of Genetics, Breeding and Feeding of Agricultural Animals, Specialty: 204 'Technology of production and processing of livestock products'. I participated in various conferences and published articles. Everything went according to the planned schedule. But unfortunately, because of the war, I had to leave everything I had worked on in recent years.

No one wanted to believe that a neighbouring state attacked us, but the reality was that we gathered what was necessary and left for Bulgaria. We hoped that we would soon be able to return home, but events in the country told us otherwise. Two months have passed since we left our native home, and we have not seen the end of this terrible war, so after consulting, we decided to fly to the UK. And already on 3 May 2022, we flew to our relatives. I didn't even know where to start and how to live on. All around me is a different country, the language of which I hardly know and the people of which I do not understand. It is very difficult, having everything in one moment, to be left with nothing. You feel despair and loneliness.

Thanks to the London Borough of Sutton and Sutton Salvation Army church, we managed to unite and create a good community. Thanks to this support, I was able to find the strength and determination to live on. At regular drop in meetings at TSA I met the representative Council Mayor, who helped find a school for my daughter. This was the first stage of the beginning of a new life.

My daughter Sofia really liked school, but she didn't know the language at all and missed her home and friends very much. At first it was very difficult for her, she longed for communication with her peers, but they did not understand her, just as she did not understand them. It was a very stressful time. But the school and teachers did everything to make her feel comfortable. Now she is a confident and happy child and has many new friends. Now I study ESOL courses at Sutton College. The next stage in our adaptation and socialisation was the search for housing and work.

Finding housing was not so easy. We had no job, no money for a deposit and no credit history in this country. The council helped with the deposit and the first month's payment for housing. And finally we rented our own house. Without knowing the language, it is difficult to find a good job, but this is not the last problem. Everywhere I am asked about my work experience in the UK. In Ukraine, I have enough experience and skills. I have a good educational base, work experience and in the near future I was supposed to become a teacher at the Odessa State Agrarian University. And here I need to start everything from a clean sheet.

After some time, I found a job in a household store as a basic store assistant. This is a small victory for me. After all, I was able to overcome everything that was impossible at first glance. So life goes on.

Unfortunately, the situation in my country is still not easy, our enemy hopes to seize the country in his cruel hands. The south of Ukraine, including my native city of Odesa, is a delicacy for Russia. Almost every two weeks, there are massive attacks by cruise missiles on the country's energy facilities. As a result, Ukraine lacks capacity to supply electricity to the population, which is why emergency power cuts are carried out. In some regions, there is light for only a few hours a day. Because of this, the entire industry and animal husbandry as a whole suffers greatly. Herds are reduced, factories are closed, as they cannot work at full capacity due to power outages. Against this background, scientific activity also suffers. We cannot create research groups on farms.

I don't know how long this war will last and what will happen next. Will we return to Ukraine? I really want it, but unfortunately I don't see it in the future yet. I am a mother and I must think about the safety and future of my child. I will do everything so that she remembers who she is and where she comes from. And one day she will again see an independent and free Ukraine, which will be even better than before. What do I plan to do next? I plan to live and work for the future of my family. This is all I have left from my past life. For this I need to study a lot and maybe in time I will find my place in this new world. Of course, I would very much like to continue my scientific activity. I hope that later I will be able to continue my work and further develop in this direction.

2 October 2023

Unfortunately, the situation in our country is not getting better, and dreams of ending the war are becoming less and less realistic.

Despite all the difficulties and homesickness, we still became more confident in ourselves and in setting our goals. So, we decided not to wait for the end of the war, but to continue building our lives in the UK. Of course, one of the factors that influenced my decision was my visit to Ukraine. This spring I visited my hometown of Odesa for just one week and realised that nothing would be the same, that people had become completely different … no, they are not bad – they are devastated, accustomed to living one day at a time and this is the worst thing! They cannot dream, plan and build the future. Their eyes are empty, there is only pain and fear in them.

When I was in Ukraine, I was amazed at how children of different ages talked about the war. It's terrible that this has become the norm for them, this is the first thing they talk about … not about a new cartoon, nor about walks with friends and plans for the future. The word WAR became the first word for many children. My seven-year-old niece knows more about safety measures in the event of a rocket attack or atomic bomb explosion than I do at 35.

I understand that now most of all I need to invest in my education and further development. To do this, I still continue my studies at college and do additional work with volunteers, improving and replenishing my vocabulary.

This really helps. If we compare the time when I first arrived and now, I can say with confidence that progress has been great. I can contact the GP if necessary and this does not horrify me from not understanding, and I can also find out the information I need at school regarding my daughter's education. I independently made her an appointment with the dentist and visited him safely. Perhaps for some this is a small thing, but for people like me this is a huge achievement. All this would not be possible if it were not for the enormous support that I receive from the people around me (Sutton TSA) and the state (Sutton College and Council).

Regarding my work, I also feel my growth within the company and the support of my colleagues.

Of course, not everything is as wonderful as we would like; no one can cancel the difficulties. For example, we thought even more about what would happen after the expiration of our visa, because this is a huge factor influencing our entire life and action planning. This also affects my daughter's life, because she began growing up here.

Sofia has adapted very well to life in this country. She went to school here for the first time, made friends, and conscious goals, dreams and interests appeared. She attends a ballet class and plans to take up gymnastics. She no longer knows any other life except this one. And now it would be very difficult for her to return to Ukraine and go to school there, because everything there is different and not familiar to her. I can't say that education in Ukraine is better or worse, it's just different … different approach, different society and views. She cannot understand children who live every day in a state of fear and stress, and they cannot understand her.

Case Study 12.3: Supporting Ukrainian refugees in the community: the role of volunteers
Nick Baum

In this section, we delve into the critical role played by the Volunteer Centre Sutton in promoting the successful integration of Ukrainian refugees within the Sutton community, as reviewed in this chapter. As we explore this multifaceted process, we will emphasise various aspects that were instrumental in the overall success of the integration efforts. These components include securing adequate funding, the range of services offered, and the comprehensive, holistic approach adopted by the Volunteer Centre Sutton.

The influx of Ukrainian refugees into the Sutton community brought with it an array of challenges and opportunities. Navigating these complexities required a concerted effort from various stakeholders. Our examination will unveil the strategic allocation of financial resources that enabled Volunteer Centre Sutton to provide essential services, empowering refugees to rebuild their lives and contribute to their newfound home.

Furthermore, we will investigate the diverse set of services that were offered, spanning from language and vocational training to mental health support and cultural orientation. These services were tailored to address the unique needs of Ukrainian refugees, thereby building a sense of belonging and self-sufficiency (see vcsutton.org.uk/ukraine/).

A central theme running through this chapter is the holistic approach employed by Volunteer Centre Sutton. By considering not only the immediate needs of the refugees but also the long-term aspects of their integration, the centre played a pivotal role in creating a supportive and inclusive environment for the Ukrainian community in Sutton. Our exploration will shed light on the strategies employed, the challenges faced, and the invaluable lessons learned in this journey of integration.

Holistic support and cultural preservation

This section sheds light on the comprehensive support offered by Volunteer Centre Sutton, demonstrating how these services were instrumental in integrating Ukrainian refugees in Sutton while concurrently preserving their rich culture and heritage. By creating layers of support that addressed diverse needs across all age groups, from individuals to groups, the integration process became not only a bridge to a new life but also a means of maintaining the vibrant Ukrainian culture within the Sutton community.

A diverse array of services

The success of Volunteer Centre Sutton's integration efforts can be attributed to the broad spectrum of services they provided. These services were tailored to cater to the varied and evolving needs of Ukrainian refugees. From language and vocational training to mental health support and cultural orientation, a diverse array of services contributed to the holistic support of the community.

- *Language and vocational training*: Recognising the importance of language proficiency and employability, the centre offered language classes tailored to different age groups and proficiency levels. Simultaneously, vocational training programmes equipped refugees with the skills needed for employment, thereby enhancing their self-sufficiency.
- *Mental health support*: Many Ukrainian refugees arrived with the emotional and psychological scars of their past experiences. Volunteer Centre Sutton collaborated with mental health professionals to provide counselling and support services, aiding refugees in coping with the challenges they faced.
- *Cultural orientation*: To facilitate cultural adjustment, the centre organised cultural orientation programmes. These initiatives introduced refugees to British customs, values and social norms while also celebrating and preserving Ukrainian culture. This approach was instrumental in helping refugees find a balance between their heritage and their new home.

Preservation of Ukrainian culture

The integration efforts in Sutton played a vital role in keeping Ukrainian culture alive and flourishing within the community. Cultural preservation was achieved through various means:

- *Cultural events*: Volunteer Centre Sutton organised and promoted cultural events and celebrations that allowed refugees to share their traditions and customs with the wider community. These events not only preserved Ukrainian culture but also promoted cultural exchange, fostering understanding and acceptance.
- *Language and heritage programmes*: The centre established language and heritage programmes that ensured that Ukrainian language and traditions were passed down to the younger generations. These programmes aimed to help children maintain a strong connection to their Ukrainian roots.

Developing social ties and community-building

The services provided by Volunteer Centre Sutton extended beyond basic needs, promoting social ties and community-building among the Ukrainian community members themselves. Volunteer Centre Sutton encouraged friendship and collaboration among refugees through:

- *Community groups*: Volunteer Centre Sutton supported the formation of various community groups, creating spaces for refugees to come together, share experiences and provide mutual support. These groups served as a source of solidarity and camaraderie.
- *Cultural exchanges*: The centre facilitated cultural exchange programmes, allowing Ukrainian refugees to learn from each other's experiences and share their unique cultural aspects. This exchange enriched the community's social fabric.

In conclusion, this section underscores the critical role that holistic support played in the integration of Ukrainian refugees in Sutton. The well-rounded services not only met immediate needs but also upheld the Ukrainian culture and fostered strong social connections among refugees. Through these efforts, Volunteer Centre Sutton ensured that the Ukrainian community in Sutton thrived and continued to contribute to the diverse tapestry of the region while maintaining their cultural identity.

Diversity of support services provided

This section highlights the extensive range of services offered by Volunteer Centre Sutton to address the multifaceted aspects of integration and support for Ukrainian refugees. These services can be categorised into three primary categories, each of which played a pivotal role in ensuring the successful integration and wellbeing of the refugee community.

Cultural services

One of the key components of the services offered by Volunteer Centre Sutton was the preservation and celebration of Ukrainian culture. Volunteer Centre Sutton recognised the importance of maintaining cultural ties while adapting to an unfamiliar environment. Several services fell under this category:

- *Saturday morning school*: This programme catered to 50–60 children from the Ukrainian community, offering a unique opportunity to engage with their cultural heritage. The Saturday morning school provided a space for young Ukrainians to learn the Ukrainian language, customs, traditions and history. Through a rich curriculum, children could maintain a strong connection to their roots, ensuring that the Ukrainian culture continued to thrive within the Sutton community.
- *Mentoring programme*: Recognising the need for a sense of belonging and guidance, Volunteer Centre Sutton introduced a mentoring programme. Young Ukrainian refugees were paired with local adult mentors who not only offered support and advice but also developed a deep sense of belonging. This programme aimed to help the young refugees adapt to their new environment, build meaningful relationships and navigate the challenges of integration (vcsutton. org.uk/ukraine/).

Wellbeing services

The wellbeing of Ukrainian refugees was of paramount importance to Volunteer Centre Sutton. To address the physical and mental health needs of the community, a range of services were offered:

- *Arts activities for children*: Volunteer Centre Sutton organised creative activities for children, nurturing their talents and promoting cultural awareness. These activities allowed young refugees to express themselves, build their self-esteem and maintain a strong connection to their culture. By participating in arts and crafts, music and dance, children were able to embrace their Ukrainian identity and develop new skills.
- *Wellbeing activities*: To promote physical and mental health, Volunteer Centre Sutton organised activities for adults, including walking and yoga sessions. These sessions not only improved physical wellbeing but also provided opportunities for social interaction and support. In building a sense of community and connection, these activities contributed to the overall wellbeing of the Ukrainian refugee population.
- *Counselling services*: Volunteer Centre Sutton recognised that many Ukrainian refugees had experienced trauma and mental health challenges. To address these unique needs, the centre offered counselling services. These services provided vital support, enabling refugees to cope with past experiences and build resilience. The provision of specialised mental health services played a significant role in helping individuals on their journey to healing and integration.

In summary, Volunteer Centre Sutton's diverse range of services catered to the cultural, wellbeing, and psychological needs of Ukrainian refugees. These services were instrumental in ensuring that the Ukrainian community in Sutton not only adapted to their new environment but also continued to celebrate their rich cultural heritage and maintained their wellbeing, fostering a sense of belonging and resilience within the community (vcsutton.org.uk/ukraine/).

Conclusion to Case Studies 12.1–12.3

The project outlined in this chapter focuses on the successful integration of Ukrainian refugees in Sutton through the efforts of Volunteer Centre Sutton and support from Sutton Council. It comprises a multifaceted approach, including a unique funding model that streamlined resource allocation, a wide array of services catering to cultural preservation, wellbeing and mental health, and a holistic approach that empowers refugees for long-term self-sufficiency. This project not only ensured the integration of refugees into the Sutton community, promoted by a

Ukrainian working with the Voluntary Centre (see Case Study 12.1), but also maintained their cultural identity and wellbeing, fostering a sense of belonging and resilience, ultimately serving as a model for effective community-based refugee support. Displaced people from Ukraine with professional and academic links (see Case Study 12.2), provide added value by maintaining active links with Ukraine.

Conclusion to Chapter 12

Insights from a London borough in this chapter demonstrate that, despite the financial difficulties faced by local and national government in the second decade of austerity (see Chapter 1), working in partnership with voluntary groups and communities provided relational added value in addressing human need. *Relational dividends* emerge from the *functional roles* and *relationships of the partners*, the *financial arrangements* promoted within the concept of *relationalism* (see Simmons, 2023, and in Chapter 20 of this volume). Understanding the *structural* and *intermediate* determinants of health will be considered in more detail in Chapter 19 and in the Conclusion from the perspective of the *Conceptual Framework for Action on the Social Determinants of Health* (see Figure I.1, Introduction, this volume).

Fundamental *structural* determinants, such as housing policy at an EU and national level, need to be addressed, as critically reviewed by Barrington (a former EU Commissioner), from an EU perspective, in the next chapter.

References

Ambitious for Sutton. London Borough of Sutton. Available at: https://www.sutton.gov.uk/ambitiousforsutton

The Bartlett Development and Planning Unit, UCL (2018) A comparison of community sponsorship and government led resettlement of refugees in the UK: perspectives from newcomers and host communities. Available at: https://www.ucl.ac.uk/bartlett/development/research-projects/2023/feb/role-communities-refugee-resettlement-comparing-resettlement-schemes-uk

Crane Linn, E. (2022) Examining the impact of community sponsorship on early refugee labor market outcomes in the United States. *Journal on Migration and Human Security*, 10(2): 113–133.

Homes for Ukraine: Council Guides, Department for Levelling Up, Housing and Communities. Available at https://www.gov.uk/government/collections/homes-for-ukraine-council-guides

Hong Kong British Nationals (Overseas) Welcome Programme – Information for Local Authorities, Department for Levelling Up, Housing and Communities. Available at: https://www.gov.uk/guidance/hong-kong-uk-welcome-programme-guidance-for-local-authorities

Open letter to Secretary of State for Levelling Up, Housing & Communities, 26 March 2022. Available at: https://www.refugee-action.org.uk/wp-content/uploads/2022/03/Letter-To-The-Rt-Hon-Mr-Michael-Gove-MP-Homes-For-Ukraine.pdf

The Sutton Plan. Available at: https://www.suttonplan.com/

Sutton's Strategic Needs Assessment (2023) *Borough Profile*. Available at: https://data.sutton.gov.uk/strategic-needs-assessment/

13

Health, housing and the international financial framework

Anne Barrington

Introduction

'Home is about emotional roots: culture, food, implicit values, the warmth of familiarity. You belong there. It has its rituals that mark the passage of time and give it meaning' (Ressa, 2022: 35). The 2021 Nobel Peace Prize winner Maria Ressa is here talking about her country of birth, but the sentiment could be transported easily to the unique space that we call our home.

Why are so many people locked out of the possibility of ever having a home to call their own, of having that sense of belonging, across Europe? Why are younger people finding it more and more difficult to leave their parents' home and set up an independent life in decent affordable housing? Why is it that many people are paying exorbitant rents if they are lucky enough to eventually find a place to live? Why is it that when there is growing evidence that 'insecurity of tenure (e.g. private market rental accommodation) and anxieties around rent and mortgage payments have … been shown to negatively impact mental and physical health' (ESRI, 2023: 2) there appears to be so little political will to tackle the issue?

Those who have a vested interest in the housing sector will give responses to these questions dependent on their perspectives. For some it is the price of land, especially in cities. For others it is the cost of building materials and labour and the inflation in costs that is the culprit. Yet others blame the slowness of the planning system in delivery. Some blame the lack of supply during the economic recession from 2010. And the fact that the government, over a prolonged period of time, sold off its public housing stock. No doubt all these factors play a part. But very few look outside the national framework at the wider financial system for answers. But it is in the wider international financial framework that we should start to find reasons why decent housing has become unobtainable for so many in the developed world.

The dominant philosophy

But first a little history that is relevant. When UK Prime Minister Margaret Thatcher and US President Ronald Reagan began their efforts to deregulate, or more accurately 'reregulate' (Raworth, 2022: 82) and privatise, few realised how successful they would become in changing mindsets. As Oreskes and Conway (2023) show, this neoliberal mindset and philosophy was a long time in fermentation. Initially conceived by big business in the wake of the Great Depression as a counterweight to Keynesian economics and as an attempt to undermine the New Deal, the neoliberal agenda at first faltered. However, over time and with the rise of anti-communism in the United States neoliberalism succeeded in equating government with everything bad and the markets with freedom. It got to the point where an attack on the market, in the form of regulation, became equated with an attack on freedom itself. Neoliberalism and blind trust in markets received a further boost with the collapse of the Soviet Union in 1989. Francis Fukuyama (1992) could proclaim the end of history in so far as liberal democracy and the free market had, it appeared, won the Cold War.

It was from around that time that post-Second World War constraints on capitalism to prove that it was a kinder system were removed. The economic philosophy of Milton Friedman and the Chicago School of economics became the dominant force driving the decisions of central banks and ministries of finance across the developed democratic world. In its crudest form, neoliberalism means that the state's role should be reduced to providing security and protecting property rights (Oreskes and Conway, 2023). Redistribution and equality policies were sidelined. Growth for its own sake became the be all and end all of economics and touted as a solution for all social ills. Structural adjustment programmes for indebted countries in the developing world became the norm. Growth was prioritised at the expense of health and education systems, environmental protection and labour laws. Taxes for the rich were reduced (Hickel, 2020: 172).

Then the banking crisis happened or, rather, was caused by the egregious failures of financial markets and the 'invisible hand' of the regulators. It became apparent that nobody, including the regulators, quite understood what the banking sector was up to. Blind faith in the market to rectify itself was found to be wanting. The prevailing neoliberal philosophy informing international and national institutions continued, however, and imposed austerity measures which, in many countries in the developed world, shifted public goods (such as education, health and housing services) from public into private ownership.

At the same time central banks began a process of quantitative easing or printing money to shore up the financial system. This coincided with a period of unprecedented low interest rates. So, there was a lot of money in capital markets and this money was looking for a return. With low interest rates prevailing, however, one of the few areas which was actually giving a significant return to investors was housing.

This is what happened in Dublin and in some other cities around Europe: governments had no money to invest in social and affordable housing and had, in any event, privatised much of their public housing stock. So, when international investment funds came offering to invest in housing they were welcomed in and given significant tax incentives to do the job.

These funds invested mostly in build-to-rent apartments in cities. Then, the investment funds leased some of the apartments to the state, in the form of local authorities, at 'market' rates with no option to buy at the end of the lease period of 20 to 30 years. The others they rented directly to tenants at 'market' rates. These rates were and remain for many not receiving state subsidies far more than the recommended 30 per cent of net pay that should be spent on all aspects of housing, including rent, energy and maintenance, making them unaffordable. That is not to say that international investment funds don't have a role to play in the housing market. They do. But their role should not be dominant, especially in the social and affordable housing sectors, and the state should work to shape the market to the needs of the citizens it serves (UNECE and Housing Europe, 2021).

Where is the European Union?

The European Committee of the Regions (ECR, 2017) was the first European Union (EU) body to tackle the housing issue. It issued an Opinion in December 2017, some ten years after the sub-prime market failure. The ECR pointed to the direct link between housing costs and the ability of individuals and families to invest in private consumption and spend on education, health and retirement, all of which are factors for economic and social wellbeing. They pointed out that the implementation of many EU objectives such as economic stability, tackling climate change and social inclusion and the implementation of many EU policies such as regional policy, the Urban Agenda, competition, energy and social policy affects housing policy on many levels and depends on them. The Committee called for greater coordination in these areas. And it called for investment in housing to be seen as a long-term investment that should be recognised under the regulatory framework and rules of the European System of Accounts 2010. The Committee also called for thought to be given to introducing conditions that facilitate non-volatile, non-speculative investment channelled to the private-sector investors (for example, insurance companies) which have similar long-term interests. Finally, the Committee emphasised the importance of a European Agenda for Housing that combined a cross-cutting approach to EU policies that are directly and indirectly linked to housing with a territorial approach that compares local policies for promoting and financing the provisions of affordable housing (ECR, 2017).

This wasn't very much but at least it was a start and it identified some of the structural issues confounding efforts to deliver affordable housing in Europe.

Then in 2021 the European Parliament adopted a report on the housing crisis in Europe. The report, titled *Access to Decent and Affordable Housing for All*, looks at the many EU aspects that have contributed to the housing crisis in member states. It was drafted by Dutch Green MEP Kim Van Sparrentak. Drawing on the Charter of Fundamental Rights, the UN Universal Declaration of Human Rights, the Sustainable Development Goals as well as the European Union's foundation treaties, the report addressed the multifaceted nature of housing and what needed to be done to address the issues.

For example, operative paragraph 31

> calls on the Commission and the Member States to ensure that no EU or Member State funds will be used for housing projects leading to segregation or social exclusion; calls on the Member States to always consider the quality of housing in terms of urban development, architecture and functionality so as to improve well-being for all; calls on the Commission and the Member States to promote programmes and incentives that foster and strengthen intergenerational ties enabling people, in particular older people, who have to leave their homes for financial or health reasons to find new accommodation that meets their needs without having to leave their communities.

The European Parliament also called on the European Commission and the member states to make sure that the right to adequate housing was recognised and enforceable as a fundamental human right through European and national legislative provisions; it joined up thinking on how housing underpins access to energy and sanitation and supports vulnerable groups and disadvantaged households to protect their health and wellbeing. It focused on the European Green Deal for a socially just transition to a climate-neutral economy. It called on the European Commission to prioritise the Renovation Wave in the multiannual financial framework and Next Generation EU. It called also for greater coherence across the EU in tackling homelessness, including among vulnerable group such as women, children, Roma and people with disabilities.

Significantly, and for the first time for an EU institution, the European Parliament report focused on ensuring security of tenure and inclusive housing markets. The report noted 'with concern the increased financialisation of the housing market ... whereby investors treat housing as a tradable asset rather than a human right'. It called on the Commission to assess the contribution of EU policies and regulation to the financialisation of the housing market and the ability of national and local authorities to ensure the right to housing. And it called on the member states and local authorities to put in place measures to counter speculative investment, to adopt policies favouring long-term investments in the housing market and to develop urban and rural planning policies that favour affordable housing, social mix and social cohesion.

The report stressed that transparency on real estate ownership was vital to preventing distortions in the housing market and to preventing money laundering. It pointed out that the expansive growth of short-term holiday rentals was removing housing from the market and driving up prices.

This European Parliament report has contributed to changing the narrative of the housing crisis at European level from housing as an asset to housing as a fundamental requirement essential to building healthy families and sustainable communities. It is an effort to introduce European values into the dialogue on housing that has been dominated for far too long by financial markets, property interests and transactional relationships. The report is also an effort to show the inextricable link between the macroeconomic framework in which the housing market works and the effects this market has on the lives of real people in Dublin, Berlin, Helsinki and Paris.

The report was adopted by the European Parliament in 2021 commanding the positive votes of all 13 Irish MEPs. It could be argued that now that we in Ireland have a national agenda for housing in *Housing for All* (Department of Housing, 2021) we have also, to a degree, a Europe-wide agenda in the European Parliament's report. And this Europe-wide agenda has cross-party support already in Ireland and across Europe. The European Parliament needs to follow up on this report and put pressure on EU institutions and on the member states to deliver.

European Union housing ministers meet

It is telling that, despite there being a housing crisis in the EU for over a decade, European ministers for housing held their first meeting in nine years in March 2022. Indeed, a resumption of meetings of ministers for housing was one of the many issues that the European Parliament report had called for (European Parliament, 2021). The aim of this informal meeting was to discuss the provision of 'affordable, sustainable, decent and resilient housing that ensures the [sic] quality of life' (Nice Declaration, 2022).

The ministers' Declaration called for 'better coordination of [housing] policies' and for 'homes of good quality which are well constructed ... situated in mixed-use, compact and dense areas with high-quality living environment and which are close to working areas'. The Declaration also called for 'increasing the affordability of housing', 'reuse of abandoned and unused buildings', increased 'industrialisation and standardisation', increased 'education and training at all levels of the construction and renovation value chains'. The ministers touched on the 'challenges and opportunities' in the use of platforms for the tourist sector and agreed to hold regular meetings of ministers responsible for housing. The ministers 'invited the European Commission to support their efforts to promote the development of participatory and inclusive housing solutions based on sustainable strategies for the use of urban space' and specifically referred to community land trusts as a useful tool for some member states. They asked the Commission 'to carry out a comparative study on the different mechanisms in place in the EU to curb the increase in rents and sale prices of housing'. Finally, the ministers asked the Commission 'to facilitate access to information on European funding dedicated to the housing and construction sector' and they asked the European Investment Bank Group to continue and develop further its financing and advisory services.

While it is encouraging that ministers for housing got together after nearly a decade and agreed anything, what is striking about the declaration is its timidity. The mantra that housing and construction policy is an exclusive member state competence is repeated, which nobody disputes. But there is no attempt to put housing in a wider framework. There is no mention of the role of the financial sector, other than the European Investment Bank Group, and the concept of financialisation of housing and the role of international institutional investors is avoided. The policies of the central banks, of economic and finance ministers (ECOFIN) or the regulatory role of the Commission are avoided too, as are any other parts of the structural framework within which housing policy is formulated and delivery is set. Policies in finance, environment, energy and industry all have an impact on housing and construction policy. And while the environment and energy each got a mention, there is precious little evidence of any real joined-up thinking. Instead there is timidity and fragmentation.

While the approach remained timid at the next EU ministers for housing meeting in November 2023, and there was no recognition of the financialisation of the housing market, there was a small development. On this occasion ministers invited 'the European Commission to assess the definition of social housing that can be considered a service of general economic interest in order to facilitate the application of state aid in housing policies'. Here, for the first time, was an explicit acknowledgement by EU ministers that the prevailing policy of the European Commission was having a negative impact on the provision of housing – to be discussed later. Also ministers for the first time expressed 'the will and the desire to be ambitious in the response to homelessness' (Gijon Declaration, 2023). Though what these ambitions were was not spelled out.

What needs to be done

First, we have to identify the problem. If we accept that the European Central Bank (ECB)'s policy of monetary easing helped fuel international investment in housing markets in the EU and has played a role in the unaffordability crisis we now experience then we must tackle that issue. Central banks will say that it is not their role to achieve stability in housing markets but only in financial markets. Fair enough, in so far as it goes. But when financial markets, through ECB policies, have been fuelling a housing crisis then it is incumbent on central banks to at least disincentivise financial markets from investing in speculative enterprises at the expense of ordinary citizens. At the same time central banks should incentivise financial markets to invest in the productive economy instead. Now, as interest rates are rising and international money markets seek out higher yielding returns there is an opportunity for central banks and other European and national institutions to shape the market to the needs of its citizens.

Second, we saw what happened during the COVID-19 pandemic. The member states of the EU tore up the rule book and fiscal rules were suspended when the public interest and public good required it. ECOFIN ministers are currently redrafting the rules of the Stability and Growth Pact. The outcome of that process must be that state provision of funding for housing must be on the balance sheet, allowing the state to get back into the core business of supporting the building of social and affordable homes. ECOFIN is also working on the future of banking union and capital markets union. These frameworks too will have an impact on how the EU will deal with finance for housing.

Each member state is part of the EU's single market. The single market has rules which must be interpreted and adhered to. Some housing interests have argued that EU state aid rules prohibit the state from getting involved in affordable housing. There is an opportunity here for the Commission, as called for by EU housing ministers in November 2023 to address the definition of social housing that can be considered a service of general economic interest (SGEI) in order to facilitate the application of state aid rules in housing policy. Or the European Commission should make it perfectly clear that housing is and remains a sector of general economic interest and as such state aid rules do not apply. There must be no real or perceived impediment to the state providing social and affordable housing when needed as in the crisis we are experiencing. We should go back to any market imperatives. The EU must ensure that it is not used as the excuse to justify rules that can be changed over fundamental principles established in treaty law and covenants.

The European Commission also has an additional role to play in shaping the housing market in the EU, a key determinant of health. It should set the provision of social and affordable housing as an essential policy goal. Within the European Semester the Commission has already highlighted the importance of affordable housing. In addition, as the European Parliament has pointed out, as a SGEI, housing is exempt from state aid notification requirements. However, social housing is the only sector in the SGEI Decision for which the European Commission mentions a target group. This Decision restricts 'housing for disadvantaged citizens or socially less advantaged groups, which due to solvability constraints are unable to obtain housing at market conditions'. There is no such definition for other social services. Such a definition for housing is restrictive and has been used within member states and more broadly to prevent public authorities from providing social and affordable housing when it is clearly needed.

The provision of housing should be principally decided by national, regional or local authorities. The Commission should adapt the target group definition of social and publicly funded housing in the rules of SGEI to allow national and regional local authorities to support housing for all groups whose needs for decent and affordable housing cannot easily be met under market conditions. In addition to articulating a clear position that state aid rules do not apply to the delivery of social and affordable housing the Commission should highlight the overlapping and connected policy areas within its competence and focus on how these affect the delivery of decent and affordable housing.

How the international financial framework has played out in Ireland

Ireland, like many countries in Europe, has suffered a severe housing shortage since the financial crash of 2008. As an indication of this, between 2015 and 2019 Ireland within 15 European countries analysed saw the largest rise in the share of young adults aged 25–34 remaining in their family home (Disch and Slaymaker, 2023: 69). House prices and rents have spiralled – and, for a large sector not receiving state support – these rents are out of proportion to increased pay and salaries. Ireland also has one of the biggest gaps in homeownership rates between younger and older generations (Disch and Slaymaker, 2023: 54). And, 'homeownership has been shown to increase individuals' sense of security and self-esteem, reduce stress and anxiety and improve mental and psychological wellbeing'

(ERSI, 2023: 2). In addition, homelessness has doubled since 2021 and reached over 13,500 people in 2024, over 4,000 of whom are children (Department of Housing, Local Government and Heritage, 2024). Housing supply and the current housing stock is insufficient to meet needs (Russell et al, 2021).

The government, in its *Housing for All* policy document of 2021, estimated that 33,000 units of housing would be required annually to the year 2030. However, this estimate did not take into account the increasing population of the country due to net immigration, to an extent influenced by Brexit. Also, the estimate could not take into account the reception of over 90,000 Ukrainians fleeing the war initiated by Russia's invasion of that country in February 2022, of which number, approximately 70,000 have been housed with state support.

A number of commentators have estimated that the actual number of housing units that will be required up to 2030 and beyond is double the government's estimate. Indeed, the government's own appointed Housing Commission, which reported in May 2024, has estimated that Ireland has a current deficit of 235,000 homes. The Commission has estimated also that average annual housing requirements 2024–2050 will range from 42,800 to 60,800 based on an average household size of 2.2 persons(*The Irish Times*, 2023).

In accordance with Council Decision (EU) 2022/382 of 4 March 2022, and despite the ongoing housing crisis, Ireland has made good progress in ensuring adequate protection for those Ukrainians fleeing Russian aggression – including in the housing area. This Council Decision activated for the first time Council Directive 2001/55/EC of 20 July 2001, which waives the need to examine individual application for asylum and enables Ukrainians to enjoy harmonised rights across the EU. Once admitted Ukrainians can move freely within the EU.

It is the Department of Children, Equality, Disability, Integration and Youth and not the Department of Housing, Local Government and Heritage that takes the lead on housing refugees in Ireland. Which begs the question: how can one arm of government manage the accommodation of 70,000 people in under 24 months while another arm of government is unable to manage the 13,500 and growing homeless people and provide them with adequate accommodation in a crisis that has lasted nearly 20 years? Is it because of the prevailing neoliberal ideology where the market rules dominate domestic discourse to an even greater extent than in the EU?

This chapter has been critical of the EU in its lack of action to take the lead in areas of its competence to address the housing crisis in member states. However, when it was confronted by the COVID-19 pandemic and the Ukrainian refugee emergency, the EU was quick to react, avoided getting trapped in ideological straitjackets and did the right thing in providing the necessary help to populations at risk of the pandemic and refuge and accommodation for many millions of Ukrainians. Ireland too played its part. Perhaps it is now time for the member states to take the lead in their own jurisdictions, overcome the outdated legacy of neoliberal market ideology and deliver sustainable housing in mixed communities that is of a decent standard, adheres to human rights obligations and is fundamental to the health and wellbeing of our societies. As the EU has shown, where there is political will there is a way. To solve our housing crisis we need political will both at international and national level now.

Conclusion

This chapter examined the influence of macroeconomic policies that shape the housing market in member states of the European Union and especially as they relate to Ireland, which has had a housing crisis since the financial crisis of 2008. The influence of neoliberal ideology on policy formulation within the EU and its institutions, the ECB, the European Parliament, the European Commission, the Council of Ministers as well as the member states is examined and found to be inadequate in tackling the issue. The solution proposed is for the member states and the European institutions to be more hands-on in shaping the framework within which housing is delivered – much the way that the EU and the member states reacted to the COVID-19 pandemic and the Ukrainian refugee crises.

Case Study 13.1: Republic of Ireland response to the Ukraine crisis
Agnieszka Cieciura-Miszczak

This case study provides an insight into the response of the Republic of Ireland, a member of the EU, to very significant challenges to its long-term housing crisis highlighted by the need to support people displaced from Ukraine. Ireland has one of the biggest gaps in homeownership rates between younger and older generations, however the hospitality of host families has provided 17,466 Ukrainian refugees with accommodation with support from the Accommodation Recognition Payment scheme. This is a significant contribution to ensuring adequate protection for those Ukrainians fleeing Russian aggression.

The Republic of Ireland remains a member of the European Union, unlike its neighbours in Northern Ireland, England, Wales and Scotland. In the EU Ireland has one of the biggest gaps in homeownership rates between younger and older generations and homelessness has doubled since 2021 and reached over 12,500 people in 2023, over 4,000 of whom are children (Department of Housing, 2021). Housing supply and the current housing stock is insufficient to meet needs and has not benefited from the late and underdeveloped EU Housing framework, reviewed in the next chapter (Chapter 14). Despite the long-term housing crisis faced by Ireland, over 90,000 Ukrainians fleeing the war initiated by Russia's invasion of that country in February 2022 have been received into the country. Approximately 70,000 have been housed with state support.

Between the years of 2018 and 2021 the Republic of Ireland observed a steady influx of persons granted refugee-like humanitarian status, and people provided temporary protection. Comparison data for the Republic of Ireland in terms of refugee statistics shows the following trends:

- Total presentations in 2022 was 81,256, a 748.98 per cent increase from 2021.
- Total presentations in 2021 was 9,571, a 5.93 per cent increase from 2020.
- Total presentations in 2020 was 9,035, a 15.91 per cent increase from 2019.
- Total presentations in 2019 was 7,795, a 29.66 per cent increase from 2018.

The Temporary Protection Directive (2001/55 EC) was activated on 4 March 2022 by EU Council Decision EU 2022/382, to provide immediate protection in EU countries for people displaced by the Russian invasion of Ukraine that began on 24 February 2022. As part of the EU, the Republic of Ireland made a commitment to provide Ukraine with humanitarian, political, financial and non-lethal material assistance. According to the Central Statistics Office there were 96,338 Personal Public Service Numbers given to arrivals from Ukraine between March 2022 and 8 October 2023, under the Temporary Protection Directive.

Women and men, aged 20 and over, made up 46 per cent and 22 per cent respectively of arrivals to date, while 32 per cent were people aged under 20. Of all arrivals to date aged 18 and over, 63 per cent of males and 50 per cent of females were married or cohabiting. There were 12,108 arrivals enrolled in further education and training courses on 1 October 2023, of which 9,425 enrolled in further education English language courses. As of 8 October 2023, 36,620 arrivals had attended an employment support event arranged by Intreo Public Employment Services. Of those, 61 per cent (or 22,351 persons) noted that English language proficiency was a challenge in securing employment. Of the 36,620 arrivals that attended an Intreo event, 17,504 had recorded previous occupations, with professionals being the largest group at 31 per cent (or 5,343 persons). Of the 26,174 persons where the highest level of education was recorded, 62 per cent had achieved an NFQ level equivalent to 7 or higher (see Figure 13.1).

The initial policy response to the accommodation and provision of services for Ukrainian people fleeing conflict has been led by the Department of Children, Equality, Disability, Integration and Youth. The Department has been working at capacity and is now

Figure 13.1: Age at entry of arrivals from Ukraine (data is cumulative)

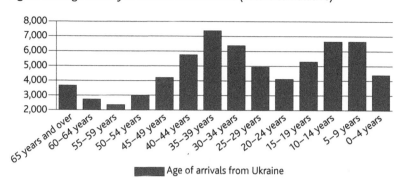

responsible for accommodating more than 96,000 people (including refugees from Ukraine and international protection applicants). A combination of hotel and guest house accommodation, accommodation provided by the general public, and emergency rest centres have been used. Of the 96,000 people who have arrived in Ireland from Ukraine, more than half have been accommodated by the state and through the generosity and compassion of the people of Ireland. As of 8 October 2023, 17,466 arrivals from Ukraine were living in private accommodations, where 7,852 hosts were in receipt of Accommodation Recognition Payment for accommodating people from Ukraine. Additional information on hosts and arrivals, such as age bands and sex, can be found in Table 13.1.

The figures for ARP may also include accommodation obtained via the 'Offer a Home' scheme, Irish Red Cross pledges and privately arranged accommodation. As of 12 October 2023, 13,947 arrivals from Ukraine were living in local authority/Irish Red Cross/Department of Children, Equality, Disability, Integration and Youth pledged accommodation, of which 5,044 were living in accommodation under the 'Offer a Home' scheme.

The substantial influx of refugees and people seeking protection exacerbated the crisis the state is experiencing in relation to limited accommodation options considering the growing number of domestic homeless presentations; the consequence of this has been declining capacity within the Housing Department.

The Irish Refugee Council, along with other non-profit organisations, recognises that emergency measures put in place through government first response should not be allowed to become permanent features of the international protection system. It is noted that while it is essential to make people as comfortable as possible while living in temporary structures, focus should be put on finding solutions to accommodation that are more permanent and appropriate.

Table 13.1: Number of hosts currently in receipt of Accommodation Recognition Payment and arrivals from Ukraine living in accommodation provided by these hosts as of 8 October 2023

Number of hosts	**7,852**
Male	4,099
Female	3,753
Under 30 years of age*	228
30–44 years of age	1,846
45–59 years of age	3,167
60 years and over	2,611
Number of arrivals from Ukraine hosted	**17,466**
Male	6,176
Under 18 years of age	2,298
18 years and over	3,878
Female	11,290
Under 18 years of age	2,283
18 years and over	9,007
County of residence**	**17,466**
Carlow	274
Cavan	503
Clare	639
Cork	1,290
Donegal	1,036
Dublin	2,902
Galway	912
Kerry	844
Kildare	663
Kilkenny	370
Laois	287
Leitrim	478
Limerick	657
Longford	294
Louth	405
Mayo	780
Meath	559
Monaghan	214
Offaly	292

Table 13.1: Number of hosts currently in receipt of Accommodation Recognition Payment and arrivals from Ukraine living in accommodation provided by these hosts as of 8 October 2023 (continued)

Number of hosts	7,852
Roscommon	420
Sligo	325
Tipperary	775
Waterford	658
Westmeath	354
Wexford	988
Wicklow	547

Note: * Current age; ** missing values combined with largest category

Source: CSO (2024)

References

CSO (2024) *Arrivals from Ukraine*. Dublin: Central Statistics Office.

Department of Housing, Local Government and Heritage (2024) *Monthly Homelessness Report*, February. Available at: https://assets.gov.ie/268

Disch, W. and Slaymaker, R. (2023) *Housing Affordability Ireland in a Cross-Country Context*. Dublin: ESRI. https://doi.org/10.26540/rs164

Economic and Social Research Institute (ESRI) (2023) *Housing Tenure, Health and Public Healthcare Coverage in Ireland*. ESRI. https://doi.org/10.26504/BP202402

ECR (European Committee of the Regions) (2017) *Towards a European Agenda for Housing*. Opinion. COR-2017-01529-00-01-AC-TRA(FR)2/9

European Parliament (2021) *Access to Decent and Affordable Housing for All*. Available at: https:/www.europarl.europa.eu/doceo/document/A-9-2020-0247_EN.html

Fukuyama, F. (1992) *The End of History and the Last Man*. New York: Free Press.

Gijon Declaration (2023) Available at: www.spanish-presidency.consilium.europa.eu

Hickel, J. (2020) *Less is More How Degrowth Will Save the World*. London: Penguin Books.

The Irish Times (2023) Research indicates annual need for 62,000 new homes. 26 January.

Lyons, R. (2022) Why Ireland's housing bubble burst. *Works in Progress*, 6, 21 January.

Nice Declaration (2022) Available at: final-declaration_finale-version-em_en_approved-20220308_vf.pdf

Oreskes, N. and Conway, E. (2023) *The Big Myth: How American Business Taught us to Loath Government and Love the Free Market*. New York: Bloomsbury Publishing.

Raworth, K. (2022 [2017]) *Doughnut Economics: Seven Ways to Think Like a 21st-Century Economist*. London: Penguin Random House.

Ressa, M. (2022) *How to Stand Up to a Dictator: The Fight for Our Future*. London: W.H. Allen.

Russell, H., Privalko, I. McGinnity, F. and Enright, S. (2021) *Monitoring Adequate Housing in Ireland*. Dublin: ESRI and Irish Human Rights and Equality Commission (HREC). https://doi.org/10.26504/bkmnext413

UNECE (United Nations Economic Commission for Europe) and Housing Europe (2021) Monitoring adequate housing in Ireland. Available at: Housing2030 study_E_web.pdf

14

Relational collaboration in supporting refugees in Norway: an organisational development perspective

Petra Kjellen Brooke

Introduction

Working with refugees and migrants is an important issue for The Salvation Army (TSA) in Norway and a strategic area for response (see Case Study 8.1). The work is primarily a consequence of the war in Syria and the ongoing war in Ukraine. Norway as a country has responded by taking in a high number of refugees from both conflicts.

This chapter begins with a brief description of immigration policy and refugee response in Norway followed by an outline of the timeline for how TSA has responded to the two major increase of refugees and migrants to Norway in 2015 with the war in Syria and in 2022 after the invasion of Ukraine and the following situation of war. After presenting the timeline, the *relational* aspect of the work in light of *relational theology* will be discussed. The timeline and TSA response is based on internal documents made available and the personal involvement of the author with the work during both of these periods.

Norwegian immigration policy and refugee response

Asylum centres in Norway are run on behalf of UDI (the Norwegian Directorate of Immigration). UDI's mission is to facilitate legal immigration, provide protection to those who qualify for protection, offer accommodation to people seeking asylum, care for minor refugees and asylum seekers, and asylum seekers between 15 and 18 years of age, prevent misuse of the immigration policy and law, facilitate effective return procedures for those without legal residency, contribute with professional and evidence-based knowledge to immigration and refugee policy, be responsible for the foreign directorate internal control systems, exchange of information with other public authorities, and oversee European Union (EU)/Schengen agreements.[1]

UDI works on behalf of the state and is governed by policy as described by the political administration in charge of the country. The aims and mission of UDI, noted on its website, are: 'We want to carry out our social mission in a correct and considerate manner, with great awareness that there are people who are strongly affected by the work we do').[2] The current Norwegian political administration (2023) is upholding a strict and regulated immigration policy using procedures for application and process procedures based on immigration laws and direction.[3] Searching for information on immigration and integration on the main governmental website (www.regj eringen.no), the text introducing information on this topic can be interpreted as reflecting the strict immigration policy: 'The government is working to reduce the number of asylum seekers without the need for protection, faster settlements of persons who receive residence, and faster return of persons without legal residence in Norway' (Regjeringen, nd).

2015: war in Syria

Asylum centres in Norway are run by various different providers, municipalities, for-profit companies and non-profit organisations.[4]

In 2015, TSA Europe felt the effects of refugees crossing the Mediterranean Sea to flee war and conflict in their home countries.[5] Because of the war and unrest in Syria and parts of Africa, migration and refugees became much more visible as they entered Europe in high numbers. TSA Greece responded in a practical way to the masses of people suddenly sleeping on the doorsteps of the TSA churches in Athens (Reliefweb, 2015), and Norway, like other countries, had to build capacity for welcoming people quickly using alternative methods and places to do so.

In 2015, with the need to expand the capacity to shelter refugees, UDI made an appeal to voluntary organisations and churches and asked if they could provide emergency accommodation. At this point, Norwegian authorities had reduced the capacity due to low numbers of refugees and migrants over some time, so the need was urgent. TSA was contacted directly by UDI and was asked about providing emergency accommodation for refugees in transition. The head of Social Services for TSA at the time gathered a small group to discuss the possibilities. At that point, TSA owned a large piece of land with a previous school and office building, situated in Oslo, and the decision to use it to house refugees was quickly made. TSA opened the first refugee shelter in April 2016, offering 250 places. After a short while a second emergency accommodation was offered on the southwest coast of the country where TSA rented available space to provide 150 places.

The agreements between TSA and UDI were generous and TSA could employ staff and provide good services to the refugees. National media had, at this time, a strong focus on how much money the state was spending to accommodate refugees. As journalists investigated all the different providers, figures showed that there were big differences in costs between the providers. Demonstrating low cost to provide good quality care for refugees, TSA's emergency accommodations came out as one of the best in the country, according to UDI. When the need for emergency accommodation eventually receded in 2016, TSA also gave unused funds back to UDI, something UDI had never experienced before.

2017–2022

In the years before the first emergency accommodations were open, TSA provided activities done by local churches in several existing long-term asylum centres These activities had a focus on integration and inclusion. A person was appointed to work on these issues at the TSA territorial headquarters. Cooperation with and project funding from UDI was not new to TSA. For several years TSA had worked with UDI to provide correct information to people who has decided to remain in the country after their application had been denied. The agreement between UDI and TSA was based on providing information about the option to return to their home country assisted by UDI and the International Organization for Migration, to people that TSA encountered. In the years leading up to 2015, and onwards, TSA had both been receiving funds to do this information work, but had also, at times, such as when UDI required statistics over how many had accepted the offer of information, decided to step out of the agreement based on ethical dilemmas regarding restriction of freedom to criticise decisions of deportation and immigration policies. Dialogues with UDI were always respectful and helpful, but there were, however, times when the gap between the mission of UDI and the mission of TSA was too wide to continue a collaborative relationship.

In 2018 the appointed person and the position of working with inclusion and integration in TSA was no longer part of the overall budget. The responsibility to keep focus on integration and inclusion was transferred to projects and centers who met refugees and asylum seekers in their daily work. This resulted in less organised work with these issues in the coming years. Contact with UDI was also less frequent in the years to follow.

2022: war in Ukraine

Moving towards more recent times and the currently ongoing conflict in Ukraine, TSA was, based on previous good relationships with UDI and successful deliverance of services, again asked to run emergency accommodation as refugees started to come to Norway. Just as in 2015, the capacity and places for refugees and asylum seekers had been reduced due to low numbers coming to Norway, so again the authorities needed to build their capacity urgently and effectively as the refugees started to fill up the reception centre at the border. This time, TSA was asked to run an emergency accommodation housing up to 700 refugees in a building, an old college, provided by UDI. TSA presented its offer, and the agreement was made just over a week after the question was asked by UDI. Within three weeks of receiving the request to open a new centre it was taken over by TSA staff in March 2022. One hundred and twenty people were interviewed for staffed positions and volunteers were recruited to serve the refugees coming to the centre. The centre has, by autumn 2023, housed over 4,000 Ukrainian refugees in transition.

As a consequence of increased contact and collaboration with UDI, TSA decided to respond to a competitive tendering bid to support regular asylum centre provision (this required the operation of regular long-term centres for all asylum seekers). In July 2023, TSA was successful and was awarded one centre located in a TSA building, a boarding school closed only two years previously located next to a corps, the training college and TSA course centre.

2023

The most critical discussions within TSA related to how TSA should respond to calls from UDI, such as the centres described earlier. Basing all work with migrants and refugees on the TSA mission statement as well as TSA International statement on refugees (TSA International, ndb) and recognising that this is an area that is both appropriate and important for TSA's mission, internal discussions have included whether this is the type of work TSA should be doing long-term. Discussions following the decision to open a permanent ordinary asylum centre has been, amongst other things, how to deal with refugees asking for additional support from churches where TSA handed out food. It has also been debated if it is appropriate for TSA to deliver services with very limited requirements for basic provision and if this is something TSA can accept. However, the main reason for the relatively lively discussion surrounding whether or not TSA should make an offer in this competitive tender was the placement of the building intended to be used. This building was a previous school traditionally used for camps and retreats as well as being next to a TSA church and the training college.

With the experiences made in TSA Norway relating to the development of work amongst asylum seekers and refugees, I will explore how the response to changing migration patterns, increasing ethnic diversity and hardening of both narratives and government policy around refugees and asylum seekers has affected TSA language and potential standing as a social justice protest movement.

Theological foundations of The Salvation Army

Following on from Chapter 4, this chapter promotes *relational theology* and reflections regarding God's interaction with creation (Oord, 2015). The relational aspect of God can also be seen in how the physical world is never disconnected from the spiritual world or the God who created it. This is grounded in the biblical description of the word becoming flesh, meaning that the physical and spiritual world can never be separated (Myers, 2011). For TSA, this aspect and acknowledgement of the relational character of God and the consequences for how God interacts with creation is reflected in TSA theology and organisation with its high level aim: Love God, Love Others.

TSA Mission Services are person-centred, and support people in the community and contracted services by loving relationships.

The consequence of this relational attitude must be reflected in all TSA action and response and align with the character of authentic Christian community, described as *covenantal, mutual, respectful and inclusive* (Oord, 2015; Bonner, 2022).

Covenantal

> The word 'covenant' has a Latin origin, 'con venire,' which means the coming together of individuals or parties to make a bond (Groningen, 2017). God made a covenant of promise with Noah and his descendants, along with all living creatures after the great flood to not destroy the earth by a flood again. By making this covenant, God protects humankind and reveals His character of justice and mercy. (Cross, 2023)

Covenantal thinking is central in TSA theology and has consequences for the practice and actions taken by TSA. One such consequence of covenantal theology can be how TSA in later years has introduced the model 'Faith Based Facilitation' (TSA International, n.d.)[6] as a model for strategic thinking and project planning. Ingrained in the model is the focus on deep relationships. This focus is important for long- and short-term engagement with people but becomes challenging as we engage with people that have an unresolved resident status. It becomes challenging because the emotional risk of hurt and brokenness is present in all relationships with refugees. It is also challenging because of the fear of the unknown and can come out in the worst cases as xenophobia. Fear of the unknown, combined with bad press about asylum centres located in built up areas, has led to a public debate regarding immigrants and especially those with an unresolved status to be hostile and full of prejudice. As TSA moved towards opening a permanent asylum centre for all categories of immigrants, not just Ukrainians, this public tendency of fear was also felt in discussions with both people in TSA and people outside, such as neighbours and public institutions (schools, health centres) affected by the asylum centre. One of the central debates, but perhaps not the most vocal, was the relationship to UDI and the description of the service they were willing to offer. As the two previous and the one ongoing emergency accommodations have a different economic framework and more generous funding than regular asylum centres and the one now considered, the relationship between UDI and TSA had not previously not been challenged to the same degree. Now, TSA faced having to make more long-term commitments to conditions for refugees that some felt were below acceptable standard, and others felt were acceptable. Included in these discussions were also the nature of the relationship to the surrounding already existing institutions (corps, officer training college and course centre) and their role or expectant role in the lives of the refugees. The issue of refugees and the need for practical assistance was already discussed as hard economic times in Norway have resulted in increased amounts of people collecting food from local corps, migrants and refugees being one major group accessing the food handout service. Local TSA church ministers and volunteers were already experiencing that their mission and calling to build deep relationships were challenged and now, for the local TSA church becoming neighbours to the asylum centre in particular, the expectation for them to cater for this group with limited resources felt concerning from a relational point of view. Having relational issues as core values in TSA, working with UDI that has no expression of relationism connected to their aims or goals, the tension between the two organisational (TSA and UDI) goals and missions became clear in the discussions regarding opening this centre.

Mutual: non-hierarchical and equal in the sense that, although there is order and process, everyone has an equal place around the table

Another interesting part of the recent developments within the TSA refugee and migrant work is how the organisation moves towards describing working with refugees as one of its core activities. There are many reasons for this decision and one is to demonstrate to external funders that TSA is a committed partner. The question is, will this commitment to the refugee work be toned down if the need for asylum centres and emergency accommodations goes down? Will TSA, by making the work a core priority, equip the organisation and staff to act as they work with this topic?

Another part of demonstrating a mutual *relational* attitude is how TSA communicates its engagement with people in marginalised situations, both internally and externally. Immigration policy is very much a 'hot potato' in the Norwegian public space and by making this topic one of our specialities, the need for addressing issues connected to refugees and migrants grows. By growing the engagement as well as making it a core activity TSA also gains more knowledge in the organisation as well as knowledge to address these issues in the public space. But, can this new focus and core area and the experiences TSA has had, as an organisation, from working closely with refugees and with UDI, help it to change policy or the public agenda to ensure a more human treatment of refugees and migrants in the future?

Another tension that has become clear and that relates directly to the 'mutual' understanding from a *relationism* perspective, is the tension lingering between the TSA churches and programme level of the organisation of the TSA social services. The pushback to not open an asylum centre on a more permanent basis was primarily voiced by the corps and programme level. It is important to point out that this was not based on xenophobic views. To better understand some of the concerns raised by the members of the TSA church, in this case regarding the church becoming a close neighbour of the centre, looking at it from a relational perspective can help. TSA church and programmes within the TSA programme department work closely with individuals having experienced what they describe as unfair treatment from UDI. TSA churches are often confronted with people experiencing being sent out of the country despite needs to stay, children being taken out of their homes in the middle of night to be transported by police to the airport or transit centres. Ethical considerations regarding having formal contracts and agreements with UDI has been mentioned earlier. Other aspects for the hesitant response from the corps can be based in how an increased pressure from immigrant groups needing food and other services makes corps feeling helpless and not being able respond due to limited resources.

On the other hand of the tension is the professionalised TSA social services. They have long experience of working with partners that in many cases can be seen as controversial, such as the child protection services that have been criticised in both national and international media and court systems and navigate some of the relational issues connected to this. For the TSA social services, the objections from neighbours and internal local people were familiar reactions when starting projects and institutions. TSA social services also have the privilege of being able to see the bigger picture, having access to other sources of information as well as having the personal relationships to individuals in contracting services such as UDI. The organisational tension between the programme and social work department in TSA Norway is unexplored and how this affects overall organisational development for future activities and engagements is an important topic to investigate as it has an effect on how TSA move forwards as one, or as a fractured, organisation.

Respectful: honouring difference and diversity

One important aspect of any engagement TSA has is asking the question 'why' it should have this project or programme. The question 'why' facilitates a deeper conversation including values and faith (see Chapter 5) and can guide towards an understanding of respect despite differences of opinion. TSA is good at the 'how'. Practical engagement is easy and in many cases this is what is required but when the engagement goes beyond the 'how', situations of injustice or malpractice might be revealed and TSA needs to know how to respond. TSA has decided to deliver services to refugees and asylum seekers based on the fact that it is different from the traditional providers. The question will then be 'Why are we different?' What makes TSA different? There might be an easy answer to the question, that we can provide many volunteers to help or that we have knowledge regarding topics like human trafficking and child protection easily available and that there is a high level of engagement and idealism creating much value for money. Although all these arguments are valid, the question will still be what it is that TSA can bring to the table to change what can be seen as bad practice or injustice as Norway accepts refugees and migrants. By engaging with external partners such as UDI that functions on behalf of political governance, is TSA daring enough to become politically critical and is there enough courage to push back as we experience injustice or bad practice? I will give one example of what I mean. As part of the process for any refugee coming to Norway, the adult refugee needs to be interviewed to map their need for protection in Norway. This interview takes up to six hours and happens on one of the first days after their arrival. TSA has accepted the role of hosting a small number of 'regular' refugees in its emergency accommodation. Unlike the Ukrainian refugees who are granted a one-year stay as they enter the country, the 'regular' asylum seekers must apply. So, parents must travel over an hour to the UDI office to be interviewed and they are not allowed to bring their children. The children are expected to be left behind, with people they just met in a country where they do not speak the language, to see their parents go. The strain on the children is immense and also for the carers who are looking after the children for many hours. This practice is thought of as harmful from a perspective of the child. How can TSA voice this concern, challenging a system and still deliver services that requires TSA to adhere to such practices? The pressure on the staff is great, and the overall discussion of values and whether TSA can quietly adhere to such practices is relatively muted.

Experiencing the tension between the TSA mission statement and the focus on deep relations with the people its encounters on one side, and the UDI's need to build relationships with the voluntary sector that had previously been few in this field on the other side, begs the question regarding values. How, if there has been an adjustment of values to fulfil a wish to contribute to an important cause, and if the reasons for this value adjustment is mission aligned or because of previous bad examples of care delivered by profit-based actors. The question as to whether TSA should move forwards with further tender competitions within this sector or not, remains. Is the acceptance of standards for how people live and how they are provided for that are lower than the standards of services we provide for other groups is less important if the alternative is not to provide the service? There is no easy answer to this question or to the question of how practices can possibly shift values. TSA Norway has described its values in mostly faith-neutral terms, making them accepted by both staff of non-faith and secular partners, but elements that can be described as ways for TSA to challenge existing social injustices are still possible. Some would say that the fact that TSA now runs the only asylum centre on a more long-term basis that has staff available 24/7 has been part of pushing back when our values have been challenged, and some would say that accepting very small sleeping quarters and to accommodate many people in one space could be said to having accepted an erosion of TSA values in a negative way.

Inclusive: where all are invited to join in the relationship

Under the heading 'Salvation in community' the relations aspect of TSA theology is described as follows:

> Furthermore, salvation in the biblical sense does not only concern individuals and communities but affects the entire world order. We are promised 'a new Heaven and a new earth'. All history is moving towards the fulfilment of God's purposes for the entire universe, 'to bring all things in heaven and on earth together under one head, even Christ' (Ephesians 1:10). (TSA International, 2010: 152)

Working according to TSA theological understanding of salvation as being relational and communal and including the entire world order, working with social justice issues like refugees and migrants can be seen as a natural faith-based consequence for TSA. Many groups in our societies are experiencing exclusion and standing on the outskirts of society, but as a refugee and migrant you are by definition placed on the margins of communities, social provision and legislation. Many refugees and migrants experience long waits in limbo for answers regarding permits to stay, and sometimes even with permits they have to wait to be accepted by municipalities in order to find a place to stay. This perspective of marginalisation is sometimes at odds with the services TSA provides that are aimed at people in the local community suffering from injustice and social needs. Marginalisation is challenging the *relational* character of any project and organisation, and the question regarding 'why' TSA chose to engage again becomes relevant. Because, relating to people on the margins can become a provocative activity for the surrounding context. One example of this is when TSA Norway engaged services directed towards Roma people begging on the streets. Publicly scrutinised, this group was asking for basic provision and help. TSA responded and was consequently also scrutinised. People giving money in the Christmas collection asked if any of the money would go to support Roma people, and if so, they would give to someone else. Becoming a voice for someone has implications for other parts of the organisation, in this case the collection of money.

As TSA moves towards a more permanent response among refugees and migrants, the aspect of protest and inclusion of people and opinions in all projects must become a relevant and open discussion. There must be an openness for those who reflect on refugees and migrants as groups too complex for TSA to work with, and the fact that the risk of constant broken relationships and friendships endanger the resilience among the carers. Being inclusive does not always mean being in agreement about all things but building inclusive relationships and communications is important for all TSA activity, including how to respond to refugees and migrants.

Conclusion

The discussion in this chapter, focusing on responses to societal crises, *intermediate* determinants of health, provides a critical insight into TSA strategy, encompassing both church and charitable dimensions of TSA in Norway and the other 161 TSA territories. The TSA is expected to respond when society needs help, both due to its standing in the Norwegian public space, but also due to its mission. This expectation will put TSA and other faith-based organisations in situations where both internal and external tensions emerge. Rather than only create learning by looking back and evaluate it is important to reflecton ongoing organisational challenges and changes to provide new knowldege, see Double loop learning in Chapter 19. This is important in future responses to new challenges, particularly where global origins and consequences are involved. TSA needs to have an organisational robust structure and value base that means that we know when to say 'yes' and when to say 'no' based on those values. There is an important aspect of living 'in' the world, but not 'of' the world. *Relationism* can provide TSA with some important aspects on how to navigate organisational development and values on the move, as mapped onto the conceptual framework of the social determinants of health (see also Chapters 5 and 19).

Notes

1   www.udi.no
2   www.udi.no
3   Immigration law and policy will be experienced differently by different groups. Ukrainians have been granted different immigratory rights to all other asylum seekers, making the policy experienced less strict. However, this might be changed as there are high numbers of refugees from Ukraine coming to Norway.
4   A complete updated list of providers can be seen at https://www.udi.no/en/asylum-reception-centres/ayslum-reception-centre-addresses/
5   For more detailed information on the refugee situation in 2015 see https://www.unhcr.org/statistics/unhcrstats/576408cd7/unhcr-global-trends-2015.html
6   See https://www.salvationarmy.org/fbf for more information.

References

Bonner, A. (2022) *The Theology of Relationalism*. Internal review. TSA.Internal document used by permission. Salvation Army UKI Territory.

Cross, N. (2023) *A Biblical and Theological Understanding of Covenant*. Conference contribution on TSA Covenant theology presented at the International Principal's conference in Kenya October 2023. Internal paper, used by permission by the author.

Groningen, G.V. (2017) Covenant. In *Baker's Evangelical Dictionary of Biblical Theology*. Logos Bible Software.

Elwell, W. A. (1996). Baker's Evangelical Dictionary of Biblical Theology. Grand Rapids, MI: Baker Cook House Company.

Myers, B.L. (2011) *Walking with the Poor: Principles and Practices of Transformational Development*. Orbis Books.

Oord, T.J. (2015) *The Uncontrolling Love of God: An Open and Relational Account of Providence*. Downers Grove, IL 60515-1426 New York InterVarsity Press.

Regjeringen (nd) *Immigration and Integration*. Available at: https://www.regjeringen.no/en/topics/immigration-and-integration/id918/

Reliefweb (2015) The Salvation Army across Europe assists refugees. Available at: https://reliefweb.int/report/world/salvation-army-across-europe-assists-refugees

TSA International (nda) *Building Deep Relationships*. Available at: https://www.salvationarmy.org/fbf. Accessed 16 August 2024.

TSA International (ndb) *The Salvation Army International Positional Statement Refugees and Asylum Seekers*. Available at: https://s3.amazonaws.com/cache.salvationarmy.org/b098ace2-8430-4db0-b89f-87db8b8b5c58_English+Refugees+and+Asylum+Seekers+IPS.pdf. Accessed 23 November 2023.

TSA International (2010) *The Salvation Army Handbook*. London: Salvation Books.

PART IV

Responding to the war in Europe

Introduction to Part IV

Peter Hain

Continental Europe has over the last few centuries experienced more wars within it than any other part of the world and also triggered the only two world wars – so far, at least.

But sadly, the peaceful era enjoyed by most in the world since 1945 is fairly unique historically, the barbaric Russian attack on Ukraine, and it's devastating impact – especially upon children and women – an ugly reminder of the horror that human beings are capable of unleashing upon each other.

Together with the centuries-old conflict on the island of Ireland and the horrific 2023 escalation in the long-running conflict between Israelis and Palestinians – with all its destabilising regional and global consequences – the turbulence, terror and carnage of recent times invites the question: how to end it and what are the lessons of successful conflict resolution?

First to note the complexity of geopolitics in our era. When the UN General Assembly voted in 2022 overwhelmingly to condemn Vladimir Putin's invasion of Ukraine, only Eritrea, Belarus, North Korea and Syria dissented – hardly an endearing group.

But 35 countries, including India and China, abstained, along with the once Nelson Mandela human-rights standard bearer, South Africa, joined by 16 other African countries.

The Ukraine war has magnified a shifting geopolitical dynamic. Russia has enjoyed expanding influence in the Middle East after its decisive role in the Syrian war, with former steadfast US allies, Saudi Arabia and the United Arab Emirates (UAE), breaking ranks with the West.

Many African leaders and other leaders from the South remember the post-Second World War US imperialism that invaded Vietnam, propped up dictators in Latin America and helped sustain apartheid.

Then there was the 2003 invasion of Iraq, launched on false intelligence that its brutal dictator had weapons of mass destruction, and which provoked regional bedlam. In bypassing the United Nations, the United States and the United Kingdom encouraged other countries to ignore international law and invade when *they* chose. The Iraq war destroyed trust in the West and left many Africa leaders reluctant to jump to America's attention over Ukraine.

A 'double standards' scepticism reinforced because Israel has remained protected whatever horror it unleashes on the Palestinians.

Also, although the old European colonial ties and subsequent investments still count a lot in Africa, new money and new influence from Beijing and Moscow counts too.

Beijing has been buying up Africa on a large scale, especially its resources, somehow avoiding being charged with economic colonialism. Moscow doesn't have anything like the same money or share of trade, but Putin has used his mercenary force, the Wagner Group, especially in the Sahel, Libya, Sudan, the Central African Republic, Mozambique, Zimbabwe and Madagascar.

The deal Wagner has been offering is security in return for lucrative mining concessions, especially gold because, with diamonds, it can evade sanctions by selling and exchanging them outside the regulated banking sector.

Elsewhere in the world, things are on the move too, as the old alliances come under pressure.

The UAE has been diversifying its strategic partnerships, continuing to host US troops and US Navy ships, while aligning with Russia in Africa. Dubai has also become an important hub for Russian sanctions-busting, with over 4,000 of its companies based there.

In Africa the UAE has increased investments on the African Continent, especially in ports, and works with Wagner Group mercenaries to combat and eliminate Islamic extremism and jihadism. The UAE president has also established himself as a power-broker in the Middle East region, aiming to undermine Islamic fundamentalism for example through forays into Libya, Sudan, Ethiopia and Yemen.

For its part, Saudi Arabia defied Washington by cutting oil production during the Ukraine crisis and has been edging closer to China on security cooperation amidst rising tension between the United States and China. North Atlantic Treaty Organization member Turkey has shown similar waywardness in US eyes over closer Russian relations.

The emergence and enlargement of the BRICS countries – Brazil, Russia, India, China – to include countries in Africa, the Gulf and elsewhere in Asia poses a challenge to Western hegemony in a polarised world.

Significantly, the UK's former head of National Security, Lord Sedwill, wrote in *The Economist* in February 2023:

> Much of the world is rediscovering the appeal of non-alignment. So the West should reinvest in its relationships with countries such as Brazil, India, South Africa, Turkey and the Gulf states. Although many countries fear aggressive neighbours and few support Mr Putin's invasion, they also complain of Western arrogance and double standards. Old friends we have neglected welcome China's investment and its boundless appetite for the raw materials on which the modern economy and green transition depend. More private Western investment in the 'global south' could be unleashed if underwritten by political investment in sustained and stable relationships. (Quoted in Hain, 2021)

Today we take for granted Nelson Mandela's 'rainbow democracy'. Yet the defeat of apartheid was painful, bitter and long, until finally once-evil oppressors settled into government with those they had imprisoned or tortured.

It's also hard to recognise that Northern Ireland was comparatively recently a theatre for such horror and barbarity, hate and bigotry. But could lessons from ending that horror offer hope to other areas of the world locked in bitter conflict, violence and terrorism?

Of course, no one would suggest that there is a 'one size fits all' model coming out of Northern Ireland. But there are some fundamental lessons that reward a closer look, while conceding that there is still an ongoing process in Northern Ireland which will take some time – probably generations – to complete: self-government has been precarious since 2017, segregation is still widespread in schools and housing, prejudice and divisions remain, and there is still violence albeit isolated and spasmodic where once it was continuous.

Similarly, the joy of a non-racial democracy in South Africa since 1994 has not by any means abolished the awful legacy of apartheid: poverty and unemployment among the Black majority remains horrendous, and there has been terrible corruption driven from the very top.

Three objectives guided Prime Minister Tony Blair's approach to peacemaking in Northern Ireland over ten years intensive years between 1997 and 2007. They were: the necessity to create a space without violence during which politics could begin to flourish; the identification of individuals with the courage and intention to lead their communities; and the search for a political framework which could accommodate the needs, aspirations and scope for compromise by all involved.

Tony Blair consciously took risks to achieve and maintain the Irish Republican Army (IRA) ceasefire, because the absence of conflict was an absolute prerequisite to progress.

What is so destructive about terrorism and violence is not just the wrecking of lives but the impact on the psychology of a community. With 3,000 murders and about 35,000 serious injuries in a Northern Ireland population of just 1.7 million, almost every family felt the horror of 30 years of 'The Troubles'.

Above all, terrorism obscures the natural desire of the majority for peace by entrenching bitterness and creating an entirely understandable hysteria in which constructive voices can no longer be heard.

It is desperately hard for people to focus on politics when they are under attack: when, in the case of Republicans, their communities felt under assault or siege by agencies of the state, and in the case of Unionists, many friends and relatives were murdered or maimed under the constant shadow of IRA attacks.

This, for Tony Blair's government, meant making concessions that went deeply against the grain, not only for Unionists, but also for much mainstream British opinion.

An example was the controversial and painful Republican and Loyalist prisoner releases at the time of the Good Friday Agreement, including individuals who had committed unspeakable atrocities.

But it was essential to show paramilitary groups that a commitment to peace brought gains which could not be achieved by violence.

Thereafter, continuously moving forward with small steps was to some extent an end in itself because time was critical: the longer the cessation of violence, the stronger the desire for peace could grow, and the more difficult the return to conflict could become.

To 'keep the bicycle upright and moving' was a key objective and required constant intervention, and even more constant attention of a forensic nature, from the very top.

The transition to peace had to be completed. But this could only be achieved through relationships of some trust with leading Republicans who had themselves been party to terrorist attacks, including in Britain.

One of Tony Blair's core beliefs was that people and personalities matter in politics, and that building relationships of trust, even where deep differences remain, is vital.

This may seem very obvious. But it is surprisingly often relegated to a place well below 'issues' in resolving conflict. It is also notable how political enmities can block the way to even tentative contact – just look at virtually all the main conflicts across the world today, especially between Israel and the Palestinians.

The key challenge for Tony Blair's government was to identify the positive elements within the opposing communities and to encourage and sustain them.

That meant establishing a *relationship of trust* (see Part III of this volume) with the individual leaders and understanding the pressures on them from within their own movement or party, as well as from outside. Ultimately this meant making judgements about the extent to which those pressures were real or tactical.

But judgements about the good faith and courage of individuals ultimately have to be political and personal, based on instinct, and at crucial junctures, the product of private conversations between the prime minister, his secretary of state and individual leaders.

The consequences of those judgements about individuals have been far-reaching: most of the decisions taken by the British government after 1998 were coloured by the need to build or *maintain confidence* in one community or another, or to allow one leader or another space to manage their sometimes–intransigent constituencies.

Judgements about key leaders within Northern Ireland were complemented by the alignment of international interest. Tony Blair was prepared as British prime minister to devote unprecedented time and energy to solving the problem as a real priority, and came into power to find a strong, confident Irish government, led by Bertie Ahern, and a US president in Bill Clinton who felt a strong personal attachment to Ireland and who was influenced by the large and politically significant Irish American community, and open to providing positive intervention or support.

Crucially, all three were prepared to work to a shared strategy, all were prepared to be bold.

As other parts of the world have discovered, these alignments of leadership and circumstances do not come along often: failure to seize the opportunity can mean condemning another generation to conflict.

It is one thing to feel that a dispute – whether in Northern Ireland or the Middle East – will eventually be resolved, but another to grip it in such a way that resolution does not wait for generations, with all the intervening violence and turmoil.

There is no inevitability about the timescale of a conflict, however ancient, however bitter, however intransigent. Northern Ireland was emphatically all three.

On Israel/Palestine, the conflict has never been gripped at a sufficiently high level, over a sufficiently sustained period. Efforts and initiatives have come and gone, and violence has returned to fill the vacuum – the 2023 horror following a decade when no meaningful international diplomacy or peace negotiations occurred to resolve matters, leaving a vacuum which violence predictably filled.

Periodic engagement led to false starts and dashed hopes. International forces have never been aligned as they were over Northern Ireland and dialogue has been stunted. Preconditions have continued to be a block against progress.

But Palestinians and Israelis cannot militarily defeat the other; there will have to be a negotiated solution which satisfies Palestinian aspirations for a viable state and Israel's need for security.

Just as legitimate grievances in Northern Ireland fuelled Republican sympathies, Palestinian grievances provide fertile territory for extremists. Addressing people's grievances – from security to ending discrimination against Catholics in jobs and housing – as we did in Northern Ireland, can undercut the extremists who seek to inflame and exploit them, so creating more fertile ground for a political process to complement engagement.

This overview of conflict since the Second World War clearly demonstrates the geopolitical *structural* determinants underpinning approaches to peace and reconciliation. The World Health Organization's *social determinants of health conceptual framework* (see Figure I.1 in the Introduction to this volume) provides an historical and contemporary context with reference to those people most at risk due to *social class*, *gender* and *ethnicity*. A brief insight into the changing impact of the war on people, their communities and economic development is presented, by commentators in Ukraine, in Chapter 15. These *intermediate determinants* are discussed in various parts of this book. In the case of the Balkan wars the consequences of conflict are long-lasting, as reviewed in Chapter 6.

From the perspective of *culture and societal values*, Chapter 4 provides a review of the role of religion in conflict, historically, and specifically in the Russian-Ukrainian conflict. In Part IV of this book the role of faith actors, public engagement and social justice is reviewed by Emma Tomalin, with reference to the war in Europe, in Chapter 18. The role of a faith-based organisation in addressing *locally led emergency* and *developmental* responses, by The Salvation Army in Europe, to the invasion of Ukraine by Russia is explored in Chapters 16 and 17.

Geopolitical *structural determinants* of health and wellbeing are influenced by international, national and regional governmental organisations. Chapters 17 and 19 critically review the role of non-governmental organisations (NGOs), such as the International Salvation Army, in working with governmental organisations. The added value of understanding needs from *locally led* activities, organised within an international organised NGO, in partnership with other organisations, should promote effective *emergency responses* which lay a other drivers of health and wellbeing. *Relational partnerships* and the *added value* of working together with trust, confidence are critically reviewed by Richard Simmons, and TSA collaborators in Chapter 19. This analysis builds on chapters in previous volumes in this series.

Reference

Hain, P. (2021). Africa caught in a geopolitical bind. *African Business*, 6 January. Available at: https://african.business/2023/05/politics/africa-caught-in-a-geo-politics-bind

15

War in Ukraine: perspectives from Ukraine

Lada Tesfaiie and Iryna Shepelenko

Introduction

This chapter is written by a freelance journalist (LT) and academic (IS) working in Ukraine. They work with a community of Ukrainian and international activists to support a network of leaders to provide effective help, in the immediate response and rebuilding of Ukraine. This international platform, Support Ukraine Now, is an ecosystem of diverse projects in the civil sector, and economy-promoting diplomacy and welfare.[1] As part of her contribution to Support Ukraine Now, LT visited the UK in the early part of 2023 with a view to understanding and connecting with the Homes for Ukraine scheme in the London Borough of Sutton (see Chapter 12).

Further input to this chapter includes interviews undertaken by Svitlana Semaniv, a psychologist currently employed by the London Borough of Sutton to support Ukrainians continuing to support families in Ukraine affected by the war (see Chapter 6).

In this chapter, insights from academic, political, community and psychosocial perspectives from Ukraine, in 2024, are provided, following interviews with people living in the war-torn country. These first-hand *in situ* contributions complement the commentaries informed by the threats to world peace and the cultural and religious identity resulting from the invasion by Russia of Ukraine in Chapters 4 and 12, and contextualised by the psychosocial view of the long-term impact on people following the Balkan war (see Chapter 6).

Education and research in Ukraine

On a daily basis, the international news media presents videos and photographs of the devastation of homes, businesses and civic buildings in the various regions of Ukraine, resulting from Russian aggression. However, the most severe casualty of war is the loss of education and cultural impact on the current and future generations of children (see Chapters 7 and 8 in this book). Educational institutions, teaching and research are paused, as in the case of Yanina, whose PhD is now paused or stopped due the physical damaged cause to buildings.

Yuriy Dmytrovych Boychuk, a doctor of pedagogical sciences, professor, corresponding member of the National Academy of Pedagogical Sciences of Ukraine, and rector of the Kharkiv National Pedagogical University, named after H.S. Skovoroda, Ukraine, commented in an interview on 1 November 2023, that:

> The effectiveness of conducting research is doubtful at present, as the active phase of the Russian-Ukrainian war continues. The state of war increases the level of uncertainty in society, so the results of research risk losing their relevance until its (the war's) conclusion. Comprehensive research is likely to be more appropriate after the finalisation of the armed conflict when it becomes possible to objectively assess Ukraine's human losses, the state of infrastructure, security factors, economic indicators, international developments, and so on.
>
> Connections with universities in Ukraine and universities in other countries could help support Ukraine's academic infrastructure and enrich the evidence base for long-term support. Connections in the areas of scientific and scientific-methodical cooperation, internships, academic mobility, and grant activities, will all help to maintain and develop the cultural, economic and political capacity of Ukraine.
>
> The university has its own experience in such support through cooperation with Cardiff Metropolitan University (UK) since May 2022. According to the Memorandum of Cooperation signed on June 28, 2023, between the Kharkiv National Pedagogical University and Cardiff Metropolitan University, among the main directions of support and long-term cooperation between our universities is ensuring the continuity of research and scientific work based on the British university, cooperation in technical support for distance education, collaboration in the fields of pedagogy, arts, sports, and physical education, as well as student self-government cooperation for exchanging experiences and more. Starting from July 2023, partner universities have discussed practical proposals and begun implementing further avenues of cooperation in the educational, scientific, and cultural fields.
>
> It should be noted that all these directions are very important for Ukrainians because the assistance and moral solidarity of such a powerful ally as the United Kingdom give confidence in Ukraine's future and bring our Victory closer.
>
> Support from the United Kingdom is highly significant for Ukraine. The active involvement of the UK Prime Minister at the beginning of the full-scale invasion contributed to a reassessment

by the leadership of Western states of their strategy for providing military and financial assistance to Ukraine. Since February 2022, the United Kingdom has consistently supported Ukraine and condemned Russian aggression. The United Kingdom's government provides infrastructure for the training of Ukrainian military personnel, and effective technical, financial, and military support. Alongside military assistance, humanitarian support for the population of Ukraine remains highly relevant, especially in the fields of science, education, and culture.

Business and economic development

Yashunin Yuriy, 39 years old, was born in Crimea, Ukraine, and has lived in Kharkiv City (Figures 15.1 and 15.2) for the last 20 years, together with his wife and young daughter. He is an IT entrepreneur, developing and supporting the Ukrainian startup ecosystem:

It's almost 600 days of full-scale invasion and almost ten years of Russian–Ukrainian war started from the Crimea occupation, so, we as human beings adapt. I stay optimistic and keep pushing hard to increase

Figure 15.1: Kharkiv. Architectural monument, designed by Iliodor Zahoskin, built in 1915, before the invasion.

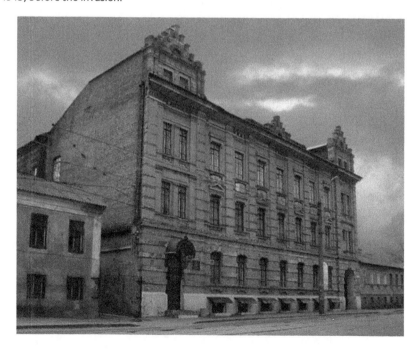

Figure 15.2: Kharkiv. Architectural monument, destroyed by a Russian strike drone on the night of 3 November 2023.

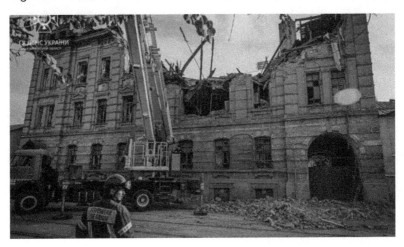

our chances of winning this war and de-occupy all our territories. Our morale is up and down, every new Russian shelling and explosion near my home, near my family and daughter is quite stressful.

As an IT entrepreneur, generally, my business is progressing well, as we can continue our business and sell our services and products globally. I have no right to complain compared to other Ukrainians who have lost their homes, businesses, jobs, etc.

I appreciate the true leadership of the UK's support for Ukraine. The UK was the first country to begin sending anti-tank guided missiles NLAW to Ukraine, just before the full-scale Russian invasion in February 2022.

It was very helpful during the first months. It helped to destroy a lot of Russian tanks and save the lives of both military and civil people, then the UK was the first country who provided us with a Storm Shadow [long-range air-launched cruise missile]. It was a real game changer – the Ukrainian Armed Forces were able to reach 200–300km goals. So, Ukrainians find the UK as a top supporter and first mover all over the world.

Support of Ukraine in the UK mustn't depend on elections, political parties in the UK, the US and other supporting countries. [Boris Johnson, Ben Wallace and Rishi Sunak are very good friends of Ukraine. I'm sure we will see a lot of streets in honour of these guys in Ukraine].

I live with my family in Kharkiv city. British architect Norman Foster had kindly agreed to lead the post-war rebuilding of Kharkiv.

The likely progress of military and diplomatic progress in the war is a hard question. Ukraine could not give up and just freeze the current frontline, as millions of Ukrainians would be left on the temporarily occupied territories.

Many people have been killed by Russians. For what goal? Was it all in vain? I hope not. If a stalemate existed on the frontline in Ukraine, Russia would have time to accumulate its military resources and definitely would start a new full-scale invasion after 5–7 years.

The ideal optimistic scenario for Ukraine is to de-occupy all our territories and become a NATO member. This will only be possible with the ongoing support of our allies and partners. Without that, it's impossible to resist Russia's military capacity maintained by 'oil money'. Millions of Russian people want to erase Ukrainian identity and culture.

Ukrainians have demonstrated their ingenuity and resilience on the battlefield. This technical agility is also seen in the IT industry, which provides IT support globally for commonly used software packages such as the PDF Expert software supported by Readdle based in Ukraine.

On the night of 3 November 2023 the enemy struck the city of Kharkiv with the fourth 'Shakhed' kamikaze unmanned aerial vehicle. The building of the Kharkiv College of Transport Technologies was also damaged. The enemy strike destroyed the second and third floors, the roof of the building, and structural elements were also on fire. The college building was more than 100 years old, it was built in 1915 according to the project of architects Zagoskin and Korneenko.

However, more visible and unprotected areas of the economy have been devastated, such as agriculture (see Figures 15.3–15.7).

Agriculture has been a very significant part of the Ukrainian economy, but also has global relevance as demonstrated by the impact on food scarcity in Africa and global prices of grain, which affected the cost of living in countries across the world.

Ukraine: breadbasket of the world?

Tatiana Pushkar, Professor at Odesa State University:

At the beginning of the COVID-19 pandemic, the Moodle [online teaching] platform was created. It was loaded with all the information of each discipline, including lecture and laboratory-practical material. We have been working online for almost two years. Then, on February 24, we woke up to repeated explosions. The youngest son called, he worked in the police and was on duty and said that the war had started. The same day we left for a safe place. When we arrived at our place of

Figure 15.3: Cattle feeding at the Agrosvit company farm. Kharkiv region, Vovchansky district, village Shestakov.

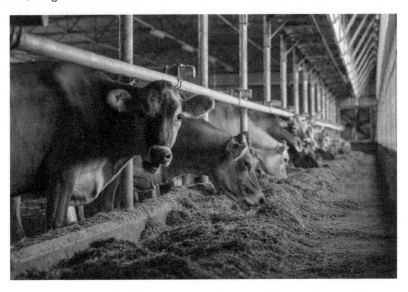

Figure 15.4: Corpses of cattle after bombing of the Agrosvit company

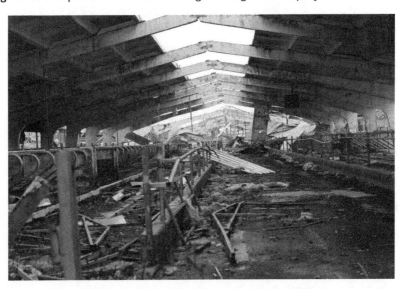

stay, my husband immediately went to the military office and signed up as a volunteer for the armed forces of Ukraine.

All television and radio channels broadcast that a full-scale invasion of the Russian Federation into the territory of Ukraine had begun.

Figure 15.5: Leonid Logvinenko in the ruins of the bombed-out Agrosvit farm

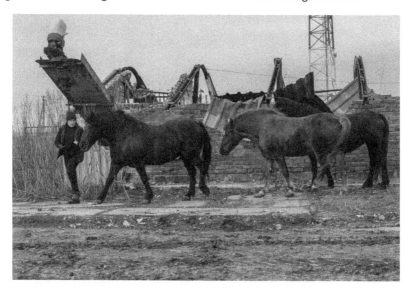

Figure 15.6: Leonid Logvinenko looking after horses not killed in the bombing of the Agrosvit farm

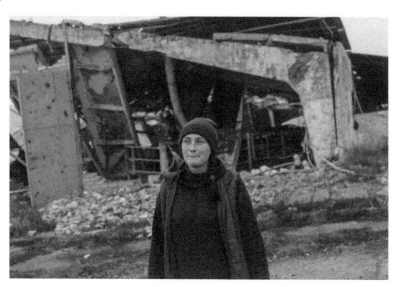

Figure 15.7: The Agromol dairy farm, in the Kharkiv region, damaged by an air raid on 28 February 2023

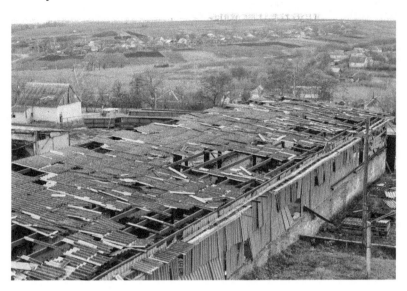

The Russians destroyed military facilities throughout the country with rocket attacks. Power and fuel outages began. Every day the situation worsened, and the occupiers were getting closer to Odesa. In the first battle with the subversive and reconnaissance group, the younger son and his colleagues entered, on the approaches to Odesa, which we learned about after a certain time. The town where we were was being prepared for defence by the military together with the citizens. Fortifications were built, roadblocks were organised, trenches and dugouts were dug, and hunters were on duty around the clock in the villages. Young people poured an incendiary mixture of 'cocktails'. With our funds and labour, we supported the defence of the city and the armed forces.

When there was a threat of nuclear power plant explosions, it was decided to evacuate women abroad. I went to Bulgaria together with my daughters-in-law and granddaughter. We were safe there. After some time, I returned to Odesa.

The situation is getting worse every day. Almost every week, the Russian Federation conducts a massive missile attack on the entire Ukraine, on infrastructure, power plants, water canals, bridges, residential buildings, hospitals and maternity homes.

Currently, it is practically impossible to conduct classes in the city due to problems with the electricity supply. It is most critical in Odesa. Light is given at an interval of eight to two (eight hours without light and two hours with light). Food prices rise, life becomes more expensive, and wages decrease. In the first days of the war, classes were not held. Many teachers left the city and the country. According to the decision of the administration, which provided for the safety of students and teaching staff, it was decided to continue online classes.

Students' whereabouts were monitored daily. A certain number of students were in the occupied territories, which were cut off from the Internet, but thanks to mobile networks, were familiar with their conditions of existence. Some students went abroad but attended online classes. Some students went to defend the country, there are also volunteers. Most of the students stayed in Ukraine. During an air raid, classes are interrupted and we have to go to the shelter.

Unfortunately, there are casualties among students, they gave their lives for our future, taking up arms to defend the country. They died from the repression and violence of the aggressors.

Despite all the problems and difficulties, we do not lose hope for victory.

In two months, I, together with my colleagues, organised and held an international scientific and practical conference, planned even in peacetime. Despite rocket attacks, power outages, and repeated postponements to other dates, we were able to hold it. This conference was attended by scientists from Slovakia, Italy, Bulgaria, France and Azerbaijan. Adapting to wartime conditions after peacetime is very difficult. Rocket attacks were on civilians and infrastructure. As a result, there is a lack of electricity and water for several days.

It is difficult to live in the countryside, but we have already adapted. Due to the lack of electricity, the water supply does not work and water must be taken from wells. We prepare food only when there is light, mostly at night. The same with washing. The fact that there is furnace heating in the house and you can warm up at least a little helps a lot. In a city without light, life seems to stop. It is impossible to keep warm or cook food in the houses. You need to keep a supply of water all the time because there are also problems with it.

It is difficult to talk about the future of the university because we do not know what will happen tomorrow. But we all believe in a happy future and the development of science and continue to plan future conferences, research, and work on scientific articles.

Until 24 February 2022, Agromol cultivated 25,000 hectares of land in the Kharkiv region. The company grew winter wheat, sunflower and sugar beet for its own sugar factory in Chuguyiv district. A small elevator with a capacity of 110,000 tons of simultaneous storage.

But Agromol was better known to Kharkiv residents for its dairy products, which it produced under the Agromol brand. Modern dairy farms in the village served as the raw material base.

The breeding and genetic centre, the creation of which was carried out as part of the 'Village of the Future' project. The average milk yield per cow in the farm is about 7,000kg of milk per year, the milking process itself is maximally automated. The farm also specialises in breeding calves of the Ukrainian red-spotted breed.

The company's farm was damaged by an air raid on 28 February and was then constantly subjected to artillery fire. Here, out of a herd of 3,000 thoroughbred cows, about 2,000 died (see Figure 15.7).

Media perspectives from within Ukraine

Vira Sverdlyk is a journalist and TV presenter:

Psychologically, physically, economically, we (Ukrainians) are going through the most difficult times in our history. It would be unfair to say that it is easy for us, but at the same time, we are strong and united more than ever. Morally we are unbreakable. Physically, we are very hardy. This is proven by our soldiers at the frontline, our medics, rescuers, energy workers who work overtime, by every Ukrainian who, despite sometimes sleepless nights, gets up in the morning to go to work and this way brings our victory closer. Economically, we are holding up. Ukrainian entrepreneurs show great will. At the same time, it is impossible not to thank international donors and countries that support us. It is difficult to talk about the social wellbeing of Ukrainians in the classical sense of this definition. Social wellbeing includes many factors particularly in relation to personal security. But the war showed that the greatest value of the nation is independence and freedom. We have plenty of this. Ukrainians are a free people!

The UK is one of the main allies of Ukraine, it is the second country after the United States in the volume of aid to us, more than 10 billion euros. The UK is a clear leader in making progressive decisions on the issue of military support to Ukraine, being the first country to provide us with lethal weapons, long-range Storm Shadow missiles, Challenger 2 tanks, and was the first to train Ukrainian pilots on F-16 fighters. British humanitarian, sanctions and energy aid to Ukraine are also necessary. London is perceived by Ukrainians not only as a strong ally, and a reliable partner but also as a friend who is one hundred per cent on your side and has no common interests with the enemy.

From the perspective of ongoing support for Ukraine, dialogue, equality and mutual support, in my opinion, are the key to long-term international relations. Bilateral negotiations at the level of central and local authorities and expert experience exchange would contribute to effective long-term cooperation between the two countries. Ukraine is currently gaining invaluable practical experience of fighting, using Western weapons in real battles, using and synchronising different types of weapons. Ukraine needs military, economic and humanitarian support. Infrastructural and economic reconstruction of Ukraine is an integral part of our victory in this war.

Both military and diplomatic ways are important in achieving victory in war. Effective, equal diplomatic negotiations are not possible without success on the battlefield. Just like success at the frontline and the provision of the troops depends on diplomatic work in particular. Consolidation of other countries is important in the fight against an aggressor-state. Strong alliances with third countries are a matter of diplomacy. The only thing where diplomacy is powerless is dialogue with terrorists. Golda Meir is reported as saying, 'You cannot negotiate peace with someone who has come to kill you'.

It is important not to get tired of war. Do not agree to compromises with evil. Support Ukraine, Ukrainians and Ukrainian culture. Every, even the smallest, action is important! The victory of Ukraine is the victory of Europe and European democratic values. (Vira Sverdlyk, personal comment)

Insights from psychologists working in Ukraine

These interviews were undertaken by Svitlana Semaniv, a psychologist currently employed by the London Borough of Sutton to support Ukrainians continuing to support families in Ukraine affected by the war (see Chapter 6).

Victoria Khromets is a psychologist, trainer and PhD candidate in sciences in public administration.

How the war affects the practice:

Currently, all work is organised in an online format. When working with military personnel, consultations may sometimes be conducted through messaging, as they cannot speak freely. In each client meeting, we always agree on what to do in case of an air raid. Efforts are made to set up a workspace in a secure part of the house.

How the war affects people in Ukraine:

Before the war, people had plans and priorities. With the onset of the war, these plans and priorities have changed. In the initial months, the focus was on critical conditions, followed by more inquiries about how to live in this war and how to support oneself. Local people are building daily plans for the short term, with adjustments for various emergencies. They experience a high level of fear and anxiety, and we work on creating instructions for different situations. For instance, a mother might plan and prepare for what her children should do if she passes away. The emotional burnout cases have increased due to the fatigue of living in such conditions.

Working with military personnel is a distinct aspect. It's challenging for them to adapt to normal life after returning from the front, especially for those who were not military before and held various other positions. It's difficult for them to transition into a military mode and accept the fact that they have to kill. Working with military personnel is a specialised field, and we also educate civilians on ecological interaction with the military to facilitate their adaptation.

Olena Maksymiak is a psychologist, supervisor and trainer.

How the war affects the practice:

All work is conducted online for the safety of everyone involved. It was challenging during power outages. Sometimes, to work, I had to drive around the city searching for places to connect to the internet, working from my car. When there is a threat of a missile strike, consultations are conducted from shelters or other secure locations. The war hasn't significantly impacted my practice since I've been in a war context since 2015. I have been working with people from affected areas and military personnel for a long time.

How the war affects people in Ukraine:

For civilians in Ukraine, there aren't many requests about the war at the moment. The war has become a part of Ukrainians' lives, intertwining with stories of love, pregnancy, family planning, and divorce.

Conclusion

The war in Ukraine affects the entire world community. Since the war in Ukraine began, the European Community has consistently seen an increase in defence spending across Europe. This has occurred at a time when European public finances are recovering from the COVID-19 pandemic era and are under enormous pressure from demand for public services such as healthcare, when energy and food prices have soared, and when they are grappling with significant political challenges.

The current political situation is beyond the understanding of traditional theoretical imperatives and classical theories of general and regional development. An analysis of modern political science and sociological literature demonstrates the contradictory approaches to assessing real political and economic events. No theory is the ultimate truth, its conclusions can be questioned and corrected by social practice. A real social process often depends to a decisive extent on very specific actions, it depends on not always well-thought-out decisions and, sometimes, on the irrational motives of the participants in the events themselves. Of particular interest is the reflection of direct participants in military events, and their assessment of their economic and social situation. We interviewed university teachers in Kharkiv, Ukraine. The interview concerned both personal perceptions of what is happening and the fate of education in Ukraine as a whole. Articles by scientists on this issue were also analysed.

From the interviews, the respondents highly appreciated the UK's assistance to Ukraine, especially in the early days of the war, when it was practically impossible to survive without outside help. They note that the UK's supply of several air defence systems, including Starstreak to destroy low-flying air targets at close range, Challenger-2 tanks, artillery systems, multiple launch rocket systems, armoured vehicles and hundreds of thousands of shells and other military equipment allowed the Ukrainian Armed Forces to repel enemy attacks, protect cities and villages, and critical infrastructure from destruction. The UK's support for our military, the provision of military material assistance, the training of command personnel and the supply of necessary modern military equipment indicates that the UK is Ukraine's leading European ally in NATO. Without a doubt, we are very grateful for the understanding of the situation and quick assistance of the former British prime minister, Boris Johnson, in the first, decisive months of the war, for the continuation of the policy of unity with Ukraine by the current prime minister, Rishi Sunak, for the support of British citizens who sheltered more than 100,000 refugees from Ukraine. Our colleagues, who were forced to migrate with the outbreak of hostilities and personally experienced the hospitality of citizens of the UK, are sincerely grateful to them for material and psychological assistance and the creation of favourable opportunities for work and study for their children and ageing parents. They also highly value the responsibility of state authorities for their destiny, for setting an example of high standards of work in a democratic country.

Professor of the Yaroslav Mudryi National Law University, Doctor of Political Sciences Igor Polischuk notes that close contacts between scientists and universities in our countries are aimed at expanding scientific research, forming and strengthening the basis of Western European integration, and supporting the scientific community of Ukraine.

Thus, the significant and multilateral support of Ukraine by Great Britain in such a difficult time for our society, aimed at resisting the military aggression of the Putin dictatorship, is highly valued by Ukrainian citizens and gives confidence in victory.

Comment from Svitlana Semaniv:

From my experience working with Ukrainians inside Ukraine and those living abroad, I can say that those inside Ukraine are coping with the war better. Ukrainians in Ukraine can react to fear and stress during bombings, taking actions like hiding and following instructions. Those abroad struggle as they cannot react when they read and see the news.

There is an increase in inquiries about military personnel from both Ukrainians inside Ukraine and in the UK. People want to know how to address them, what reactions to expect, how to keep them safe, and how to help them. People are experiencing fatigue, but it doesn't affect their zest for life and development. Ukrainians show a commendable trait – adaptability. Despite all obstacles, people continue to move forward.

Note

[1] https://supportukrainenow.org

16

Non-governmental/faith-based approaches to addressing poverty and social exclusion in Europe

Cedric Hills, Johnny Kleman and Raelton Gibbs

Introduction

In the previous volume of this book series, *COVID-19 and Social Determinants of Health: Wicked Issues and Relationalism*, a number of examples of relational partnerships demonstrated the added value of government and non-government organisations (NGOs) working together. These *relational dividends* include financial, administrative, legal and social dividends. Examples of these relational benefits can be seen in partnerships to address poverty, homelessness, human trafficking, domestic abuse, adverse childhood experiences and other wicked issues. Community organisations and small charities are important in addressing these issues, however, as was seen during the COVID-19 pandemic, their viability can be compromised due to reliance on volunteers and charitable funding (O'Leary and Chadha, 2023). During and after COVID-19, there was a haemorrhage of both volunteers and voluntary donations. Large and small charities have struggled, and this led to the fear that thousands of smaller charities across the UK could cease to exist in 2021.[1]

Anchor organisations are large organisations whose long-term sustainability is tied to the wellbeing of the populations that they serve (Anon, 2021). The Salvation Army (TSA) is an anchor organisation from the perspective of more than 150 years of working within communities supporting people at the margins of society (Bonner, 2006). It is currently operating in 135 countries and therefore is particularly well positioned to respond to the global impact of wicked issues such as poverty, climate change adaptation, migration and the flow of refugees from the global south and war zones such as Ukraine. TSA is a faith-based movement and provides the added *relational dividend* in promoting and supporting relationship building and helping people to discover or, in many cases, rediscover a sense of belonging, self-worth and wellbeing.

In 2023, the 135 countries in which TSA operates are managed within 53 territories within five zones: Africa, Americas and Caribbean, Europe, South Asia, and South Pacific and East Asia. TSA has legal registrations in those countries where it works with governmental and other NGOs. The global perspective of Salvation Army-related partnership working will be explored in the fifth publication of this Policy Press series, *Global Determinants of Health in an Unstable World: Drivers of Climate Justice.* In that volume, collaborative working between TSA and world-leading universities will provide a unique insight into a relational approach to promoting health and wellbeing across this divided world, via The Salvation Army International Collaborative University Network.

The Salvation Army in Europe

This chapter will focus on the European zone and TSA's role as a faith-based anchor organisation at a time of increased political and social change in Europe, linked to the direct and indirect impact of the war in Ukraine. TSA, working in the Eastern Europe region, was reconfigured in the early 1990s, however historically TSA in Europe has been addressing the *wicked issues* of poverty alleviation, social and health exclusion, housing and homelessness, migration and refugees since the inception of its work in the UK (1865).

The two world wars, the war in the Balkans, and waves of legal and illegal refugees and human trafficking have all shaped the organisation and its response to changing sociopolitical situations in both the global north and south. This is reflected in the commencement, withdrawal and recommencement of TSA in Europe (see Appendix B).

For some time, TSA activities have taken account of the tension between its work in Russia and the Ukraine. Throughout this period, TSA in both countries has always worked to provide the best support for local communities. This is reflected in changes of administrative support and boundaries with a view to maintaining TSA's objective of giving support where it is needed. TSA has had to practically work out its response to war since the Boer War. From this time through the world wars, it has had to work through that tension between patriotism and internationalism. In trying to steer its way through the many challenges of the wars it was clear that it was pragmatic as well as principled. In an attempt to ensure the internationalism of the movement, 'their refusal to risk giving offence or take sides conveyed at times an impression of moral as well as political neutrality' (Clifton, 2015: xii). This now puts TSA in the unique position of understanding the spiritual and material dimensions of the people it supports, and so the ability to work on both sides of the current conflict, acknowledging that not everybody supports conflict or are free to express their objection. As a movement it has always struggled with the exploitation of the marginalised, both in times of peace and conflict. TSA is unable to practically resource the work in Russia although remaining in constant communication. Its officers and members continue to experience periods of uncertainty, face new challenges, and yet demonstrate a desire to serve their local communities both spiritually and practically.

From an historical perspective, across Europe there have been different responses to the refugee situation influenced by a particular government's response plan, as discussed in other parts of this book. The number of people in transit has presented challenges in how to deal with both those that are passing through to other destinations and those that are settling locally whether for a short or longer term. This chapter will provide a context for TSA response to the war in Europe presented in this chapter. Included are also short case studies to give some context to the current situation.

Soup, soap and salvation, 1914–1945

During the First and Second World Wars, TSA, through its internationalism, provided an 'ambulance unit' in France, canteens to support armed forces in combat and demobilised soldiers and distressed people whose homes had been bombed. It also provided spiritual and practical Christian ministry to German civilian internees, to German military forces and to German prisoners of war all over Europe (Clifton, 2015). This has continued in the movement's response to conflicts throughout the world. In Iraq, for example, TSA, in cooperation with the coalition Provisional Authority, hired contractors to restore more than 50 schools (*All the World*, 2004: 17). When the time came to withdraw in 2003 due to security issues it worked with local employees to form the Iraqi Salvation Humanitarian Organisation, which it continued to mentor for a number of years, ensuring its long-term future.

War in contemporary Europe

A critical reflection of a local–led international response to the war in Europe is presented in Chapter 17. That chapter provides an insight into the direct and strategic response of TSA to the war, underpinned by many conflicts across the globe where TSA has mobilised resources and worked with established TSA community services. Figure 16.1 provides a view of TSA's ongoing country-based support networks in 29 countries around Europe in the TSA Europe zone, with respect to the basic needs of people affected by war – poverty alleviation, housing and homelessness, children and families.

With reference the *social determinants conceptual framework* (see Figure I.1 in the Introduction to this book), poverty, housing and homelessness, support and protection of children and families, and people in transition may be regarded as *intermediate determinants*.

Figure 16.1: Salvation Army activities in Eastern Europe

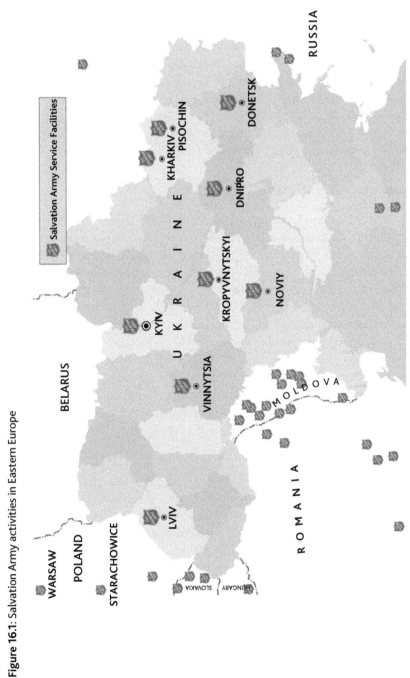

Source: From Salvation Army website, with permission

Poverty alleviation

In these days of economic hardship following the COVID-19 pandemic, a rise in inflation due to conflict and other factors, along with the movement of people, TSA has continued to provide resources for those in poverty. Often in partnership with other organisations it has been important to maintain a balance of support between those moving into an area due to conflict and the local population who are also struggling to survive. During economic crises, studies show that strategic innovation, to support people and communitiestakes place to unexpected threats and situations (Martin-Rios and Pasamar, 2018). Warm welcome spaces and the development of a voucher system in partnership with Sodexo, allowing families to receive goods appropriate for their needs, are examples.

Housing and homelessness

Throughout Europe TSA has developed a comprehensive network of social services, which in many countries have significant expertise working with the homeless. Facilities range from the traditional 'hostel' to 'housing first'. The Netherlands, for example, provides accommodation for 5,267 people, with an additional 70 beds for those seeking substance misuse services. Across the zone, while operating independently in each country, networks meet regularly to share good practice and to develop holistic perspectives of the unique elements of practice offered by the movement.

Children and families

Throughout its existence, TSA has seen the family unit, whatever form it takes, as important, and particularly the welfare of children and young people. Within Europe one of the most excluded groups of people are the Roma. In Slovakia, TSA has developed preschool, kindergarten and community centres close to the Roma settlement in Plavecký Štvrtok, attempting to provide accessibility to preschool education, afterschool activities and social work to both Roma and non-Roma children and families. In the case studies that follow there is strong theme of working with children and families.

Case Study 16.1: Eastern Europe Territory response to the Ukraine War

The Eastern Europe Territory (EET) is made up of five countries, Bulgaria, Georgia, Moldova, Romania and Ukraine. Moldova and Romania border Ukraine and Georgia shares a border with Russia. When Russia invaded Ukraine on 24 February 2022, TSA in Eastern Europe responded in helping both internally and externally displaced people from Ukraine. The work has varied in each of the countries depending on a number of factors, including the size and capacity of TSA in each location, and the spread of where displaced people are located and their needs. There were a number of areas of work that we focused on, which are discussed next.

Meeting the immediate needs of refugees

This includes vouchers, provision of food and cooked meals, practical items (such as blankets, clothing and bed linen), anti-human trafficking information, shelter and a safe place to gather also see Chapter 17.

Children and families

In terms of meeting the needs of children, both immediate needs and activities for children such as camps, clubs and afterschool programmes have been developed. Most of the people that left the country or are displaced are women, children and the elderly, as men aged between 18 and 60 years could not leave and martial law was imposed. Our work focused on meeting their needs for items such as food, including baby food/formula, hygiene items (including nappies and feminine hygiene) and other practical items such as blankets, linen and clothing.

The assistance provided changed over time. At first it was the provision of food and hygiene parcels, but as the war continued vouchers became the major way of providing humanitarian aid in the countries of the EET, with the exception of Ukraine. This was a new way of working in some countries. In Moldova there were limited vouchers available and with the divisional leaders working with companies they were able to source vouchers not only for food and hygiene items, but for clothing, household items (such as linen) and electrical items. In Georgia there was no voucher system that existed and through the work of TSA, this is now in place for food, clothing and hygiene items. With Romania and Bulgaria being European Union (EU) countries, vouchers were in place and therefore easily accessible.

Having vouchers was beneficial to recipients as they were able to purchase what they needed to suit their individual situations. TSA did not need to store items or create packages for people, which saved time and money. The recipients liked the vouchers, particularly if they needed specific items due to dietary requirements or items for babies who had allergies to certain formulas. The vouchers gave people dignity and empowered them to make choices for their families that met their needs.

Children became a focus and, where possible, children were invited to come to existing programmes such as scouts, afterschool and kids' clubs. This was true for Moldova and

Georgia, as they share Russian as a common language. It was more problematic in Romania and Bulgaria as the languages and alphabets are completely different. However, children and adults have been invited to share in existing programmes that some have chosen to do and found very beneficial.

Some programmes were developed specifically for children from the Ukraine, such as summer/winter camps and afterschool clubs to learn the local language and culture.

TSA in Georgia has held camps specifically for Ukrainian children, one in the summer and one in winter. The camps had great impact for those who attended. There is a story relayed from Georgia regarding a child who was very unsettled, not sleeping well, had feelings of isolation and was angry due to leaving home and friends. As they attended the camp, they met other children who shared similar experiences. They gained new friends and continued to keep contact after the camp, so the feelings of isolation diminished. The parents reported that their child was more settled and slept much better and was less angry after attending the camp. This is only one story, but it has been reported by a number of parents the impact the camps had on their children and that it was more than just having a good time. It helped them settle into their new life and the sense of isolation and frustration at the circumstances lessened and they were coping much better.

Activities for women have been expanded. In Bulgaria, while children's activities are going on, there has been a place for women to share in crafts. They have found it good to meet with other women and share similar experiences where they can find a safe place to talk about and gain assistance in finding solutions to presenting issues.

Due to the small size of TSA in the EET, volunteers have helped with the work undertaken in assisting refugees. A number of Ukrainians have now volunteered to assist in this capacity. They help with sorting donated goods as well as in the distribution of vouchers. At one TSA community church in Chisinau (Moldova), Ukrainian volunteers not only helped with the distribution of vouchers, they helped local children by purchasing and donating toys for Christmas. This is helping to build strong relationships in the communities that TSA is working in. The impact of the work of TSA may not have been seen for many years. Children who have attended activities, whether they are a one-off, or longer-term activities such as afterschool programmes, have become more settled in the country they are living in and have found friends who share similar situations. This has helped both their physical and mental health. Women who have shared in activities have also found friends, a safe place to gather and are feeling less isolated. They feel that they are more able to cope with situations they find themselves in. They have somewhere to go to chat about things and know that their children are enjoying activities.

People in transition

Within Europe the large movement of people has led to different political responses, and while this is a constantly changing picture, the following case studies outline TSA experience in Poland and Latvia.

Case Study 16.2: The Salvation Army Poland region response to the Ukraine refugee crisis

The invasion of Ukraine by Russia has led to a humanitarian and refugee crisis on a massive scale. Sharing a 500km land border with Ukraine and situated on the far side of the country and away from the immediate area of conflict, Poland was an obvious choice for families fleeing danger.

Poland is the largest country on the North Atlantic Treaty Organization's eastern flank. It is quite easy for refugees to move freely in both directions and many Ukrainians have friends or family in the country. On 24 February 2022 Poland was transformed into a country hosting one of the largest refugee populations in the world. In March 2022, the International SOS organisation stated that '[t]he Polish border has the highest transit rate and the most simplified document requirements. Entry is permitted to anyone fleeing armed conflict in Ukraine, even without documents'. Not surprisingly, therefore, United Nations High Commissioner for Refugees figures of July 2023 report that over 13 million Ukrainians have crossed the border into Poland since the start of the conflict. Checkpoints at border crossings are mainly located in the Subcarpathian area, southeastern Poland. There are as many as nine of them, facilitating entry into Poland by car, on foot or in some cases by trail. While more than 11 million have since crossed back into Ukraine, the huge number seeking either temporary or permanent refuge and safety in the country represent great need and diverse challenges. In context, Poland's pre-conflict population was around 40 million.

TSA in Poland is small, just four corps (churches) with a handful of officers (ministers) and few volunteers. The officers and members quickly found themselves facing a situation they had neither prepared nor trained for. Feeling initially overwhelmed, TSA in Poland was delighted to receive support from a small number of experienced emergency workers, deployed from the organisation's International Headquarters (IHQ).

One of the early deployees, Major Bill Barthau (Canada), recognised that the displaced community in this conflict were largely female, mothers, the elderly and children. Along with local TSA members, Bill visited the border where trains were arriving with refugees and watched as they disembarked in confusion. They made their way out of the station, where tents had been previously erected to offer food and clothing. Other tents offered a place to rest for those who had nowhere to go. Bill went with a Polish TSA officer to a church which was sheltering 90 refugees where some had arrived wounded, needing first aid.

Another member of the early international team, Captain Matthew Beatty (IHQ), also witnessed the efficiency of the set up at the border, reporting that the Polish border reception centres for refugees were well run and well stocked with food.

The methodology of TSA is usually to assess needs, identify gaps in provision and focus on, in coordination with other agencies, those unmet needs. With the initial needs of incoming refugees apparently met by government, other organisations and agencies, TSA began to help in a different way. Due to the flexibility of EU regulations, Ukrainians entering Poland were permitted to seek employment and apply for social security benefits. New arrivals could access a one-time cash payment through the UN refugee agency before commencing the registration process with the Polish social security system.

The first emergency payment was processed quickly and efficiently, but approval to access the social security system could take up to two months, leaving families waiting in limbo for their second cash payment. There was a significant gap in between, leaving families temporarily vulnerable. A study conducted by the University of Warsaw's Centre for East European Studies and the EWL Foundation for Support of Migrants on the Labour Market showed that 78 per cent of Ukrainians in Poland were employed.[2]

Others had destinations outside of Poland in mind, so used Poland as a temporary staging point before moving on quickly. To support those choosing to remain, and who found themselves without work or other means of support, TSA quickly established a cash voucher distribution programme.

The initial (rapid response) emergency grant from IHQ supplied the four TSA centres with US$20,000 each in store vouchers that they could allocate to families or individuals. These vouchers were purchased through the international supermarket chain, Lidl. With branches located throughout the country, refugees could shop as they wished, purchasing items that they themselves prioritised, giving them the dignity of personal choice, and the same flexibility as members of the local population. During the ten-month period (March–December 2022) 14,600 individuals were provided with Lidl shopping vouchers.

Other important non-food items included hygiene items, clothing, shoes, infant supplies, blankets and toys. Supplies of these items were either purchased or collected and more than 15 shelters/refugee camps were visited and assisted with supplies.

The Polish city of Rzeszów is located only 85km from the Krakowiec checkpoint on the border with Ukraine. The TSA church leader, Captain Ryszard Potocki, and church members regularly visited neighbouring refugee shelters. Potocki reported:

> On June 25, we visited a refugee centre in Radymno, near Przemyśl. The shelter accommodates more than 200 people, adults and children. We could see immediately how great the needs are to support such a large group of people. We bought items in one of the local supermarkets, mainly food and cleaning products for the residents of this shelter, along with our Lidl food vouchers. Our help is highly appreciated. As always, there is an opportunity to talk to the residents and bring words of hope and comfort.

As the conflict continued, inflation of almost 15 per cent[3] contributed to the challenges of supporting refugees. Increasing costs, combined with public donor fatigue and reductions in statutory assistance, exacerbated the difficulty of sustaining support to refugee families. In this context, the grocery card programme, which continues to this day (July 2023) has been warmly welcomed.

At this time (February 2024), food assistance continues and, in Starachowice, 300 Ukrainian refugees receive food packages every month. In Rzeszów, following a distribution of pillows, sleeping bags and hygiene kits, TSA received a civic award, acknowledging the support provided to the refugee shelters in the area. Special regulations, introduced very quickly into the conflict, provided refugees with access to social security, the labour market and healthcare. Additionally, many families receive additional support through being permitted to apply to nurseries and schools. These measures, provided by the Polish government, supported refugees in finding some normality in this far from normal situation.

The TSA church (corps) in Warsaw has a unique advantage in that the corps leader, Captain Oleg Samoilenko, is a Ukrainian national who moved to Poland with his Polish wife just a few years ago. As a Ukrainian, his recent experience of relocating meant he was able to empathise with the challenges of official bureaucracy. A translation service was established, which ran alongside the Polish language classes. Each application for paperwork must be supported with photographs, so a project has been created with a local photography studio to provide official photos. The TSA family centre that was established just a few hundred metres from the corps building in the Prague district of Warsaw became a haven for confused families, while also being inundated with enquiries and requests for help. Captain Oleg testified to the emotional challenges he faced when confronted by families from his hometown, or people registering home addresses that he personally knew. His own extended family was impacted, with his mother and aunt making their way across the border to join them in Warsaw. These family members now work along Oleg in caring for Ukrainian families.

As the TSA anti-human trafficking contact person, Captain Oleg worked with local contacts to organise five anti-human trafficking workshops for Ukrainian women. Alongside the workshops a photo exhibition was set up in the shopping mall of Warsaw, featuring photos depicting the theme 'I work in Poland legally'.

The goal of providing a 'home from home' for those viewing their time in Poland as temporary, or the challenge of helping newcomers to integrate and develop long-term roots, was readily grasped by our four corps (churches).

Despite the congregations being small, each of the TSA churches organised activities for Ukrainian refugees. These included children's clubs, meetings for ladies, Polish language classes, information points and afterschool programmes. In addition to psychosocial counselling, TSA has been pleased to offer spiritual support. The small congregations have been boosted by the influx of worshippers from Ukraine, with some becoming formal church members.

One unexpected problem was created by the uniforms and official insignia. As the national name of TSA is Armia Zbawienia, uniforms in Poland bear the letter Z on epaulettes. As this letter has been adopted by the Russian military for their vehicles, the sight of uniformed workers wearing a 'Z' was quickly felt to be unhelpful. Therefore, all 'Z' logos were banned in Poland, with salvationists switching to the more internationally recognised 'S' symbol!

Reflecting on the experiences of the previous 18 months, several lessons have been learned.

A coordination workshop involved TSA strategic leaders was held in January 2023, see Figure 16.2. Training of officers and workers is vital if they are to respond effectively at times of disaster and emergency. A training course held in September 2023. With good planning and organisation, significant work can be undertaken – even by a small team.

Figure 16.2: Planning workshop, 27–28 January 2023

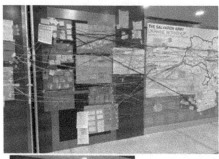

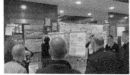

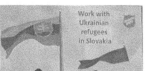

TSA is one part of a larger response, you cannot help everyone, but coordinating with others allows opportunities to maximise the impact.

At times of disaster, TSA is not alone, the support given by the international network of TSA territories has proved invaluable. Nurturing those relationships and developing good communication links is vital. Refugees are not simply communities requiring support. They come with their own strengths and resources. We harness those, and integrate them into their surroundings, and they can greatly enhance our churches and communities.

Case Study 16.3: The Salvation Army in Latvia and assistance of Ukrainian refugees

Stage 1

Latvia is a former Soviet Republic with borders to both Russia and Belarus and the Polish border not far away. With that geographical position, Latvia quickly became a common destination for refugees, particularly from the eastern part of Ukraine seeking shelter when the Russian full-scale invasion of Ukraine began. Since a large percentage (around 30 per cent in the country, and higher in the capital city of Riga) of the population are native Russian speakers, Latvia became an attractive country of escape where the refugees knew there was a possibility of making themselves understood and where there was a higher possibility of finding work in their own language. TSA in the Latvia region began helping Ukrainian refugees when members of the public began donating food, clothes and hygiene products at the regional headquarters in Riga. The regional leadership quickly took the initiative to let officers and other staff, many of whom speak Russian, take turns in distributing the donated goods to the Ukrainian refugees. At the same time TSA was able to make available some of its apartments for refugee families needing emergency accommodation. Because of this immediate response, word quickly spread that TSA was caring for Ukrainian refugees and soon both the donations as well as those seeking help increased dramatically. A small team of volunteers, mostly made up of Christians from different churches in Riga, were soon organised to assist with the distribution of clothes, hygiene items and food. By the end of March 2022, TSA in Riga was granted financial support from the International Salvation Army to be able to purchase food and hygiene items, since the donated food was no longer enough to meet the demand from the many thousands of Ukrainian refugees arriving in Latvia.

Stage 2

In May 2023 the next step of the Ukrainian refugee work began when a person, herself a Ukrainian refugee, started helping as a volunteer, again thanks to support from the

International Salvation Army, and was employed to coordinate the growing assistance programme. Starting around this time a programme was developed where refugees could get help with food, hygiene items and clothes. Being Ukrainian herself, the new coordinator had a wide reach, and was able to recruit many volunteers (themselves refugees from Ukraine) who, on a rotational basis, took turns sorting clothes, packing food products into bags and helping with the distributions. Volunteers who previously had worked as hairdressers were also recruited and organised to offer free hair-cutting appointments for refugees. As the work and time progressed, it became clear that the needs were not limited to the basic things such as food and clothes but there was also a need for emotional and psychological support – particularly for those who had been living in Latvia for a longer time and were slowly realising that they probably would not be able to return to Ukraine as soon as they had first hoped to. To tackle the psychological issues many refugees were facing, a psychologist, also a Ukrainian, was employed to offer free counselling for any refugees who so desired. The psychologist has been able to help many who are dealing with issues such as survivor's guilt, post-traumatic stress syndrome and other issues caused by the often-traumatic escape from the war. As well as beginning to offer psychological help, TSA noticed that there was a growing need to help with the more practical needs of those who needed to set up a new life for themselves in Riga, developing the work to also include distributing furniture, child strollers, kitchen utensils and bedding – often things donated by the public.

As of September 2023, many thousands of Ukrainian refugees have received help, physically, emotionally and psychologically through the TSA refugee centre in Riga. We have also seen some of them attending the corps (church) Sunday services where relationships develop with their spiritual family.

Future activities

The current work with Ukrainian refugees will come to an end by December 2023, due to both changing needs and less funding from abroad. Discussions regarding how to transform the work into a longer-term community programme, focused not only on catering to immediate needs but also on longer-term integration, has been ongoing.

Conclusion

Building on William Booth's vision

In the previous publication of this series, *COVID-19 and Social Determinants of Health: Wicked Issues and Relationalism*, McCombe and Pallant (McCombe and Pallant, 2023) provided a review of TSA operating as a church and charity to provide faith-based response to contemporary *social evils* in the UK, including innovative approaches to welfare reform and debt advice, unemployment, human trafficking and modern slavery, homelessness, supporting people with drug and alcohol problems in the community, children and youth priorities and providing for older people's care. TSA Mission Service Units, with the capacity to respond to the complex multiple issues experienced by many of the people, have been working with the *whole person perspective*. The social evils, addressed by William Booth in the landmark publication, *In Darkest England and the Way Out*, are now recognised as *wicked issues*.[4]

From the perspective of the *social determinants conceptual framework*, the need for the (soft) *intermediate* structures, provided by organisations such as TSA, to work with the hard *structural determinants* of public and private partnerships in promoting health and reinvigorating communities was highlighted by Chasteauneuf et al (2020). Many years of providing *relational support* by TSA has resulted in the development of psychologically informed environments to understand a person's real needs and agreeing on a journey of recovery with a focus on their personal strengths, based on an asset-based approach to supporting people in their communities.

The tradition of TSA has core Christian values (see Chapters 5 and 15), maintaining a stance that its services are offered without discrimination. The faith-based elements, while not suggesting it is better than traditional services, does offer a framework that is attractive to communities where faith is an integral part of their society (see Chapter 18). It is legitimate to indicate that people have benefited from traditional services but with the opportunity to explore religious and spiritual issues, there is the opportunity to understand and address mental health issues. This enhances the outcomes and assists in their integration back into society (Gibbs, 2013).

Social justice

Ongoing research led by Sir Michael Marmot[5] clearly shows that health and social disadvantage in people at the lower end of the social gradient are exacerbated, particularly during the COVID-19 pandemic, by low self-esteem and poor self-image, significantly impacted by adverse childhoods, employment opportunities, poverty and other socio-environmental factors. TSA aims to have a strategic voice to advocate for promoting human dignity and social justice. The TSA Europe zone is tasked to resource, support and bring together those on the front line to participate in making a difference. The support of the other four TSA zones (Africa, America and the Caribbean, South Asia and South Pacific and West Pacific) enables this international organisation to play a significant role with other NGOs and faith-based organisations in addressing global issues such as the war in Europe.

The next chapter provides a *structural determinant* perspective of *locally led* initiatives, providing *intermediate* support, from an international organisation, The Salvation Army.

Notes

[1] https://www.bbc.co.uk/news/uk-54754902

[2] https://tvpworld.com/69902996/nearly-80-of-ukrainian-refugees-in-poland-are-emplo yed-survey

[3] https://www.worlddata.info/europe/poland/inflation-rates.php

[4] '[D]ifficult or impossible to solve because of incomplete, contradictory, and changing requirements, and not resolved by traditional "technical" managerial approaches to the provision of public services' (Rittel and Webber, 1973; see Chapters 1 and 2 in *COVID-19 and Social Determinants of Health: Wicked Issues and Relationalism*).

[5] https://www.ucl.ac.uk/news/2022/sep/marmot-review-thousands-will-die-and-milli ons-will-suffer-humanitarian-crisis-fuel-poverty

References

All the World (2004) April–June.

Anon (2021) *The Health Foundation*. Available at: https://www.health.org. uk/news-and-comment/charts-and-infographics/the-nhs-as-an-anchor-institution.

Bonner, A.B. (2006) *Social Exclusion and the Way Out*. Chichester: John Wiley and Son.

Chasteauneuf, T., Thornton, T. and Pallant, D. (2020) *Local Authorities and Social Determinants of Health*.

Clifton, S. (2015) *Crown of Glory, Crown of Thorns: The Salvation Army in Wartime*. London: Salvation Books, pp 282–307.

Gibbs, R. (2013) *Standing in the Shadows: Faith, Homelessness and Troubled Lives* [Professional Doctorate Thesis]. Tavistock and Portman NHS Foundation Trust.

Martin-Rios, C. and Pasamar, S. (2018) Service innovation in times of economic crisis: the strategic adaption activities of the top EU service firms. *R & D Management*, 48(2): 195–209.

McCombe, D. and Pallant, D. (2023) Wicked issues: a faith-based perspective. In A. Bonner (ed), *COVID-19 and Social Determinants of Health: Wicked Issues and Relationalism*. Bristol: Policy Press.

O'Leary, C. and Chadha, R. (2023) Volunteering and small charities. In A. Bonner (ed), *COVID-19 and Social Determinants of Health: Wicked Issues and Relationalism*. Bristol: Policy Press, pp 258–268.

17

A critical reflection of a locally led international response to the war in Europe

Joanne Beale, Damaris Frick, Richard Bradbury and Ivor Telfer

Introduction

When Russian forces invaded Ukraine in February 2022 The Salvation Army (TSA), having been in the country since 1993, responded not only in Ukraine but also to TSA operations in 29 countries around Europe which received refugees or offered cross-border support. Many more TSA territories in countries across the world offered financial assistance to these initiatives. This was a natural response for an organisation which, being both a church and an international movement, has justice and care for the vulnerable at the core of its mission. TSA has notably responded to the Rwandan genocide, Gulf War and the world wars. However, the world has changed since the movement began in the 1860s in the east end of London and we are now more acutely aware than ever of the need to listen to local voices and facilitate locally led and locally skilled initiatives.

Through the lens of Linking Relief, Rehabilitation and Development (LRRD) this chapter will reflect on the response of TSA to the war in Europe. Exploring lessons learnt from previous responses to the situation of forcefully displaced people, it will explore how lessons learned influenced TSA's response to the Ukraine situation. Following on from Chapter 16 this chapter presents the localised response to the war in Ukraine and the bordering countries. This strategic focus will be reviewed in Chapter 19, from the perspective of resourcing and capacity development required to enable adequate action and analyses how the breadth of programmes tries to respond to various stages of the LRRD spectrum. It will look at the establishment of a Ukraine Response Unit at TSA International Headquarters (IHQ) and how the TSA International Emergency Services (IES) team and International Development Services (IDS) team are collaborating with those closest to the war to provide the international perspective to a localised response.

A global movement

TSA is active in 134 countries across the world. In countries that are financially independent (meaning they can raise the funds they need to operate in their home country) social services and community initiatives are mostly managed within the structure of the organisation in that country. However, in countries that require external support to maintain their operations to run projects, a more complex network of stakeholders emerges. The General, the global leader of TSA, is based at the IHQ and is supported by staff and other TSA ministers (officers). IHQ facilitates the distribution of funding across the world, coordinating those who should contribute and those who should receive support. In IHQ the Programme Resources department houses the IES and IDS teams which exist to coordinate and facilitate, among other things, the 2,000+ active externally supported projects across the world with a portfolio value of almost US$200 million. The two teams by necessity have different ways of working: In an emergency the focus is on releasing funds as quickly as possible to countries where the emergency has occurred based on a rapid needs assessment in order to enable a rapid response to disaster events. In a development context, however, the focus is on rigorous and appropriate programme designs which meet the long-term needs of communities and catalyse lasting change with projects supported by technical specialists in the countries providing the financial support for projects, managed financially via IHQ. It is unusual for IES and IDS to work together as closely as they had to in the first two years following the Russian invasion in Ukraine and this chapter aims to reflect on that.

Within TSA, countries with a smaller presence are grouped into territories for the purpose of management and coordination. TSA Eastern Europe Territory (EET) comprises the countries of Ukraine, Moldova, Romania, Bulgaria, and Georgia. The work of TSA in these countries has developed more recently than in other European countries (see Appendix B). Work in Ukraine and Georgia commenced in 1993, with Moldova in 1994, Romania in 1999 and Bulgaria in 2023. TSA in EET is still small, with 38 churches offering community work, just over 2,000 members and 94 officers across these five countries.

As an international church and charity, TSA IES works with other organisations, in the case of Romania this includes the Bucharest municipality, UN organisations such as UNHCR, other international and local NGOs such as the International Federation as well as business and the private sector such as IKEA. These organisations include the International Federation of Red Cross, World Vision, Salvati Copii, Good Neighbours Japan, Hebrew Immigrant Aid Society, Save the Children Community Organized Relief Efforts and IKEA.

TSA is a member of ACT Alliance, a global faith-based coalition organised in national and regional forums operating in more than 120 countries.[1]

Case Study 17.1: Locally led responses to forced migration, 1970–2024

Since its establishment TSA has been responding to the needs of forcefully displaced people. The organisation has a long history of providing practical, emotional and spiritual assistance to people fleeing conflict, violence, persecution, natural disasters and poverty. In 1896 it responded to the Armenian crisis, it supported displaced people through both world wars, the Spanish Civil War and also welcomed and assisted people fleeing Vietnam and arriving in the UK in the late 1970s (The Salvation Army International, 2020).

The genocide in Rwanda and TSA's response to it resulted in the creation of a specialist section at IHQ which was initially named International Emergency and Refugee Services. In Europe the work of this section included the response to the conflict in Bosnia and the support to returning internally displaced people from 1996 to 1999. Over three and a half years, TSA implemented a multifaceted emergency and recovery programme, including emergency feeding and clothing programmes, stove distribution, home and livelihood reconstruction, school and clinic rehabilitation, various agricultural inputs and micro-credit schemes. When hundreds of thousands of refugees poured into Albania from Kosovo in 1999 TSA responded with immediate food and non-food items at the border crossings. A bit later TSA teams were deployed to refugee camps in Tirana, Korce and close to Durres to provide hot meals. Close to 50,000 refugees were being fed by TSA.

In 2015:

> [T]he influx of refugees and migrants [into Europe] had reached staggering new levels ... dominating headlines and prompting stormy political debate. The main route shifted from the dangerous Mediterranean crossing from Libya to Italy, to what would prove to be an even deadlier crossing from Turkey to Greek islands like Lesvos. Tragedy propelled the issue to centre stage on the European agenda, and the sheer weight of numbers ... kept it there for months. (Spindler, 2015)

TSA in other countries in Europe responded as well but a lot of attention was on Greece, a country where the organisation only had a small presence in Athens and Thessaloniki. Despite their small numbers, church leaders and volunteers in Athens immediately started to provide assistance to some of the thousands of refugees who had fled to Greece from North Africa and the Middle East. The response in Greece as well as other countries in Europe was supported by IES financially but also with the deployment of short-term relief personnel and with technical expertise and advice. In the first half of 2015 up to 1,500 people were arriving every week at the Port of Pireas, Athens, with many setting up unofficial camps in the centre of Athens (The Salvation Army, 2015). *The New Internationalist* reported:

> The Salvation Army of Athens has seen first hand the predicament of these families. It supports nearly 1,000 refugees every day, going to the main squares

and parks each morning to hand out donated food, bottled water and other essentials. In the evenings, a team of volunteers prepares hundreds of sandwiches to be distributed to impoverished people throughout the city. (Freitas, 2015)

At the beginning most refugees arriving in Greece tried to travel through the country as fast as possible in the hope of reaching countries like Germany or Sweden. After an initial phase of fairly unhindered travel from Greece to Central and Northern Europe, various countries later closed their borders and refugees were stuck in the country. Reacting to this changed situation, TSA adjusted its response from the initial provision of relief items to assist people on the move to longer-term integration support and case management.

The case workers were actively involved in tracking the trends and challenges facing asylum seekers in Greece. In collaboration with other agencies, the case workers assisted asylum seekers to find suitable shelter or assisted to cover some of the initial costs of housing.

Another focus was on maternal and infant health and nutrition. In coordination with midwives from other organisations, each mother and infant was evaluated and the best possible support, including breast feeding support or the provision of formula milk and other baby products, was determined. In partnership with local surgeons and hospital staff willing to donate their time and operating rooms after hours, TSA also assisted with referral services for urgent medical care. Often the case workers worked with family members to seek solutions and advocate on behalf of clients to other local and government agencies. Other assistance included computer and budgeting courses, sewing workshops and assistance with translation or official documentation.

Strong relationships and partnerships with other groups such as UNHCR, Apostoli, UN International Organization for Migration and Armutel ensured that TSA's focus and objectives were in line with the needs identified. The inter-agency relationships were strengthened through this response.

The atmosphere and attitude towards refugees had changed in Greece and across Europe and so had the needs, but the local TSA still did what they do best, meeting human needs of the person in front of them without judgement, expectation or discrimination.

The theory behind the practice: Linking Relief, Rehabilitation and Development

In a foreword for a 2013 study by the Netherlands Ministry of Foreign Affairs, Prof Dr Ruerd Ruben wrote:

Linking relief, rehabilitation and development (LRRD) is not a new subject. The 'gap', as it is called, between humanitarian aid and development is something which has been discussed by policy-makers, development practitioners and aid workers for decades. ... Yet, as comprehensive evaluations ... have shown, many fundamental challenges to linking short-term, emergency aid to longer-term, sustainable development still remain today. (IOB, 2013)

When commencing LRRD, any emergency includes both emergency and development practitioners. Good practice suggests that this should be the normal practice in all emergency situations, as aid given inappropriately can lead to problems in the later development phases. LRRD commences with the first delivery of aid.

However, at a TSA Community Based Disaster Preparedness Conference in Hong Kong in 2016, one of the recommendations was that Disaster Risk Reduction be included in all project proposals and all activities that take place in communities. There was an agreement that aid programmes without consideration of long-term implications can cause problems for development activities later. However, in conversations between development and humanitarian practitioners it was found that problems also arise from the other side, with development programmes not considering hazards and risk factors and therefore contributing to a population's vulnerability towards disasters. Disaster Risk Reduction will be more successful if the components of LRRD noted earlier are implemented as part of all community development programmes. In this way, when a disaster strikes, resilience is already being built up and will enable the community to respond more effectively to the impact of the disaster.

The diagram in Figure 17.1 was created in 2021 and shared internally within TSA. Before the theory could be debated further the opportunity to put it into practice was presented through the war in Europe. The main strands of LRRD and the definitions used by TSA are shown in the figure. The figure shows the 'pathway' for LRRD – it is not a straight line and steps will not automatically follow one another as communities will be starting the LRRD process from different points. Additionally, the pathway will never end, as prevention, preparedness and mitigation will continue after each disaster and will in turn be included in community development programmes, continually building increased resilience. Embedding this pathway in the way TSA approaches its work will require a more *agile and adaptive* management approach, which is able to flex to the constantly changing environments and timeline in which it is operating.

In the case of the response to the arrival of refugees in Greece the shift from rapid response to initial case management happened quite smoothly as TSA on the ground continued the partnerships that were built during

Figure 17.1: Linking Relief, Rehabilitation and Development

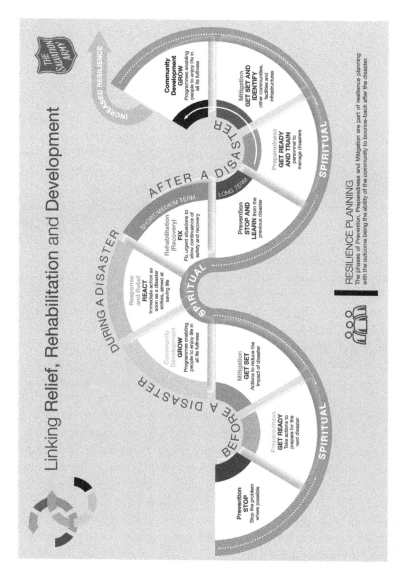

Source: Adapted from IOB (2013)

the rapid response phase. However, complications emerged later with changes of personnel on the ground, at IHQ, within other organisations and with a larger number of TSA development offices involved more directly. Different people and different offices came with different focus areas, technical expertise and expectations. In addition to this there was now less media attention as well as fewer unrestricted donations from The Salvation Army's own fundraising efforst which allowed a great flexibility during the response phase.

The Ukraine crisis: the local response

As noted in Chapter 15, '[t]he Russian invasion of Ukraine has caused civilian casualties and destruction of civilian infrastructure, forcing people to flee their homes seeking safety, protection and assistance. Millions of refugees from Ukraine have crossed borders into neighbouring countries, in addition to those displaced inside the country' (UNHCR, 2023).

Echoing the way that TSA responded in the past, and with the escalation of the 2014 Russo Ukrainian war in February 2022, TSA across Europe responded to this humanitarian crisis quickly and in many cases very spontaneously (see Chapter 16). In Romania, within a few hours of the invasion, a small team drove for seven hours from Bucharest to the Ukrainian border with supplies of food and clothing to assist refugees. Similar support was given from the other four countries of the EET as well as Hungary, Slovakia and others.

Response activities began immediately and continue until today. This includes efforts in Romania where the TSA colleagues joined the inter-agency response at border crossings to provide urgently needed relief items but also to share human-trafficking awareness information with people arriving in the country. In Moldova, TSA churches prepared their church halls and community centres with foldable beds, mattresses and bedding material to provide temporary, safe accommodation and a chance for people fleeing the war to rest, wash themselves and their clothes before continuing their journey to other European countries. In Ukraine itself the TSA utilised its eight church locations as shelters, as places of warmth and comfort, as places where people could receive hot meals and food parcels. Members and volunteers also used their kitchens at home to prepare food and snacks which were distributed and shared at train stations to people fleeing. Hundreds were provided with shelter in the early days of the war. More than 50,000 food and non-food parcels were provided in the first 18 months, together with over 4,000 children's activities, safe spaces for group conversations, online connections for schooling and many more local activities being provided in Ukraine, through these eight TSA churches (corps). TSA is typically at its best in locally-led initiatives of individuals and church groups seeing a need and responding to it very quickly and utilising all available resources. In an emergency, this would normally last for a period of weeks, perhaps months. As this is an ongoing war situation, the response phase in some areas and at some times is still necessary, as new IDPs and refugees appear. The harsh winters in Ukraine together with new bombardments and challenges with utilities cause a new influx of those in need.

To coordinate this work, on day one of the war, TSA-EET headquarters in Moldova collaborated with the five TSA country leaders, in daily briefings, guiding the centralised EET in response to the growing concern and numbers of refugees, together with internally displaced people in Ukraine.

As time went on and the immediate lifesaving activities were established, it became evident that refugees in the countries of the EET needed ongoing support. To address the provision of food, clothing and hygiene needs, and to enable the refugees to retain their dignity, a new voucher system was introduced. This was piloted in Moldova with two large supermarket chains being chosen to service the vouchers. TSA concentrated on supporting the children as other non-governmental organisations, international non-governmental organisations and churches supported in different ways. TSA gave a voucher to the mother (as most men had to remain in Ukraine) for each child which could be spent on whatever they felt was needed. This system was piloted in Romania where, because of TSA's prompt response, TSA was requested by the Romanian government to set up alongside UNHCR and government agencies in the large Romexpo building, supplying vouchers to parents for children. A similar voucher programme was then introduced in Georgia, which until that time had never used vouchers. These programmes are ongoing.

In Georgia, Moldova, Romania and Ukraine, in addition to the voucher support, children's winter and summer camps have been provided, allowing refugee children to mix with local children and commence their rehabilitation after the stresses of evacuation and war. Additional support in Georgia includes legal clinics in a TSA church, Ukrainian women cooking Ukrainian food for other refugees, and self-help and facilitated discussion groups.

Although the response of the first months had primarily been in the form of accommodation, food relief and personal items, referral services, vouchers and human-trafficking awareness, it is apparent that the destruction of homes and buildings in Ukraine is extensive (see Chapter 15). It became evident that a much more robust and comprehensive strategy to address the safety and wellbeing of the affected families was needed in the long term. In addition to emergency relief activities (which in some locations might continue for the foreseeable future) there are now already longer-term social and development activities, and, at some point, there will be the work of recovery, reconciliation and reconstruction in Ukraine, both on community level but also with regards to TSA property and churches.

Until this point all these initiatives were designed by those working on the ground who were experiencing the need for themselves and hearing from those who would be receiving support. Those people were mostly TSA ministers, not trained in disasters nor community development. It was a truly locally led response. However, as response moved to rehabilitation in some countries, TSA recognised that the activities were becoming more specialised and that there was need for external technical support.

The issue of mental health and psychosocial support (MHPSS) is high on the agenda for the Ukrainian government, UN organisations and TSA. As the conflict continues with no signs of a cessation, TSA has prioritised the addition of further MHPSS activities using an adapted version of the Pyramid of Intervention (IASC, 2007), as shown in Figure 17.2. As an organisation TSA seeks to add to the existing work in the bottom two categories of the MHPSS pyramid and also offer more focused non-specialist support.

The *response phase* is ongoing in some situations and reoccurs due to weather, increase in hostilities or country challenges. However, in addition to this support – as a community-based church – *rehabilitation and prevention* with increased MHPSS is vital. This will assist in longer-term community development and resilience when the war concludes. To be able to embrace this work EET has seen the need to recruit someone with expertise in this area to work within the territory.

Since the start of the war over 90 projects totalling almost US$14.5 million have been funded and are either completed or underway in the five countries

Figure 17.2: Mental health and psychosocial support pyramid

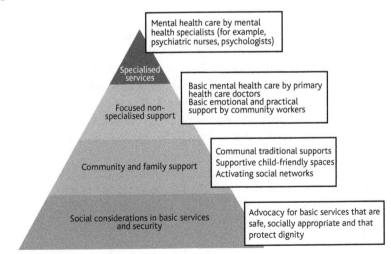

Source: Adapted from IASC (2007)

of the EET. Most of these projects are responsive, including meeting winterisation needs. However, as we move forward, the response element, which is still necessary, has been supplemented by mitigation activities to enable children to have fun, build relationships with other children from Ukraine and from host countries. Further activities including language classes and support for school requisites have also been implemented in an attempt to reduce the impact of the war on their young lives (see Chapter 7). The increased focus on MHPSS is an effort to mitigate the impacts of family separation, trauma, language challenges and stress, and has been included by giving a safe space to Ukrainians to meet each other, chat, cook and eat Ukrainian food and bring some sense of community life and normality. The volunteering of Ukrainian women to assist in food and voucher provision from TSA facilities has been a much needed help and has been very beneficial to those receiving help but also for the mental and psychosocial support of the volunteers. It has equally been important to ensure the mental and emotional wellbeing of our staff and officers and TSA internationally has helped to fund activities, such as retreats, for those implementing the response.

In the EET, from a pre-war budget of US$1.8 million and only three development projects being implemented, the considerable increase in funds coming through the headquarters posed a significant challenge for a small local organisation. This speaks to the preparedness part of the LRRD pathway. It was fortunate in this case that a development staff member had been appointed to the territory a month before the war broke out. Had she not been there, the response would not have been as large or as successful. This sudden increase in programmatic and financial responsibility in what was a very small headquarters was and still is a huge challenge. While the response itself could be locally driven it needed international support and coordination and this was provided through IHQ and the creation of a Ukraine Response Unit.

The Ukraine crisis: international coordination

From the earliest days of the crisis the TSA IES team, based at its IHQ in London, worked alongside the EET Territorial Leaders to provide the coordination, administration, technical and project support to the country leaders and responders in Ukraine and neighbouring countries. Since the beginning of the war, IES not only provided the operational support for the response, it also arranged for the deployment and management (pre, during and post) of trained and experienced international personnel to support the local relief initiatives, the logistical support regarding warehousing and transportation of relief items into Ukraine through Poland as well as the coordination of the requirements and expectations of the donors and funders.

In addition to almost daily meetings with various project/development officers on the ground, IES used a range of responses in different countries, including deploying teams and working with funders, individuals and businesses who offered to donate relief items and other stakeholders. The IES team at the London headquarters also supported the communication efforts of the response. New initiatives and programmes such as cash- and voucher-based assistance were set up in several countries and stronger partnerships with governments, local and international non-governmental organisations, church networks and other stakeholders were built. At the time of writing the international TSA supported over 120 projects in 14 countries. Many more activities and programmes are run, managed and funded locally.

As the crisis in the Ukraine grew and refugees travelled further into Europe activities in 29 (TSA) countries across Europe emerged. It became evident that the scale of the humanitarian needs and the coordination they demanded exceeded the experience and resources of local churches and initiatives. Prolonged effort to sustain the operational and strategic support for the TSA's response became unsustainable with the existing number of personnel in IHQ and it was apparent that additional support was needed.

Lessons learnt from previous major disaster operations highlighted the benefits of setting up a temporary specialist desk or unit. The Ukraine Support Unit was set up late 2022 and is situated at IHQ, providing the linkages to the other taskforces and supporting IES with the strategy as well as the administration needed for project administration, development, maintenance, closure, financial control, donor (supporting offices) relationships, and so on. For the first year, the unit had a coordinator, admin support and a communication specialist who focuses on all tasks related to public relations and communications. This was then reduced to one position, covering all responsibilities. In addition to providing additional capacity within the IES team the unit also enables strengthening the links between IES and IDS as well as other development practitioners within TSA. Regular meetings are now taking place between all stakeholders involved in the work in Ukraine, which include strategic plans for longer-term scenarios including a potential time after the war has come to an end. Some of the plans would be more on a preparedness level including considerations regarding the construction of a warehouse. Other planned activities focus more on recovery, on peace and reconciliation and on rebuilding a 'new normal'.

The focus remains on the locally led response and activities across Europe will therefore differ significantly in the various operational areas, however the specialist unit can support these initiatives with professional guidance in particular with regards to the alignment with the operational roadmap for MHPSS actions during and also after the war (WHO, 2022).

Conclusion

While the war in Europe is, unfortunately, an ongoing crisis, it is timely and necessary to reflect on the response of TSA to date and to pull out key lessons to inform the ongoing work and any future responses.

The learning from the last 18 months can be viewed through the LRRD lens that we have reflected on throughout the chapter.

Preparation

The initial response to the war was driven by local TSA officers with very little training or experience in disaster response. TSA trains its staff and officers around the world in basic disaster management and will continue to do so in order to have people in place with the right skills when unexpected events occur. However, it is impossible to plan for a truly locally led response as each context is so different – this was evident in the activities which took place immediately. Since the beginning of the war two classroom disaster preparedness, response and recovery training courses have now taken place for delegates from Ukraine, Moldova, Romania, Bulgaria, Georgia, Poland, Germany, Lithuania, Latvia and the Czech Republic. Additional, informal and online training on various subjects including cash and voucher-based assistance has been provided.

Response and relief

EET leadership immediately supported the excellent local responses and had daily contact with leaders in Ukraine and regular meetings with the other four countries which gave a strong local level of coordination from the very beginning. The international role at this point therefore was to coordinate funding streams in order to take that pressure and high communication volume away from those on the ground as well as deploying additional emergency personnel and providing technical support. As response becomes *rehabilitation* it is much more possible to have unified approaches and coordinated technical input.

TSA, being a church, has a huge benefit in being a permanent presence in the communities in which it operates. It means that the churches are already part of community life and that local networks are already established, meaning there is no time lost at the onset of a disaster. However, there was a lack of capacity to partner more effectively with large-scale programme implementers. The partnerships that were formed came much later in the *response phase* and enabled what was a relatively small organisation to deal with a large demand which had come about from the status of TSA in the community. Had these partnerships been formed earlier and more strategically it is possible that more could have been done.

Rehabilitation

It became clear as the response went on that *rehabilitation, or response,* was something that was being done without necessarily acknowledging the transition. While lifesaving actions continued to take place in Ukraine and surrounding countries more thought was being put into allowing continuance of safety and recovery, particularly for refugees. With these activities came an increase in the budget of projects and once again the lack of administrative and financial capacity locally was a challenge. The creation of the Ukraine Response Unit around this time enabled the local team to be supported in these tasks at an international level but even then TSA noted that officers and staff living in a war situation in Ukraine for so long are becoming fatigued and additional support is now being sought to try and relieve the pressure.

There was no Europe-wide strategy for the work of TSA until 18 months after the conflict commenced. This initially allowed a *locally led* response based on context, as countries in the European Union had different support facilities from those in Schengen areas and those outside the European Union. Additionally, the support by UNHCR and other key stakeholders was varied in each country and the locally led response was able to handle these different levels of support. However, as the war was ongoing, it was necessary to look at the long-term impacts and this drove the focus on the MHPSS pyramid. This strategy, while agreed locally by the affected countries, needed to be held and driven internationally, in order to ensure that those raising funds also respected this direction of work. Initially, the history of *locally led* responses presented as a resistance towards introducing a top-down strategy but over time with good coordination between stakeholders this has been more generally accepted.

Community development, or more recovery

It has been acknowledged through this experience that, in practice, it is almost impossible to define where the different elements of LRRD start and end. This was reinforced by a visit to Ukraine in 2023 by the IES and IDS team leaders and the Ukraine Response Unit coordinator in which it was noted that effective organisations can switch from *emergency* to *development* depending on the current situation or season and they can also sit alongside each other in a healthy way. TSA has discovered this almost accidently – by being a small department where both IDS and IES are able to discuss and share on a daily basis it has been possible to work organically together on the areas of work that fall in a complex space between response and community development. As a consequence TSA currently has longer term projects running alongside emergency projects in many of the countries in the EET. The challenge before the Ukraine Response Unit was created was that there was no space in either team to think about the more strategic rehabilitation aspects.

This lack of distinction between the stages of the LRRD pathway has also been noted by others. Akashi (Secretary General of the UN in 1997) referred to recipients not seeing programmes moving through *preparedness, mitigation, rehabilitation* and *development*, but rather seeing them holistically. This has been a key learning for TSA, which acknowledges that being more agile and adaptable will be a key component of any future responses. As a result of learning from the current Ukraine war the IDS and IES teams are now working more closely than before and seeing LRRD as less of a linear process and more of a complementary, concurrent approach. This is replicated at the local level, where a joint training was given to staff in the EET division to try to reinforce the development mindset even in response activities, and this is now a package that can be delivered in other countries of operation. By linking relief, rehabilitation and development together we have learnt again the benefits to everyone of focused collaboration and a joined-up approach.

Acknowledgements

The authors would like to thank the staff and officers of the EET, in particular the territorial leaders Colonels Kelvin and Cheralynne Pethybridge, the development officer, Major Elizabeth Garland, and the emergency officer, Major Galina Korenivska. They, along with many others we cannot name here, have worked sacrificially to ensure a high quality response of TSA to the ongoing conflict in Ukraine, and the resulting crises in surrounding countries.

Note

1   https://actalliance.org/who-we-are/

References

Charlson, F., van Ommeren, M., Flaxman, A., Cornett, J., Whiteford, H. and Saxen, S. (2017) New WHO prevalence estimates of mental disorders in conflict settings: a systematic review and meta-analysis. *The Lancet*, 394: 240–248.

Freitas, J. (2015) Soldiering on in Athens and helping refugees. *The New Internationalist*. Available at: https://newint.org/features/web-exclusive/2015/08/10/refugees-greece-migration/

IASC (Inter-Agency Standing Committee) (2007) *IASC Guidelines on Mental Health and Psychosocial Support in Emergency Settings*. Geneva: IASC.

IOB (2013) Linking relief and development: more than old solutions for old problems? *IOB Study No. 380*. Ministry of Foreign Affairs, Netherlands Government.

The Salvation Army (2015) The Salvation Army in Greece offers assistance to refugees. *The Salvation Army International.* Available at: https://www.salvationarmy.org/ihq/news/inr140815

The Salvation Army International (2020) *Displaced* [Film]. Available at: https://www.salvationarmy.org/ihq/displaced

Spindler, W. (2015) The year of Europe's refugee crisis. *UNHCR Stories.* Available at: https://www.unhcr.org/news/stories/2015-year-europes-refugee-crisis

UNHCR (2023) What is happening in Ukraine? Available at: https://www.unhcr.org/uk/emergencies/ukraine-emergency

WHO (2022) *Ukrainian Prioritized Multisectoral Mental Health and Psychosocial Support Actions During and After the War: Operational Roadmap.* Available at: https://reliefweb.int/report/ukraine/ukrainian-prioritized-multisectoral-mental-health-and-psychosocial-support-actions-during-and-after-war-operational-roadmap-enuk

18

Faith actors, public engagement and social justice in Europe: addressing the direct and indirect consequences of war

Emma Tomalin

Introduction

As I started writing this, the abhorrent war between Israel and Hamas in Gaza had been underway for over three weeks and it was difficult to separate thinking about what to include in this chapter from unfolding events. While Israel-Palestine is not geographically part of Europe, the 70-year-old crisis has its roots in European dynamics. These date back to the Zionist movement beginning in the late 19th century when European Jews responding to new waves of persecution sought to establish a Jewish homeland in Palestine (Avineri, 2017). This was followed by the setting up of Israel as Jewish state in 1948, in response to the genocide against Jews in Europe during the Second World War, a geopolitical move that has led to the increasing annexation of Palestinian Muslims and Christians and is at the root of the current crisis (Black, 2018; Dowty, 2018). Given the religious significance of the so-called 'Holy Land' to Muslims, Christians and Jews, alongside the fact that most people in Israel are Jewish and in Palestine are Muslim, religion is a key dimension in this conflict. While it is often portrayed as war over religion, the situation is more complex with colonial, ethnic, nationalist and territorial factors also playing a role. Indeed, faith leaders on both sides have played a role in stoking violence and nationalism, but others have been prominent in brokering peace (Freedman, 2019).

As this conflict was worsening, I was attending a long-planned three-day gathering of faith actors from different religious traditions in a major city in Europe, who work on issues of peacebuilding, humanitarianism and development. The widespread feeling among participants that 'we have to do something' was intense and occupied much of the side conversations that were taking place parallel to the actual business of the meeting. These one-to-one discussions ranged from concern and anger that the conflict was not being mentioned in public fora at the meeting – and that on the few occasions where it was mentioned by invited high level government representatives it reflected what some viewed as a one-sided support for Israel – as well as the challenges facing individuals who wanted to say something but were fearful that they would be perceived as taking sides in this unwinnable war. Participants came together and decided to not only issue a joint statement demanding an immediate ceasefire, but also a video of individuals from different faiths who were present at the meeting praying for peace, reflecting the exhortation from one participant that 'prayer is *our* decisive language'.[1] Although a collective effort, these statements were hosted and disseminated by EU-Cord, a network of European Christian organisations advocating for humanitarian action, development and peace as 'Christian organisations collaborating for a transformed, just and equal world'.[2]

During the meeting I was also keeping a close eye on media coverage, which was reporting on the direct consequences of the war for those in the Israel-Palestine region, this included the bombing of sites officially protected under International Humanitarian Law (Liyanage and Galappaththige, 2022), including Al-Ahli Arab Hospital (Al Jazeera Staff, 2023a; Saladana, 2023) and the Greek Orthodox Saint Porphyrius Church (Al Jazeera Staff, 2023b), both in Gaza City, as well as the indirect consequences for people in Europe. This included increased hate crimes linked to antisemitism and Islamophobia. In Berlin two Molotov cocktails were launched at a synagogue on the morning of 18 October 2023, where according to police, 'antisemitic incidents in the country have been rising following the violent escalation in the Middle East' (Grieshaber, 2023). At the same time, pro-Palestinian protests in Berlin were being forcibly broken up and protestors detained, a move widely interpreted as Islamophobia (Human Rights Watch, 2023; Makowski, 2023) and a product of what many see as the overcompensation of the German state to avoid any accusation of antisemitism (Bastasic, 2023). I have also heard first-hand reports of employees in Muslim and Jewish faith-based organisations receiving death threats and having to increase security measures. Widely reported also were large gatherings of Muslims undertaking *dua* (prayer) at key sites in Europe, including Downing Street in London, the home of the British prime minister. Other dimensions not so widely reported upon in the media included the behind-the-scenes advocacy, diplomacy and high-level mediation that faith actors engage in to bring peace. For instance, Cardinal Pietro Parolin, the Vatican's secretary of state, has been reported to have offered the services of the Holy See to contribute towards peace talks, as they have been doing in the Ukraine dispute. In Israel-Palestine, as well as in other conflicts, faith-based mediation is a long-established response of faith actors to war, both informally in their communities but increasingly also in formal international efforts (Holmsen, 2018; Allen, 2023; Pinedo, 2023).

It is very striking how prominent religion is in these accounts of responses to the Israel-Gaza conflict, not only in terms of the role that religion plays as a contributing factor to the war, but also in terms of mitigating and mediating it. Little over a half a century ago sociologists were predicting that religion would largely lose its public role, becoming a purely private matter or completely disappearing, as societies became more modern and enlightened (Norris and Inglehart, 2004). By the 1980s they were beginning to revise these predictions, spurred by the rise of Islamic politics in many parts of the Middle East and the Christian right in the United States, but also the important role that faith actors were playing in domestic and international social welfare with the rolling back of the state in an increasingly neoliberal world (Evans et al, 2005; Williams et al, 2012). That the world was becoming more unstable has also given rise to civil society based social justice movements around issues such as poverty, war and climate change, with faith actors playing a key role as drivers of change (Beyer, 1994).

As a scholar of religion and public life, this perseverance/prominence of religion in modern societies is my 'bread and butter' and I am strongly committed to scholarship that highlights the public role of faith actors, in ways that transcend the 'good religion'/'bad religion' binary (Orsi, 2022). There are victims and perpetrators on all sides of a conflict, where the inherent 'ambivalence of the sacred' creates a situation where religion can both mitigate and exacerbate conflict (Appleby, 2000). Given the pressing need for hope and solutions at this moment, in this chapter I do not want to unpick further the role of religion in perpetuating conflict but instead to draw attention to some aspects of faith actors' public engagement with the direct and indirect consequences of war in ways that promote social justice. While taking recent events in the Middle East as the starting point for my approach in this chapter, I will nonetheless focus on Europe, with the caveat that given the global character of many conflicts and responses to them, European boundaries are not always clear-cut. Moreover, although not directly focusing on health, reflecting the theme of this volume, the chapter can be viewed through a 'social determinants of health' lens where health is not just understood in terms of medical factors but also a whole range of 'social determinants', that is, 'the circumstances in which people are born, grow up, live, work and age, and the systems put in place to deal with illness. These circumstances are in turn shaped by a wider set of forces: economics, social policies, and politics'.[3]

In reflecting on the reactions outlined earlier to the intense situation unfolding in the Middle East, several areas of faith-related response to the direct and indirect consequences of war stood out to me and I make these the focus of the chapter: the role of faith actors in advocacy to bring about peace; the role of faith spaces as places of sanctuary and asylum for displaced people; and the role of prayer. However, I first provide some context on the 'ambivalence of the sacred' (Appleby, 2000) and the implications for war in an unstable Europe.

The 'ambivalence of the sacred': the implications for war in an unstable Europe

There is a long history of religiously inflected war in Europe, where religious beliefs, identities or motivations have played a major role in driving or exacerbating conflict. In these conflicts, factors such as differing religious beliefs, religious identities or religious institutions have been central to the causes, motivations or justifications for the conflict. This includes conflicts that have compromised peace across the region, from the Roman occupation of large parts of Europe which eventually replaced pagan religions with Christianity following the First Council of Nicaea in 325 CE, the Crusades between the 11th and 13th centuries (Bachrach, 2003), the European Wars of Religion between the 16th and early 18th centuries, following the Reformation (Palaver et al, 2016), to the more recent 'war on terror' since 9/11 (Burleigh, 2009). It also includes conflicts that have been isolated to specific regions within Europe, from the Northern Ireland 'Troubles' between the late 1960s and 1998 (Bourke, 2003) to the Balkan conflict in the 1990s (Baker, 2015). Nonetheless, it is important to recognise that these conflicts are not solely about religion *per se* and intersected with other factors, such as ethnic, political, economic or historical issues. Moreover, although religion has been an underlying factor in the dynamics that have led to conflict in Europe over the past centuries it has also provided material, moral and spiritual resources for addressing war, as well as seeking to prevent future conflicts. Thus, such conflicts are complex and multifaceted, and understanding the 'ambivalence of the sacred' is crucial for conflict resolution and peacebuilding efforts (Appleby, 2000).

Catalysed by the devastating consequences of the Second World War followed by the start of the Cold War, faith actors in Europe increasingly mobilised collectively to work for peace and reconciliation as well as to provide support to those affected by conflict. For instance, in the UK the Church of England played a large community role between 1939 and 1945 (Dochuk, 2001), in 1945 Christian Aid was 'founded by British and Irish churches to help refugees following the Second World War'[4] and across Eastern Europe churches often remained the only spaces where people could gather and were important players in facilitating the social mobilisation that led to the fall of communism (Weigel, 1992).

In Western Europe, this impetus for combined action at the level of civil society took place against the backdrop of the emergence of international peacebuilding and humanitarian efforts coordinated via the United Nations (UN) and its member states. These initiatives have involved activities that address the direct and indirect consequences of war. This includes immediate action such as conflict mediation, interfaith dialogue, addressing hate crimes, advocacy for policies that promote peace and social justice, and support for displaced people, including with respect to humanitarian assistance and psychological trauma, as well as longer term responses that address ongoing refugee crises, reconciliation processes and rebuilding communities with tools to resist future conflict. In 1970, Religions for Peace was founded in New York but has chapters in Europe.[5] Across Europe there have also been ecumenical movements such as the Taizé Community (founded in France in 1940),[6] the Conference of European Churches (founded in 1959),[7] the Community of Sant'Egidio (a lay Catholic organisation based in Rome founded in 1968),[8] and Church and Peace (a European ecumenical network of Christian peace communities, congregations and organisations set up in 1978). However, this has not just been a Christian effort. For instance, in 2012 the King Abdullah bin Abdulaziz International Centre for Interreligious and Intercultural Dialogue, headquartered in Lisbon, Portugal, was founded, following a meeting in 2007 of Pope Benedict XVI and King Abdullah of the Kingdom of Saudi Arabia.[9]

While the response in Europe has been dominated by Christian actors, other faith traditions have also played a role. This includes HIAS (originally known as the Hebrew Immigrant Aid Society), founded in 1881 in New York, 'the world's oldest refugee agency ... to assist Jews fleeing pogroms in Russia and Eastern Europe'.[10] As Europe has become more religiously diverse over the past half century or so, other faith actors have also engaged in activities to support the direct and indirect consequences of war. For instance, within the Muslim faith, Islamic Relief was founded in 1984 to address the humanitarian crisis following the famine in the Horn of Africa, and then played a leading role in supporting victims of the 1992–1995 Balkan War, where efforts continue to this day with post-conflict reconstruction and development in Bosnia and Herzegovina.[11] While other faith traditions in Europe are part of interfaith initiatives for peace, so far they have been less likely to organise distinctive faith-based organisations for peace and humanitarian relief. Instead, in addition to participating in interfaith initiatives, their activities are more likely to be organised informally within faith communities and from places of worship. This includes, for instance, the role that Hindu temples played in London in providing sanctuary for Tamil refugees fleeing the Sri Lankan civil war between 1983 and 2009 (Maunaguru, 2021).

'War knows no religion': faith spaces as places for sanctuary and asylum

The bombing of the Greek Orthodox Saint Porphyrius Church in Gaza City on the night of 19 October 2023, which was sheltering both Christians and Muslims, has been condemned as a 'war crime' that contravenes International Humanitarian Law (IHL).[12] On the one hand, under IHL places of worship are 'recognized as protected places under the definition of "cultural properties" and no armed groups should attack or destroy them' (Liyanage and Galappaththige, 2022: 402; see also Kishkovsky, 2022). On the other hand, displaced and endangered people often take shelter in places of worship, as they did at Saint Porphyrius Church and, although IHL forbids the targeting of civilians, among the hundreds of Palestinians taking refugee there, 16 or more were reported to have been killed (Berger et al, 2023). In terms of its original meaning a 'sanctuary' refers to sacred space such as a shrine or a place of worship, and over time the term has come to be used to mean any place of refuge (Rabban, 2016). In this case, and there have been others, under the brutal conditions of war, the sanctity of the place of worship was insufficient to protect buildings and people from attack: they are not inviolable. Nonetheless, although never completely safe, as a constrained choice in a time of intense crisis, a place of worship is likely to offer greater security during an armed conflict than many other locations, but also runs the risk of being viewed as a target (Glinski, 2017).

Within Europe places of worship and their accompanying buildings are being used as shelters for people in the current Ukraine war, and as in Gaza these have been targeted and civilians killed. A report from a UN Security Council meeting concerning the war in Ukraine drew attention to 'upholding the right to freedom of religion' and 'the dangers of using religion to fuel conflict', but also the specific role of 'religious sites in times of conflict'.[13] In addition to providing a potential place of sanctuary as described earlier, one contributor to the meeting also looked to the longer term where not only is it the case that 'religious leaders and communities of faith can play an important role in building peace and providing comfort during war' but also that 'places of worship are the centre of gravity for communities of faith and can serve as important platforms for post-war national healing'.[14]

Places of worship are also spaces where people displaced across borders due to war can seek sanctuary in areas away from the conflict. Churches, mosques and other religious buildings play a large role in receiving displaced people and providing them with support. However, places of worship have often provided sanctuary in contexts where displaced people are at risk of deportation. This has been an important role historically, where churches have provided a haven for those unjustly persecuted or at risk of danger. As Rabban notes, while an ancient religious practice, 'constant across cultures and millennia' (2016: 48), in the 20th century activists have built on this earlier tradition in response to the increasingly hostile attitude of their governments to receiving asylum seekers, including in countries across Europe such as in France, the UK, the Netherlands and Scandinavia (Rabban, 2016: 196ff). However, it is the German church sanctuary movement that is best known, which started in 1983 and is still active today (Rabban, 2016: 199). A Protestant church in Berlin provided refuge to three Palestinian families who were going to be deported to Lebanon and they were allowed to stay. However, the next year a church in Hamburg took in a Philippine family and the police violently evicted and deported them. The outcome of this was that, following a large public outcry, 'the police stopped invading churches to remove sanctuary seekers' (Rabban, 2016: 199) and churches increasingly provided sanctuary to those seeking legal asylum but who were being denied it. By 1994 the German Ecumenical Committee on Church Asylum[15] had been formed (Rabban, 2016: 119) and while it continues its work, as Strack reports, 'the German government takes a harder stance against asylum seekers taking refuge in churches' (2023: np).

'We have to do something': the role of faith actors in peacebuilding in Europe

Following the start of the war between Israel and Hamas, faith actors swiftly involved themselves in calling for a ceasefire, through online statements and street protests to engaging in diplomacy and mediation. As mentioned earlier, participants at the interfaith event I was attending as the war was breaking out, developed and distributed an online statement. The statement opened with the words: 'Faith leaders, faith practitioners, researchers and faith-based organisations calling for the protection of civilians in Israel and the occupied Palestinian territory, Ukraine, Syria, and other contexts affected by armed conflict, October 2023',[16] and concludes: 'Faith has been at times weaponized to spread violence, hatred and vengeance. But it has also served as a catalyst in efforts for sustainable peace, justice and protecting civilians in times of war. Protecting civilians and ending violence is our call with this statement.'[17]

While the statement was a 'heartfelt plea to leaders around the world to respect the protection of civilians and adherence to international humanitarian law',[18] one might wonder about the extent to which such efforts go beyond a gesture to satisfy people's need to do something 'there and then', as a response to their despair and helplessness. In discussing this issue with activists and academics in the light of the Israel-Gaza conflict, who are keen to justify the role of such online statements, it is clear that they are considered to have a more wide-reaching impact. For example, such statements play a role in raising awareness and in education, and can be particularly helpful in providing an example of how to articulate things in a way that is credible and legitimate in a climate where a topic is inflammatory. Additionally, they offer an important way to express solidarity with victims and to indicate that people care in a situation where they feel they have been forgotten. Indeed, while some have been concerned that there is a vicariousness to those not directly affected by the conflict speaking out and that we should be listening to the voices of the victims, one of those affected emphasised that while in some instances this makes sense ... In a political struggle. We all go in ... If you're willing to echo Palestinian demands, speak everywhere: Libraries, churches, community centres, set up a table in the market, write an oped, get on the local news, organise a reading group or a study get-together, call your reps.[19]

In addition to such indirect advocacy, faith actors are also much involved in direct advocacy and diplomacy for peace through their participation in mediation processes. While informal mediation and diplomacy is a well-established feature of faith actors' public engagement, they are increasingly brought into formal processes, through 'track 1.5' and 'track 2' dialogues: the former includes 'a mix of government officials – who participate in an unofficial capacity – and non-governmental experts' and the latter 'brings together unofficial representatives on both sides, with no government participation' (Staats et al, 2019). Their influence is often based on moral authority, credibility and their ability to build trust and facilitate dialogue. Additionally, the success of faith actors in diplomacy depends on their ability to operate in an inclusive, non-partisan and neutral manner, respecting the principles of human rights and international law.

The Quaker tradition as a pacifist church has played a key role in conflict mediation, both informally and formally, including through the Quaker United Nations Office established in 1947 (Yarrow, 1978: 44; Bailey, 1993: 101–103). At the UN in New York and Geneva it deploys different methods towards peace, including advocacy, mediation and reconciliation. Vernon-Rees (2022) writes about the method of 'quiet diplomacy' practices at Quaker houses in Geneva and New York, where officials are invited for 'off-the-record' meetings, where they are provided with a meal and a relaxed homely setting where people are 'comfortable enough to have uncomfortable conversations' (QUNO, 2019: 5). Another prominent faith-based movement involved in conflict mediation in Europe is the Community of Sant'Egidio, founded in 1968. Headquartered in Rome, with a few employees based there, it has a large cohort of volunteers in Italy and beyond (Marshall, 2023). In its 'track 1.5' engagements Sant'Egidio hosts meetings with government and other formal negotiators. In this respect, it played in large role in bringing together the warring sides in South Sudan to arrive at the Juba Peace Agreement in 2020 and continues to host peace talks in South Sudan and at the Vatican.[20] It also engages in 'track 2' diplomacy, as described earlier, as well as in what some describe as a 'track 3' approach, 'at the "grass roots", working to address local tensions and conflicts that can fuel larger disputes, building the "cultures" and mechanisms of community engagement that can take situations beyond stalemate towards common and constructive action' (Marshall, 2023: np). Writing about the Sant'Egidio Community, Holmsen argues that its 'position as a leading practitioner of religious diplomacy has gradually translated into considerable influence and leverage on ongoing negotiations over the role and meaning of religion in international politics' (2018: 14; see also Haynes, 2009).

With respect to the war in Ukraine, Cardinal Matteo Zuppi, the head of the Italian Bishops' Conference and a member of Sant'Egidio – 'the pope's favorite of the new movements which is dedicated to ecumenism and social justice, [which] has assisted in previous international peace processes' – was appointed the 'pope's designated trouble-shooter for Ukraine' in May 2023 (Allen, 2023: np). He has since met with political leaders in both Russia and Ukraine (Babynski, 2023) but also religious leaders, including the Patriarch of Moscow, Kirill, 'often considered a "soft power" ally of Russian president Vladimir Putin' (Brylov et al, 2023: 16). As Houston and Mandaville write, Patriarch Kirill 'depicted the war in starkly spiritual terms: "We have entered into a struggle that has not a physical, but a metaphysical significance." He portrayed the war as a struggle "for eternal salvation" for ethnic Russians' (2022: np; Hudson, 2023). However, there is not only tension between Orthodox Christians in Russia and Ukraine but also within Ukraine where some religious leaders are affiliated to the Russian Orthodox Church through the Ukrainian Orthodox Church–Moscow Patriarchate and are supportive of the Russian interests in the war (Brylov et al, 2023: 14). The need for interfaith dialogue in this conflict is clear, where although not a war over religion, as Brylov et al write (2023: summary, np):

> Religion and religious actors have an important effect on Ukrainian society at large, the evolution of conflict dynamics, and prospects for future peacebuilding. … Despite its clear relevance, international policymakers, humanitarian actors, and peacebuilders have rarely engaged with religion as a key factor in understanding the conflict in Ukraine, its possible evolution, or opportunities for peace.

'Prayer is *our* decisive language': considering the role of prayer in faith-based peacebuilding

It was widely reported, particularly in the Catholic press, that '[a]mid the ongoing Israel-Hamas war in the Holy Land, Pope Francis has called for a day of prayer and fasting on Friday, Oct. 27'.[21] During the prayer, he

> prayed to the Virgin Mary to 'inspire the leaders of nations to seek paths of peace' … that she would 'touch the hearts of those imprisoned by hatred; convert those who fuel and foment conflict. Dry the tears of children, be present to those who are elderly and alone; strengthen the wounded and the sick; protect those forced to leave their lands and their loved ones; console the crestfallen; awaken new hope'.[22]

Days afterwards, Vatican News posted on its website the haunting image of children praying 'fervently for an end to the war and peace for all' in the Holy Family Catholic Parish in Gaza, which 'has turned into a refuge for many seeking shelter',[23] with the sound of bombs exploring in the background:

> The two-minute video of young people of various ages shows them making the sign of the cross, praying the Our Father, the Hail Mary and the Sub Tuum Praesidium prayer (Latin for 'Under thy protection'). They thank the Pope for Friday's Day of Prayer, Fasting, and Penance for Peace in the World, and pray for him, with a closing greeting directed to everyone.[24]

While over the past 20 years scholarship on religion and war has moved beyond an emphasis on religion as solely a cause of violence, and today there is a substantial literature on religion and peacebuilding as well as how faith actors provide material and psychological support for victims of war, there are there are still gaps, including a lack of attention to the role of prayer. Neither have humanitarians and peacebuilders, outside of faith circles, supporting victims of war or engaging in peacebuilding activities, paid much attention to what many faith actors consider to be their 'decisive language'. As Schwarz writes, prayer is 'a practice neglected and largely misunderstood by scholars and FBO [faith-based organisation] funders … in agenda setting, conflict resolution, post-conflict reintegration programs, reconciliation processes, and psychosocial care' (2018: 4). Ganiel, writing about the role of prayer in addressing the Northern Ireland 'Troubles', agrees, and writes that '[g]iven that prayer matters so much to so many faith-based peacebuilders, it is surprising that previous research has not focused on this subject' (2021: 73). Indeed, according to the Community of Sant'Egidio prayer is the heart of the life of the movement 'and is its absolute priority'.[25] Both Schwarz and Ganiel view this gap as a product of a secularist bias where scholars and donors view prayer as 'largely inconsequential for "real" peacebuilding work' (Schwarz, 2018: 15; Ganiel, 2021: 73).

At its most fundamental level, prayer can be viewed, in the words of William James, as 'inner communion with the spirit thereof – be that spirit "God" or "law" – [it] is a process wherein work is really done, and spiritual energy flows in and produces effects, psychological or material, within the phenomenal world' (James, 1902: 477). This transcendental or 'intangible' dimension of prayer, dependent upon supernatural forces, is clearly at odds with the empiricist and tangible focus of a secular post-Enlightenment worldview and is likely another reason why prayer has been neglected in scholarship, policy and practice. Nonetheless, regardless of what we believe the mechanisms of prayer to be it can also be shown to have tangible impacts that are beneficial to peacebuilding processes.

Ganiel is one of the few scholars to address the role of prayer in peacebuilding sociologically. With reference to her research about Father Gerry Reynolds (1935–2015), a Belfast based Catholic priest during the 'Troubles' – who 'saw his practice of prayer and his peacebuilding work as interdependent, a perspective that is shared by faith-based peacebuilders in other contexts' (Ganiel, 2021: 724) – she 'proposes a preliminary theoretical framework for understanding the role of prayer in faith-based peacebuilding' (2021: 74). She suggests three main roles for prayer in peacebuilding: two at the individual level '(1) prompting religious identity change; and (2) sustaining hope and activism during adversity; and one socio-political effect: (3) creating and sustaining real-world initiatives' (2021: 74). She argued that despite its neglect, prayer 'may be one of the most significant faith-based resources for peace and is worthy of further and deeper analysis across contexts' (2021: 74).

Conclusion

The chapter has not directly focused on health, but the topics addressed can be viewed through a 'social determinants of health' lens. War adversely affects people's health in a range of ways, from death and serious injury, the spread of disease and the impact of trauma, caused directly by combat but also from the failure of infrastructure, including water, sanitation and the supply of food and medical equipment, the lack of medical care and the longer-term impact of rising poverty and political instability. As I was writing the chapter a war between Israel and Hamas in Gaza broke out on 7 October 2023 and was still raging several weeks later as I completed it. I took my observations and reflections on the war in the Middle East as a starting point for what to focus on here, with several areas standing out: the role of faith actors in advocacy to bring about peace; the role of faith spaces as places of sanctuary and asylum for displaced people; and the role of prayer. The 'ambivalence of the sacred' (Appleby, 2000) means that religion can both exacerbate and mitigate violent conflict and it is important to avoid essentialising particular religions or religious expressions as instances of either 'good' or 'bad' religion. However, given the need for hope and solutions, my aim in this chapter has been to draw attention to some aspects of faith actors' public engagement with the direct and indirect consequences of war in ways that promote social justice.

Notes

[1] https://www.youtube.com/watch?v=wGzZSbiwzOE

[2] https://www.eu-cord.org/about-us/core-values/; https://www.eu-cord.org/about-us/members/

[3] https://www.who.int/news-room/questions-and-answers/item/social-determinants-of-health-key-concepts

[4] https://www.christianaid.org.uk/our-work/about-us/our-history
[5] https://rfpeurope.org/
[6] https://www.taize.fr/en_article6526.html
[7] https://ceceurope.org/who-we-are/history
[8] https://www.santegidio.org/pageID/30008/langID/en/THE-COMMUNITY.html
[9] https://www.kaiciid.org/who-we-are
[10] https://hias.org/who/our-history/
[11] https://www.islamic-relief.org.uk/where-we-work/country/bosnia-and-herzegovina/
[12] The quote in the heading is from Mhawish, 2023.
[13] https://press.un.org/en/2023/sc15178.doc.htm#:~:text=Highlighting%20the%20imp
ortance%20of%20protecting,of%20faith%20and%20can%20serve
[14] https://press.un.org/en/2023/sc15178.doc.htm#:~:text=Highlighting%20the%20imp
ortance%20of%20protecting,of%20faith%20and%20can%20serve
[15] https://www.kirchenasyl.de/herzlich-willkommen/welcome/
[16] https://form.jotform.com/eu_cord/statement-sign-on-
[17] https://form.jotform.com/eu_cord/statement-sign-on-
[18] https://form.jotform.com/eu_cord/statement-sign-on-
[19] https://twitter.com/meznaqato/status/1717655032114368935
[20] https://sudantribune.com/article274625/
[21] https://www.catholicnewsagency.com/news/255808/7-ways-to-participate-in-day-of-
prayer-and-fasting-called-for-by-pope-francis
[22] https://www.reuters.com/world/gaza-war-rages-pope-francis-leads-day-pra
yer-world-peace-2023-10-27/
[23] https://www.vaticannews.va/en/church/news/2023-10/gaza-children-pray-for-peace-
and-thank-pope-francis.html
[24] https://www.vaticannews.va/en/church/news/2023-10/gaza-children-pray-for-peace-
and-thank-pope-francis.html
[25] https://www.santegidio.org/pageID/30036/langID/en/PRAYER.html

References

Al Jazeera Staff (2023a) Israel bombs Greek Orthodox Gaza church sheltering displaced people. *Al Jazeera*. Available at: https://www.aljazeera.com/news/2023/10/20/war-crime-israel-bombs-gaza-church-sheltering-displaced-people

Al Jazeera Staff (2023b) Investigations reveal discrepancies in Israel's Gaza hospital attack claims. *Al Jazeera*. Available at: https://www.aljazeera.com/news/2023/10/20/what-have-open-source-videos-revealed-about-the-gaza-hospital-explosion

Allen, E.A. (2023) Pope's designated mediator on Ukraine has history as a peace-maker. *Crux*. Available at: https://cruxnow.com/vatican/2023/05/popes-designated-mediator-on-ukraine-has-history-as-a-peace-maker

Appleby, S. (2000) *The Ambivalence of the Sacred: Religion Violence and Reconciliation*. Lanham: Rowman & Littlefield.

Avineri, S. (2017) *The Making of Modern Zionism, Revised Edition: The Intellectual Origins of the Jewish State*. New York: Basic Books.

Babynski, A. (2023) How Cardinal Zuppi's visits played in Ukraine. *The Pillar*. Available at: https://www.pillarcatholic.com/p/how-cardinal-zuppis-visits-play-in

Bachrach, D.S. (2003) *Religion and the Conduct of War c.300–c.1215*. Suffolk: Boydell Press.

Bailey, S.D. (1993) *Peace is a Process (Swarthmore Lecture)*. London: Quaker Books.

Baker, C. (2015) *The Yugoslav Wars of the 1990s*. London: Palgrave Macmillan.

Bastasic, L. (2023) I grew up in Bosnia, amid fear and hatred of Muslims. Now I see Germany's mistakes over Gaza. *The Guardian*. Available at: https://www.theguardian.com/commentisfree/2023/oct/23/bosnia-muslims-germany-gaza-ethnic-cleansing-palestinian

Berger, M., Hill, E. and Ables, K. (2023) Historic church sheltering civilians struck in deadly Gaza City blast. *The Washington Post*. Available at: https://www.washingtonpost.com/world/2023/10/20/gaza-church-strike-saint-porphyrius/

Beyer, P.F. (1994) *Religion and Globalization*. London: SAGE.

Black, I. (2018) *Enemies and Neighbours: Arabs and Jews in Palestine and Israel, 1917–2017*. London: Penguin.

Bourke, R. (2003) *Peace in Ireland: The War of Ideas*. London: Pimlico.

Brylov, D., Kalenychenko, T. and KryshtalBrylov, A. (2023) *Mapping the Religious Landscape of Ukraine*. Washington, DC: USIP. Available at: https://www.usip.org/publications/2023/10/mapping-religious-landscape-ukraine

Burleigh, M. (2009) *Sacred Causes: The Clash of Religion and Politics, from the Great War to the War on Terror*. New York: HarperCollins.

Dochuk, G.E. (2001) *I Saw Religion in Action in the Shelters: The Church of England's Experience in War-time London, 1939–1945* [MA Thesis]. Simon Fraser University. Available at: https://library-archives.canada.ca/eng/services/services-libraries/theses/Pages/list.aspx?NW_S=Dochuk,%20Gregory%20Edwin,1974-

Dowty, A. (ed) (2018) *The Israel/Palestine Reader*. Medford: Polity Press.

Evans, B., Richmond, T. and Shields, J. (2005) Structuring neoliberal governance: the nonprofit sector, emerging new modes of control and the marketisation of service delivery. *Policy and Society*, 24: 73–97.

Freedman, M. (2019) Fighting from the pulpit: religious leaders and violent conflict in Israel. *The Journal of Conflict Resolution*, 63: 2262–2288.

Ganiel, G. (2021) Praying for Paisley – Fr Gerry Reynolds and the role of prayer in faith-based peacebuilding: a preliminary theoretical framework. *Irish Political Studies*, 36(1): 72–91.

Glinski, S. (2017) Cathedral becomes refuge of last resort for South Sudan's displaced. *IRIN*, 15 August. Available at: https://www.thenewhumanitarian.org/feature/2017/08/15/cathedral-becomes-refuge-last-resort-south-sudan-s-displaced

Grieshaber, K. (2023) The German chancellor condemns a firebomb attack on a Berlin synagogue and vows protection for Jews. *ABC News*. Available at: https://abcnews.go.com/International/wireStory/berlin-synagogue-attacked-firebombs-antisemitic-incidents-rise-germany-104064043

Haynes, J. (2009) Conflict, conflict resolution and peace-building: the role of religion in Mozambique, Nigeria and Cambodia. *Commonwealth & Comparative Politics*, 47(1): 52–75.

Holmsen, J. (2018) *Believe It or Not: The New Face of Religion in International Affairs: A Case Study of Sant'Egidio* [Thesis]. European University Institute. https://doi.org/10.2870/410921

Houston, A. and Mandaville, P. (2022) The role of religion in Russia's war on Ukraine. *USIP*. Available at: https://www.usip.org/publications/2022/03/role-religion-russias-war-ukraine

Hudson, P. (2023) Zuppi meets Kirill on Moscow peace mission. *The Tablet*. Available at: https://www.thetablet.co.uk/news/17298/zuppi-meets-kirill-on-moscow-peace-mission

Human Rights Watch (2023) *Israel-Palestine Hostilities Affect Rights in Europe*. Available at: https://www.hrw.org/news/2023/10/26/israel-palestine-hostilities-affect-rights-europe

James, W. (1902) *The Varieties of Religious Experience: A Study in Human Nature*. London, Bombay and New York: Longmans, Green and Co.

Kishkovsky, S. (2022) Ukrainian churches and places of worship devastated by war. *The Art Newspaper*. Available at: https://www.theartnewspaper.com/2022/07/15/ukrainian-churches-destroyed-war-russia

Liyanage, I. and Galappaththige, T.R. (2022) Protection of places of worship during armed conflicts: the enrichment of international humanitarian law through Buddhism. *Beijing Law Review*, 13: 401–413.

Makowski, M. (2023) In Germany, historic guilt is fueling Islamophobia, anti-immigrant policies. *The Progressive Magazine*. Available at: https://progressive.org/latest/germany-historic-guilt-makowski-20231025/

Marshall, K. (2023) Navigating religion and peacebuilding: lessons from the community of Sant'Egidio. *ISPI*. Available at: https://www.ispionline.it/en/publication/navigating-religion-and-peacebuilding-lessons-from-the-community-of-santegidio-135750

Maunaguru, S. (2021) 'Homeless' deities and refugee devotees: Hindu temples, Sri Lankan Tamil diaspora, and politics in the United Kingdom. *American Anthropologist*, 123: 552–564.

Mhawish, M.R. (2023) 'War knows no religion': Gaza's oldest church shelters Muslims, Christians. Available at: https://www.aljazeera.com/news/2023/10/16/war-knows-no-religion-gazas-oldest-church-shelters-muslims-christians

Norris, P. and Inglehart, R. (2004) *Sacred and Secular: Religion and Politics Worldwide*. Cambridge: Cambridge University Press.

Orsi, R.A. (2022) The study of religion on the other side of the good religion/bad religion binary. *Journal of Religious Ethics*, 50(2): 312–317.

Palaver, W., Rudolph, H. and Regensburger, D. (eds) (2016) *The European Wars of Religion: An Interdisciplinary Reassessment of Sources, Interpretations, and Myths*. London and New York: Routledge.

Pinedo, P. (2023) Vatican calls for peace in Holy Land, offers to mediate between Hamas and Israel. *Catholic News Agency*. Available at: https://www.catholicnewsagency.com/news/255678/vatican-calls-for-peace-in-holy-land-offers-to-mediate-between-hamas-and-israel

QUNO (Quaker United Nations Office) (2019) *Conciliation in the Work of the Quaker United Nations Office*. Geneva: QUNO. Available at: https://quno.org/sites/default/files/timeline/files/2022/QUNO%20Paper_Conciliation%20Woodbrooke%20event%202019.pdf

Rabban, L. (2016) *Sanctuary and Asylum: A Social and Political History*. Seattle: University of Washington Press.

Saladana, S. (2023) In war zones, hospitals are holy ground: the explosion of one in Gaza is a tragic turning point. *America The Jesuit Review*. Available at: https://www.americamagazine.org/faith/2023/10/18/al-ahli-arab-hospital-sanctuary-gaza-israel-246325

Schwarz, T. (2018) *Faith-Based Organizations in Transnational Peacebuilding*. London: Rowman & Littlefield.

Staats, J., Walsh, J. and Tucci, R. (2019) Primer on multi-track diplomacy: how does it work? *USIP*. Available at: https://www.usip.org/publications/2019/07/primer-multi-track-diplomacy-how-does-it-work

Strack, C. (2023) German church officials face charges for helping refugees. *DW*. Available at: https://www.dw.com/en/german-church-officials-face-charges-for-helping-refugees/a-57783108

Vernon-Rees, A. (2022) *To What Extent Has the Quaker Faith Shaped the Work of the Quaker United Nations Office and Their Effectiveness at the UN?* [MA Thesis]. University of Leeds.

Weigel, G. (1992) *The Final Revolution: The Resistance Church and the Collapse of Communism*. Oxford: Oxford University Press.

Williams, A., Cloke, P. and Thomas, S. (2012) Co-constituting neoliberalism: faith-based organisations, co-option, and resistance in the UK. *Environment and Planning A*, 44: 1479–1501.

Yarrow, C.H.M. (1978) *Quaker Experiences in International Conciliation*. New York: Yale University Press.

19

Drivers of change and stability in an uncertain world: the case of the Salvation Army UK and Ireland Territory response to the war in Ukraine

Richard Simmons, Olly Thorp and Ben Gilbert

Introduction

This book uses the *Conceptual Framework for Action on the Social Determinants of Health*, proposed by the World Health Organization (WHO) in 2010 (see Figure I.1 in the Introduction to this book), to provide an operational approach focusing on people who have limited resources and resilience to respond to challenges such as war. The *structural determinants* of social class, gender and ethnicity are mapped in this framework, onto which interventions can be visualised as *intermediate determinants* of health and wellbeing. This chapter provides a strategic planning approach to *uncertainty and complexity* in order to identify demand-side *imperatives* and *drivers*, and supply-side *enablers* that could be used to support more effective interventions, in a 'Dynamic Change Model' (DCM). In reviewing both locally led and internationally supported development approaches by The Salvation Army (TSA) to the war in Ukraine (presented in Chapters 16 and 17), the significance of understanding from this model can be considered in the context of this emergency response.

As various contributions to this volume show, there are currently many disruptions to established patterns in different human contexts that simultaneously require both an 'urgent' and 'considered' response. For example, the rapid response required to the war in Ukraine has resulted in a series of interventions at different levels from international governmental organisations such as the North Atlantic Treaty Organization and the United Nations (UN), as well as national governments, and both international and local *non-governmental* organisations. Meanwhile, attempts to stabilise the situation and provide a basis for rebuilding the lives of those affected are also underway. This has resulted in numerous changes that must be managed collectively at a system level, as well as organisationally, to support communities and individuals. This chapter brings some of these insights together, identifying the dynamic tensions present in a complex and uncertain world, and how these might be addressed. First, it provides a model and theory of 'dynamic change' that can be broadly applied in the face of disruption and change, of different scopes, scales and speeds. It then applies the model to the case of TSA UK and Ireland Territory's (UKIT) response to the war in Ukraine.

Uncertainty and complexity

Uncertainty and complexity are widely acknowledged to structure the contemporary decision-making environment (Geyer and Cairney, 2015). As is widely recognised, phenomena such as bounded rationality (Simon, 1955) and wicked policy problems (Rittel and Webber, 1973) mean that 'policymakers must often act in the face of irreducible uncertainty – uncertainty that will not go away before a judgment has to be made about what to do, what can be done, what will be done, what ought to be done' (Hammond, 1996: 11). Navigating this terrain can be challenging, with the governance of problems demanding particular forms of response (Rittel and Webber, 1973; Grint, 2005; Hoppe, 2011). Such complexity and dynamism in many policy environments place a premium on not only sound judgement, but also the ability to *question, learn and adapt,* if effective progress is to be made.

As Sanderson (2009: 713) argues, 'learning is the dominant form in which rationality exhibits itself in situations of great cognitive complexity'. That is, when dealing with a complex issue, space created through the asking and answering of questions allows clarity, and fact, to inform decision-making. Often, to make any kind of progress, a key task here is to identify the 'right questions' to ask (Simmons, 2023a). Jessop (1997: 111) therefore identifies 'reflexive monitoring and dynamic social learning' as key processes: reflection, with the involved input of others, is vital. However, as Argyris (1976: 376) points out, often 'participants in an organization are encouraged to learn as long as the learning does not question the fundamental design, goals and activities of their organization'. Argyris (1976) calls this 'single-loop learning'. By contrast, Greenwood (1998: 1049) points out that:

> In double-loop learning the agent does not merely search for alternative actions to achieve her same ends; she also examines the *appropriateness and propriety* of her chosen ends. Double-loop learning therefore involves reflection on values and norms and, by implication, on the social structures which were instrumental in their development. By reflecting on the world they are instrumental in creating, human agents can learn to change it in ways that are *more congruent* with the values and theories they espouse. (emphasis added)

In terms of practice, this means considering the 'why' and 'what': why are we in the room, why are we hoping to achieve the things we have identified and what assumptions have led us to this starting point. This should be reflected upon throughout any development process. Sanderson (2009: 711) therefore characterises policy making as 'a domain of practical reason ... not just concerned with the instrumental notion of "what works" but a broader practical notion of "*what is appropriate in the circumstances*"' (emphasis added). In turn, as Cahn (1996: 31) observes, the success of any policy lies in 'frequent reassessment and repositioning to accommodate intervening influences and maintain a course, albeit an updated course toward the predetermined policy goal'. When context, inputs or resources change, the route to the intended goal, and potentially the goal itself, need to be reflected upon. Characterising policy making as 'craft' as much as 'science', Rhodes (2015: 21) therefore identifies a need for 'practical wisdom' to better understand 'what works as part of the *repertoire of governing*; of *what fits in a particular context*' (emphasis added). For Thornton and Ocasio (2008: 117) this enables institutional change processes such as 'bricolage', or 'the creation of new practices and institutions from different elements of existing institutions'.

Stability and change

Thornton and Ocasio (2008) further suggest that different underlying 'action logics' shape *stability and change*. As a result, four potential positions emerge: 'stability-positive', 'stability-negative', 'change-positive', 'change-negative'. Thus, while change and stability each have something to offer, a sensible strategy may be to acknowledge something of what each offers and claims, while recognising that neither asks all the right questions, and that any settlement between them may only be temporary.

In one reading of the relations between these positions, within *the same context at different times*, there may be a relatively linear process whereby action logics on the *'upside' of stability* create a context in which consistency and predictability are highly valued. However, in today's complex and dynamic contexts, events may push things into negative territory on the *'downside' of stability* (for example, stagnation and apathy). This may result in a search for 'progress' or 'new energy' on the *'upside' of change*, which may or may not be sufficient to provide effective solutions. If such change is ineffective, it may simply induce problems of 'inconsistency' and 'frustration' on the *'downside' of change*, to which a return to stability provides the preferred solution (Johnson, 2014). In this scenario, policy makers may be doomed to a personal sense – or accusations from others – of 'going round an infinity loop', 'reinventing the wheel' or putting 'old wine in new bottles'.

However, in a second, more dynamic reading of this process, 'more change' and 'more stability' may be required in *different but related contexts at the same time*. For example, even in the face of conformity in institutions, there may be both 'dominant and subsidiary norms' that need to be considered

(Thornton and Ocasio, 2008: 106), or multiple frames that may be needed in governing problems more effectively in the face of contextual uncertainty and dynamic complexity. In short, these insights demonstrate that policy makers' adoption and/or maintenance of a 'one-best-way orientation' often becomes untenable in anything more than the most controlled circumstances.

Finding a way forward

Dynamic Change Model

In an unstable world, there are a number of dynamic contexts in which we face various important *imperatives*. From these emerge a number of key *drivers of stability and change* that are important for optimising *stakeholder outcomes*. It is here where the opportunity to add *value and impact* is created. Pursuit of these drivers creates demand in the system that *may* be met by the *lever* of governance interventions. This chapter provides a novel DCM to identify the relationships between some of these emerging issues (see Figure 19.1).

The DCM also shows how the lever of governance interventions at the core of the model may be strengthened. This brings in two further elements of the model.

First, a series of key *enablers* of effective interventions are identified. These are:

- Technology, data and evidence: How do we use technology to communicate quickly and effectively across boundaries, as well as gather useful data and combine this with other data sources to make informed decisions on the effectiveness and prioritisation of interventions?
- Relationships: How do we build relationships with different actors to help catalyse and support more effective interventions?
- Entrepreneurship: How do we find ways to combine the capacities and capabilities of different actors (from the public, private, third and community sectors) in the supply of effective interventions?
- Strategy: What policies and guidance support more effective interventions?
- Capacity: What resources of staff, volunteers and funding are available to support interventions?

Each of these enablers are important in strengthening the ability of interventions to raise the effectiveness of the system, driving stability or change to meet the imperatives it faces, and raising the level of broader system and stakeholder capabilities. Importantly, *the stronger these enablers, the stronger the potential response.*

Second, there are a number of common criteria, or intermediate outcomes, against which interventions must be judged (including the speed, cost, risk and direct and indirect benefits of their deployment). These sit in dynamic tension with one another in which trade-offs are generally necessary, as it is

Figure 19.1: Dynamic Change Model

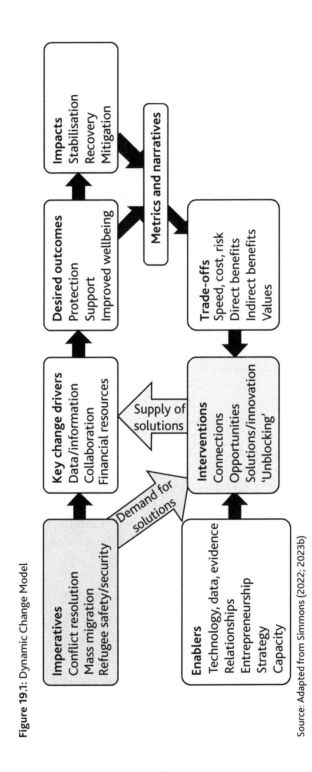

Source: Adapted from Simmons (2022; 2023b)

rare to be able to maximise them all simultaneously. Judicious navigation of these issues in managing tensions between them is then another space within which support for change and stability may be considered. Importantly, *the more difficult it is to navigate these trade-offs, the more constrained an actor's response.*

The Emergency Response Cycle

This chapter links insights from the DCM with strategies and capabilities drawn from the widely used 'Emergency Response Cycle' (ERC; National Governors' Association, 1979), a model which provides the building blocks for the TSA's in-house Linking Relief, Rehabilitation and Development model cited in Chapter 17. This encompasses a series of stages: mitigation, preparedness, response, recovery and prevention (see Figure 19.2).

This chapter moves on to explore the response of TSA UKIT to the war in Ukraine, using the combined perspectives from these two frameworks. The DCM recognises the war in Europe as a dynamic context which faces various important imperatives. As with many armed conflicts, these include safety and protection, managing the displacement of people, servicing basic needs (food, water, shelter and so on), handling of trauma, and – eventually – rebuilding, restoration, repatriation and peacebuilding. To the extent that these imperatives may be known in advance, they form a context for building ERC strategies and capabilities of *preparedness*. However, each emergency brings specific

Figure 19.2: Emergency Response Cycle

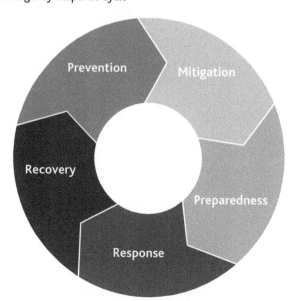

Source: Five Steps of Emergency Management, www.stlouis-mo.gov

disruptions to established patterns in different contexts that simultaneously require both 'urgent' and 'more considered' responses. Accordingly, various drivers of stability and change must be employed. In the *response* phase of the ERC, this creates demand for interventions from the system of governmental and non-governmental actors. In turn, actors such as TSA UKIT may seek to meet this demand, using their resources and connections to either create new opportunities, or help unblock the path to potential solutions. Given that different actors often have different strengths and capabilities, any single actor will rarely be able to meet this demand on their own. This means that the overall emergency response will often benefit from each actor (1) recognising 'the art of the possible', and (2) contributing to a level of collaboration and co-production within the system (whether this is deliberately coordinated or more self-organising; Groethe-Hammer and Berthod, 2017).

As patterns begin to stabilise in the *recovery* phase of the ERC, it is possible to evaluate both the effectiveness of the immediate (urgent) emergency response, and assess the need for ongoing (more considered) adaptations and recalibrations in the wider system. This is undertaken with the intention of optimising desired outcomes and restorative impacts. However, actors' ability to deliver on these outcomes and impacts may be constrained. As noted earlier in the DCM, this recognises both the inevitable 'trade-offs' in different interventions, and the strength of an actor's 'enablers'. In this way, evidence from the best available metrics, standards and stakeholder narratives may be used to strengthen feedback for the future. Such metrics include a 'combined added value' approach (Simmons, 2023a), whereby the value added by interventions may be mapped in a number of important ways: from 'functional' value (for example, calibrating activities to better fulfil the needs of beneficiaries) to 'social' value (for example, wellbeing of individuals and communities, social capital and the environment) to 'emotional' value (for example, the way people feel as a result of interventions) as well as 'financial' value (for example, cost efficiency).

This mapping framework can be used either quite quickly and intuitively, or in much greater depth, to identify gaps that help optimise 'value creation' and minimise 'value leakage'. Learning from this (and other important frameworks and metrics) can be fed into discourses around creating, sharing, transferring, adapting and embedding good practice – in turn, helping to promote effective *prevention* and *mitigation* in the ERC, and to return the system to a greater sense of *preparedness* for future events.

Facing new challenges: the case of the Salvation Army UK and Ireland Territory response to the war in Ukraine

The DCM and ERC each travel well between different contexts, providing conceptual and methodological resources in relation to the important challenges we continue to face in an uncertain world. They are discussed and applied here in greater depth in understanding the particular case of TSA UKIT response to the war in Ukraine.

Imperatives

In this crisis the focus was the timely and sustained preservation of life. For UKIT this was bounded by their Christian Mission: Love God, Love Others. The war in Ukraine prompted an unprecedented public donation response for TSA's international work from UKIT, even without a formal appeal. Managing funds by TSA UKIT posed a high-profile challenge, exemplifying a rapid and complex response to a 'wicked issue', while also emphasising the need for evolving structures and processes for future effectiveness.

TSA UKIT responded to the crisis by collaborating with other TSA entities (territories) worldwide, immediately facing challenges due to the crisis's dynamic nature and lack of an initial overarching strategy. Communication hurdles arose as the crisis unfolded rapidly. Expectations from funding territories varied and did not always match immediate on–the–ground capacity. TSA's model is not that of an international aid agency, where response teams can be landed in a crisis zone at short notice. As shown in Chapters 16 and 17, their models of working are through churches, social services and people who are already living in–country, for whom the response is often highly personalised.

Key drivers

Over time, the complexity of this situation became apparent. An ordinary emergency response would cover one specific location/territory. Here, the response was needed simultaneously across many different countries that were highly impacted by the flow of refugees. This was a challenge for UKIT, where money and projects are normally assessed and matched through a model used for disasters in one specific location (for example, an earthquake). Instead, projects and funding needed to be channelled to multiple entities throughout a complex system that was only materialising as the emergency progressed.

The public's compassionate response to the crisis, driven by a focus on humanity and the desire to bring dignity and safety to those affected by war, played a pivotal role. Generous financial giving, nearly 20 times more than typical campaigns in the initial weeks, allowed TSA to respond across Europe, demonstrating flexibility in addressing the widespread impact beyond Ukraine. Messaging to the public ensured that scope was allowed for long-term spend, and that spending was not restricted only to within Ukraine, but to all affected by the war regardless of country.

UKIT's role was to help with the distribution of funds. As identified in Chapter 16, UKIT's response is often bespoke and localised; quick, but small-scale. This is TSA's strength as an organisation, where it is a Church first and foremost. This model for the use of its own internal partnerships led to some resistance in scaling up the response by funding additional personnel and project teams, as is common practice in some international non-governmental organisations.

Interventions: connections, opportunities, solutions, innovation, 'unblocking'

The UKIT's response to the Ukraine crisis has involved two distinct strands: providing funds to TSA in Ukraine itself and territories bordering Ukraine; and TSA support within the UK for those displaced by the war. Both aimed at localised, organic support, including meals, vouchers, shelter, social integration and emotional support.

In this way, TSA is quick to respond, but through local officers, volunteers and members from a corps responding, and growing organically from there. In the early weeks of the crisis in Ukraine, the officers and volunteers from the corps were in the subways, providing hot meals, comfort and emotional support. TSA is often first at the scene if it is close by; its offices are localised to the context, and officers, volunteers and members are often local, speak the language, and can mobilise quickly to help people. Although on a local scale, this proved a huge strength.

TSA tends to be very 'hands-on', fulfilling needs that are very real on the ground. For example, it distributes vouchers, food and hot meals. But it also has considerable pastoral strengths in its church personnel and officers, providing comfort and emotional support. Internal conversations are now leaning towards supporting people where there is trauma, stress and emotional strain, taking a person-centred approach. This is not driven by hard strategy, but by more organic learning from TSA's experiences over the preceding months.

Enablers

Strategy

TSA's strategy to act locally where corps are already in-country can, however, limit work where the TSA is not physically located or cannot expand organically. Given that the crisis spanned multiple TSA administrative zones of varying capacities, scales and make-up, coordination has been challenging. As highlighted in Chapter 16, the crisis also highlighted a weakness for the organisation: working country-by-country leading to a lack of an overarching strategy and set of objectives at the zonal (regional) level. Although this strategy was emerging slowly by mid/end 2023, structures, governance and sovereignty between territorial and zonal offices probably would need to be considered and addressed if TSA were to respond more strategically at a European (zonal) level.

Another key issue is a lack of coordination for fundraising: TSA does not have a global fundraising strategy. Its response to the war in Ukraine has highlighted a weakness in terms of cross-territorial communication and decision-making processes. Territories may thus miss opportunities to leverage each other's strengths, and provide a coordinated message to the public as one organisation.

Relationships

Internal relationships have been key during the crisis response. At international level, a former European international development structure was expanded to include other funding territories, called the Supporting Office Forum (SOF). In a good example of *preparedness*, officers knew each other quite well coming into the crisis. When the SOF started meeting weekly, there was a good rapport and a positivity about collaborating. In turn, good relationships between the SOF, TSA International Headquarters and the International Emergency Services (another internal team) served to maintain a level of mutual accountability. These relationships have remained strong in working through challenges productively. SOF has moved to monthly meetings as the crisis has stabilised.

More locally to the war in Ukraine, as also discussed in Chapters 16 and 17, UKIT opted for direct spending due to TSA presence in crisis areas. TSA Eastern European Territory (EET) has been the primary responder, benefiting from live relationships and shared regional languages. As the crisis persists, transitions to longer-term strategies include increased personnel in Ukraine, extending services to encompass education and enhancing quality of life for displaced individuals both within and outside Ukraine.

In terms of external relationships, parts of TSA contribute to another faith-based organisation called the ACT Alliance. This gave UKIT the option to utilise TSA money to fund programmes with any ACT Alliance partner for people impacted by the war. Yet that option was rarely utilised, highlighting a hesitance to working with and through external organisational partners as a result of historical partnerships resulting in little perceived benefit.

Entrepreneurship

Faced with an unprecedented influx of public donations, UKIT needed to be resourceful in distributing funds. Initially, it approved a certain amount to be ring-fenced for the UK response, setting up a very simple application process for any corps/centre/department in the UKIT. It then developed a guide to what the funds could and could not be used for. Slowly, corps by corps, people applied for those funds – anything from a few hundred pounds to fund a laptop for an individual that needed to apply for jobs, to the Sundial Café in Norfolk, which employed a Ukrainian chef to help celebrate the Ukrainian culture. In the last 12 months, corps have been actively engaged. Mirroring the response in Ukraine, corps officers and volunteers are responding on an individual, family-by-family level, as opposed to a big territorially coordinated response.

Overall, a key message to the public was that UKIT was going to be part of the response to the crisis in Ukraine for as long as it takes. This long-term perspective meant that the money being raised could be spent down the line for refugees arriving in the UK. UKIT is now in the process of extending these funds to ensure there is enough money to continue to respond to these people's various needs.

Technology, data and evidence

During the first few weeks and months of the crisis data was not coming out fast enough for UKIT to be able to feed back to donors about what TSA was actually doing on the ground. Data was very limited, but also very haphazard in those initial days, brought together from whatever was available from Facebook, emails and telephone calls. As a result, a Monitoring, Evaluation and Accountability Learning Group (MEAL) was formed, made up of SOF offices and EET personnel. MEAL adopted a tool from the Switzerland territory, called Kobo, to report back on all activities: the number of meals provided, the number of people reached, and so on. No similar data was coming out of other territories, however. It is ironic that UKIT has the same struggles on its own territorial level; in the UK, getting data about what has been happening in relation to Ukraine remains very difficult.

It is also worth noting that technology has been key for document-sharing and communication across TSA's country offices during the crisis. Communicating via Microsoft Teams has enabled them to share information much more quickly. In turn, this has helped ensure the funding model was not negatively impacted, and that there has been communication back to the public on the crisis response and how they could provide further support.

Capacity

Public donations saw a significant giving response from the general public. The EET rose to the situation and organised themselves to utilise the funding that was coming in. This saw their budget rise from less than US$1 million per year on programmes to suddenly $16.4 million in a year. That huge step up in capacity has provided a strong basis for programming and the ability to deliver future projects. Nevertheless, months of high stress and emotional toil erodes people's ability to be effective, and TSA has had to build in ways of giving people rest, given the pastoral nature and time length for the response.

Trade-offs

Passions and interests

The crisis in Ukraine has raised questions about organisational identity when working in the humanitarian space. How can TSA utilise its strengths? It may need to clarify who it is as an organisation in a humanitarian response to be able to operate in external partnerships – whether it is ACT Alliance or UN cluster groups that meet in different emergency settings.

Scale of response

The common vision for preservation of life and ongoing wellbeing galvanised the TSA response throughout the globe. TSA is typically not able to rapidly upscale like some other international non-governmental organisations and charities. As its operating model is one of funding its existing local entities, it is not specialist at that sort of response modality. As a church-based movement, TSA is much more small-scale, but its presence is very long term. Thus, TSA is able to assess the trade-offs in terms of shared goals, and where it is willing to compromise. As we saw in Chapter 16, a desire to invest resources is illustrated by moving staff from administrative roles at International Headquarters to Ukraine and neighbouring countries, rather than having budget or resource to move personnel from other response projects or employ many new staff.

Internally, territories plan their own response for emergency work, and make decisions with little intervention at the zonal level. This can cause misalignment when multiple TSA entities are involved in a complex response – such as TSA's response to the war in Ukraine. The global refugee migration situation provides an opportunity for TSA to step in and assess the need for a regional strategic response, rather than just aggregating what individual countries are doing.

Speed of response

In the evolving long-term response, TSA will start looking at community development-led initiatives, while still acknowledging people have basic needs due to displacement. It is not a clean transition from one stage to the next. For example, within the same response, TSA might be handing out food vouchers in one country while the neighbouring territory is moving onto longer-term community engagement.

How money is spent

Limited capacity on the ground can cause pressures from donors. For example, restrictions on funding meant money could not be spent on purchasing TSA buildings, which some feel is a key long-term need. For some practitioners this represents a lack of appreciation of what is happening on the ground, but TSA has to maintain the spirit of the donations to respond to the crisis, and capital investment would likely go beyond that purpose.

Desired outcomes

These included clear humanitarian-care-guided project outcomes, in a family-by-family, individual-by-individual, person-centred approach, focusing on food, pastoral care and directing individuals to key agencies. While TSA's decentralised model allows locally driven services according to the context, challenges can arise over time in the prioritisation and alignment of outcomes as people move from one country to the other, without a proper system for tracking them. An excellent example of this is highlighted in the young child accessing children's camp in Chapter 16 and the emotional benefits of attending something that is not part of a linear development programme.

In examples of *prevention* and *mitigation* in the ERC, there is now a shift from emergency provision around food towards longer-term thinking. Particularly with Ukraine, TSA is looking to fund a physical team in Ukraine to support existing personnel in terms of where the programme funding is going. When the war does stop or scale down and there is an influx of people back into Ukraine, there will be another big call for funds to help rebuild, and these offices will need to have this additional capacity.

Impacts

Despite challenges in measurement, impacts are evident with a significant upscale in provision of meals, shelter and vouchers. The response within EET alone is very high: to date more than 88,000 cooked meals and over 91,000 vouchers have been distributed. Over 13,000 overnight stays have also been provided, including for children, in TSA-run facilities.

Organisational shifts, including the MEAL subgroup, have enhanced TSA's global crisis response capability. The crisis has also prompted new considerations regarding collaboration with external partners, and how TSA's strengths can combine with broader humanitarian efforts. However, in the absence of definitive outcomes or impacts, TSA may be missing opportunities to share learning and capture impact. Anecdotal evidence provides some incredible impact stories, but the extent to which they are informing TSA's approach is unclear.

Metrics and narratives

Success in UKIT's role with the distribution of funds is a key metric. More broadly, the response shows some of the complexity of agreeing direction without overarching objectives. The Kobo tool, recording and reporting on day-to-day, real-time activities, has been a very positive step. It provides real-time information for decision-makers, rather than waiting for progress or end-of-year reports. This holds considerable positive potential for TSA to both plan and respond much more quickly.

Information flows from all partners have been key to understanding the situation. However, for UKIT, data collection at the local levels within the UK has been a challenge. This presents another missed opportunity to share learning and improve what the movement does. While cultural challenges in an action-led environment mean that recording data might be seen by some as a distraction from practical activities, cycles of learning may be devised to alter this perspective.

Organisational learning

TSA has developed its systems to drill down in more depth in response to the complexity of the crisis in Ukraine. Increased use of standardised monitoring software across the EET and other partner territories offers real-time insights on the ground, increasing their capacity and ability to scale up. However, this stops short of a properly formed strategy.

Challenges in forming a strategy involve the level at which decisions are taken. One of the key principles TSA holds dear is to listen to the people who are closest to the action, rather than try to dictate things from afar. For emergency work, territories thus currently decide entirely on their own plan and response with little or no coordination at the zonal level. In terms of *preparedness* in the ERC framework, to what extent would TSA be better equipped zonally or globally to respond to future crises through more efficient ways of working and collaborating together? Moreover, how does TSA deal with partnerships with external agencies? It is important to move these things forward, step-by-step. This may mean addressing tensions related to structures, governance and territorial sovereignty within TSA's various administrative levels, especially at a European (zonal) level, so that intended outcomes and capacities can be aligned.

Learning from the Dynamic Change Model

A key practical limitation with pre-applied logic models is that the enablers, context and proposed outcomes are rarely the same, and the breadth of services undertaken by TSA (pastoral, food provision, older people services, children and youth services) is extremely broad and interwoven. In high-demand and dynamic environments, grounded definitions and 'rules of engagement' become essential tools, particularly amid changing stakeholders and potential language barriers.

Yet as an opportunity to stand back and take a more considered perspective around 'optimising outcomes' from these services, interventions and engagements, the DCM serves as a valuable framework for reflecting on completed work and guiding ongoing responses to the evolving crisis from the war in Ukraine, as well as other complex issues faced by TSA. As Simmons (2023a) notes in a previous volume on the *Social Determinants of Health*, to make any kind of progress with such 'wicked' problems, the task is often to ask the right questions rather than provide the right answers. Yet in complex and uncertain spaces, 'what is a good question?' is itself a good question. Navigating this terrain is a complex and ongoing task (Grint, 2005).

In conjunction with the ERC model, the DCM encourages actors in emergency response settings to identify and ask various questions that may have been missed or ignored. Figure 19.3 provides a worked example to address UKIT's response to the war in Ukraine. Starting from the top left corner and moving across the top, Figure 19.3 considers the DCM's key *imperatives* in relation to this complex problem, as well as some important *drivers* of change or stability in optimising desired *outcomes* and *impacts*. Important questions of prioritisation arise in each of these aspects in guiding the organisation's response. At the next level, various additional questions arise in Figure 19.3, in the demand created in the system for *interventions* that may or may not be met by TSA. The degree to which this is attempted/ achieved is then dependent on the strength of TSA's *enablers* and how *trade-offs* are negotiated. The prominent role of technology as an enabler to donations, response and communications is noted here as a key support for the data and entrepreneurialism enablers. In each case, Figure 19.3 raises further questions about the capacities and capabilities of TSA to intervene effectively across the emergency response cycle.

Conclusion

In this volume, the *Conceptual Framework for Action on the Social Determinants of Health* provides an operational approach and focus on people who have limited resources and resilience to respond to challenges (such as war, and the related issues of being displaced from their homes and their country). The *structural determinants* of social class, gender and ethnicity are mapped in this framework, including being a refugee, and living in a war zone. Interventions (such as supporting mothers and children; see Chapters 7, 8 and 12) can be understood as *intermediate determinants* of health and wellbeing.

Figure 19.3: 'Optimising Outcomes': TSA's UKIT response to the war in Ukraine

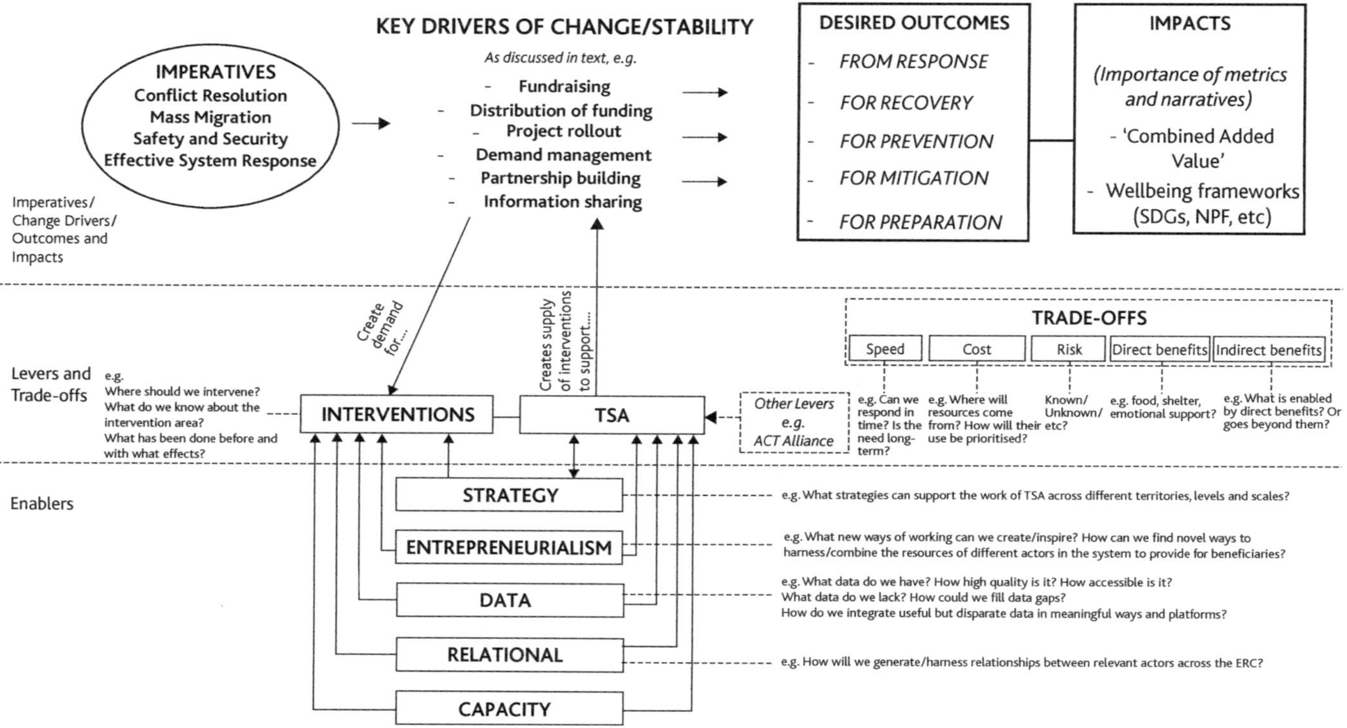

Source: After Simmons (2022; 2023b)

This chapter builds on the strategic approaches to wicked issues (as reviewed in the previous volume in this series, *COVID-19 and Social Determinants of Health: Wicked Issues and Relationalism*; Bonner, 2023), in understanding more about such interventions. Addressing immediate and longer-term developmental approaches to war in Ukraine requires an understanding of the complexity and dynamism in many policy environments, which places a premium on not only sound judgement, but also the ability to *question, learn and adapt*. This chapter has introduced a model and theory of change (the DCM) developed in two previous applied research contexts (Simmons, 2022; 2023b), which offers the potential for novel insights in numerous further settings. In combination with the ERC, the DCM has been used here to illuminate the case of TSA UKIT's response to the war in Ukraine.

The model provides a structure around which to ask 'good questions' that allow more informed planning, choices and decision-making. This takes in questions of prioritisation, as well as the design of interventions in the light of trade-offs and the strength of key enablers. It further invites organisational learning as a result of the answers to these questions. In complex environments, where the problems faced by organisations such as TSA are often located, this provides an important tool for adaptation, mitigation and innovation in navigating a path to possible new solutions, both in the immediate and longer term.

References

Argyris, C. (1976) Single-loop and double-loop models in research on decision-making. *Administrative Science Quarterly*, 21: 363–375.

Bonner, A. (2023) *COVID-19 and Social Determinants of Health: Wicked Issues and Relationalism*, Bristol: Policy Press.

Cahn, M. (1996) *Building Evaluative Models in Environmental Policy*. Northridge: California State University.

Geyer, R. and Cairney, P. (2015) *Handbook on Complexity and Public Policy*. Cheltenham: Edward Elgar.

Greenwood, J. (1998) The role of reflection in single- and double-loop learning. *Journal of Advanced Nursing*, 27: 1048–1053.

Grint, K. (2005) Problems, problems, problems: the social construction of leadership. *Human Relations*, 58(11): 1467–1494.

Groethe-Hammer, M. and Berthod, O. (2017) The programming of decisions for disaster and emergency response. *Current Sociology*, 65(5): 735–755.

Hammond, K. (1996) *Human Judgment and Social Policy*. Oxford: Oxford University Press.

Hoppe, R. (2011) *The Governance of Problems*. Bristol: Policy Press.

Jessop, B. (1997) The governance of complexity and the complexity of governance. In A. Amin and J. Hausner (eds), *Beyond Markets and Hierarchy*. Cheltenham: Edward Elgar, pp 111–147.

Johnson, B. (2014) *Polarity Management*. Amherst: HRD Press.

National Governors' Association (1979) *Emergency Preparedness Project Report*. Washington, DC: Government Printing Office.

Rhodes, R. (2015) Recovering the 'craft' of public administration in Westminster government. Paper to Political Studies Association Conference, Sheffield, March–April.

Rittel, H. and Webber, M. (1973) Dilemmas in a general theory of planning. *Policy Sciences*, 4: 155–169.

Sanderson, I. (2009) Intelligent policy making for a complex world: pragmatism, evidence and learning. *Political Studies*, 57: 699–719.

Simmons, R. (2022) *Optimising Outcomes from Procurement*. Final Report, ESRC.

Simmons, R. (2023a) Using relationalism to navigate wicked issues. In A. Bonner (ed), *Wicked Issues, Relationalism and the Social Determinants of Health*. Bristol: Policy Press, pp 41–55.

Simmons, R. (2023b) *The Value of Water: A Theory of Change*. Stirling: Hydro-Nation Chair.

Simon, H. (1955) A behavioral model of rational choice. *Quarterly Journal of Economics*, 69(1): 99–118.

Thornton, P. and Ocasio, W. (2008) Institutional logics. In R. Greenwood, C. Oliver, R. Suddaby and K. Sahlin-Andersson (eds), *SAGE Handbook of Organizational Institutionalism*. London: SAGE, pp 99–129.

Conclusion

Adrian Bonner

This book has been developed as a result of grounded research over many years into the issues faced by people at the edge of the communities related to a range of issues reviewed in previous volumes of this *Social Determinants of Health* series. Significant determinants of health include social inequality (Bonner, 2018), the role of local authorities (Bonner, 2022), the impact of COVID-19 and its impact and socioeconomic challenges for the most deprived people and communities (Bonner, 2023). The range of psycho-social domains impacting a person's vulnerabilities, and affecting their wellbeing across the life course, are mapped across the *structural* and *intermediate* determinants of health are represented by *social position* in Figure I.1, in the Introduction to this book. The previous publications have provided perspectives through which to consider the global threats of war in Europe and displacement of 6,739,400, people from Ukraine; 6,168,100 moved to Europe and 571,300 beyond Europe (UHNRC, 2024). Understanding the complexity of this quintessential 'wicked issue' and navigating through it with appropriate governmental and non-governmental strategic and governance structures, is suggested through a *relational* perspective. This should facilitate the development of appropriate responses, at a human level and with respect to interrelated public and community–voluntary partnerships. Examples of *relational* approaches to supporting displaced people from Ukraine are presented in Part III of this book.

The role of the United Nations (UN) in safeguarding human rights is being challenged by war crimes committed by Russia. As part of aggressive political posturing, global nuclear safety is threatened by Russia withdrawing from the Comprehensive Nuclear Test Ban, agreed by the UN on 10 September 1996 (see Appendix A and Chapter 3).

The war in Europe, and existential threat of nuclear confrontation, add to the complexity of navigating the drivers of change by both government and non-governmental agencies (see Chapter 19).

Since the publication of the first book in this series (Bonner, 2018), written in the *decade of austerity*, the global challenges of COVID-19 and the increasing awareness of the *climate change crisis* on human welfare are global threats to health and wellbeing which impact on people across the globe, particular those at the lower end of the social gradient (Marmot, 2020).

The main themes of this social determinants of health series are mapped out in Figure C.1, beginning, in the first volume, with social inequality and wellbeing. The *structural* frameworks of local and national communities should provide the hard structures which protect the fundamental rights to human life, peace and dignity (see the UN Charter [UN, 2023a]). However, the importance of people supporting each other and volunteering to help those less fortunate was demonstrated in the COVID-19 pandemic (O'Leary and Chadha, 2023), and in responses to supporting people displaced from Ukraine (see Chapter 12). The direct and indirect effects of conflict have both immediate and long-term effects on health. Early death and disability can result from fighting, however war has wider socioeconomic effects, as discussed in Chapters 1, 2 and 19. Socioeconomic factors can impact on health reflected in trauma and family violence (see Chapter 9), child health, sexual, reproductive and maternal health (see Chapter 6), and both infectious and non-communicative diseases (due to stress-related impairment of the immune system). In the longer term the consequences of war can be seen in human development (see Chapters 6 and 8) and the process of ageing (see Chapter 10). War-related public health issues have been reviewed by Garry and Checci (2020).

Of all of the consequences of war listed here, military aggression on children is a violation of their human rights. Multilevel, trauma-informed approaches supporting psychological and physical resilience, mitigating the distress caused by forced separation from parents, are needed to address the mental health and psychosocial intervention needs of current and future children who have remained in the war zones and those displace into receiving countries (Racioppi et al, 2022).

As part of the Ukraine National Recovery Plan, the World Health Organization has set out a set of priorities for the recovery of the health system in Ukraine (WHO, 2023). These include:

- Restoring priority health services in ways that scale up the government of Ukraine's vision for health service reform, while addressing critical health risks facing the Ukrainian people due to impacts of the war.
- Capital investment, planning for major investments in recovery and reconstruction with long-term consequences for the health system, to enable Ukraine to protect health in the near term while building back better in the long term.
- Health financing priorities to sustain essential services in the face of severe fiscal constraints and achieve more with available funding.
- Strengthening institutions – supporting the needs of central and local government health-sector institutions responsible for policy, planning, stewardship and governance functions, and governance reforms that are vital to an effective, accountable healthcare system and Ukraine's aspirations of European integration.

Figure C.1: Books in the *Social Determinants of Health* series

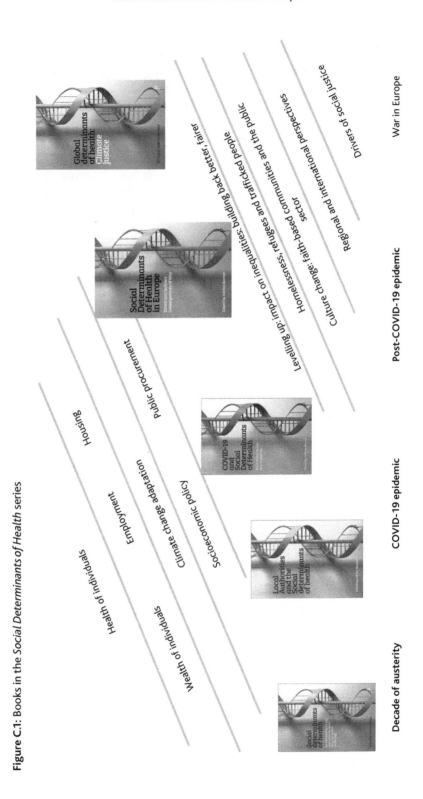

Wicked issues and barbarians

The origins and causations of war, since the emergence of early civilisations, have deep-seated existential roots, based on human insecurity exacerbated by the threat of 'barbarians at the gate'. In 2014, Barack Obama urged a united response from the Muslim world after the *barbaric* beheading of Steven Sotloff by the Islamic State (Black, 2014). The West used the term 'barbaric' to refer to acts of evil undermining a safe and secure society.

The word *barbarian* is derived from a Greek word, a term which has changed significantly since the term was used in historical discourse on the 'Roman barbarians' who attacked the ancient 'Mycenaean' who ruled a large part of Greece 3,300 years ago (Jarus, 2022; Lacey, 2022).

It has been suggested (Vlassopoulos, 2013) that 'by the archaic period [2,700 years ago]', the word *barbarian* had a linguistic connotation, related to communication issues leading to distrust and aggression groups. In the historical literature, Greeks referred to any non-Greek people using a different language (Egyptians, Persians, Indians, Celts, Vikings and Goth, and others), some producing sounds such as 'bar bar'. In the changing meaning of the term, from an understanding of geographical, social structures and customs, 'different from us', and those that do not speak our language, the term 'barbarian groups' has been used as an ethnocentric description related to physical appearance or behaviour (Dench, 2022).

From a Eurocentric view of the world in the 19th century the concept of 'civilised' and 'uncivilised' barbarians was commonly held. This underpinned notions such as admission to the 'family of nations', and the concept of *civilisation,* as distinct from the ancient ideas of civilised barbarians (developed by Mirabeau, in 1757, then Fergusson in 1767), contributed to the self-concept of European-centred international society (Bowden, 2004; Heraclides and Dialla, 2015).

In the *Something Understood* podcast, 'Waiting for the barbarians', Mark Tully debated the proposition in Cavafy's poem 'Waiting for the barbarians' that every culture needs a sense of *barbarians outside the gate* in order to give meaning to its sense of identity and civilisation, and to provide a sense of unity within a society. The existential threats of barbarians and a social value underpinned the expressed superiority of colonisers, such as the British in suppression of Indians in the Raj, and 'barbarians at the gates' has, in colonial times, motivated inhuman actions such as the Amritsar Massacre in which British troops fired on a large crowd of unarmed Indians in 1919 (Wilson, 2019).

Examples of barbarians at the gates include the besieging of Leningrad, by Germany – regarded as barbarians at the gates of the city. In an interview with Mark Tully in 2005, Derek Hawes (who worked in the School of Policy Studies, at the University of Bristol), commenting on Cervantes' comment on Cavafy's poem, noted that 'all civilisations need barbarians to allow us to assess the challenges of outsiders to our values, and allow us to judge and reassess our own way of living, strengthen and redefine our values'. Not only can we learn from the barbarians but sometime take on board new thinking and practices, and provide a better unified society. That view was supported by St Paul in early Christian philosophy, at a time when the world was unstable; Greeks were being overshadowed by the Romans, in the letter to the Colossians, 'although you all come from differ places, and have different values, *all are one* from a Christian ethical perspective'. Hawes goes on to suggest that the barbarians are no longer in the distant hills, but are within society, as seen in anti-social and sometimes aggressive activities within our towns and cities, referred to by Obama, with reference to ISIS.

Contemporary values and ideas, and insecurities, such as 'barbarians at the gates', develop from early nurturing of children and the nurturing environment reviewed in Chapter 8, and in the description of the values taught to children in Russia and Ukraine, when it was part of the Soviet Union (see Chapter 7). In the Israel–Palestine conflict, children in Gaza are being subjected to unimaginable levels of aggression against themselves, their homes and their communities. The long-term effects on children and their families from the war in the Balkans (see Chapter 6) demonstrate the fundamental existential personally held values which mitigate against peace and reconciliation, as highlighted by Peter Hain, in the Introduction to Part IV.

Culture and societal values are *structural* determinants of health (see Figure I.1 in the Introduction). In Chapter 5, Froud reflected on the mapping of *UN Sustainable Goals* onto the *social determinants of health* framework, and provided an insight into the values-drive strategy of the church and charity, The Salvation Army. This faith-based organisation has played a significant role in addressing human suffering since its origins in the late 19th century. Its activities in Europe are listed in Appendix B. Tomalin in Chapter 18 considers how faith-based organisations can make an important contribution in influencing societal values. These can be positive drivers of health and wellbeing. Conversely, division and hate can be stirred up. However, 'faith-based mediation is a long-established response of faith actors to war, both informally in their communities but increasingly also in formal international efforts'. Chapters 4 and 18 provide critical reviews of the roles of religion and faith identity in human conflict since the beginning of civilisation.

In a contemporary diverse multiethnic, multi-faith, more multicultural world, there is an increasing need to help people to understand and be proud of their differences. This view of civilisation has to take account of 'foreigners', legal and illegal immigrants and refugees coming into 'our country' (barbarians at the gates?), The increased support for far-right political parties, some, with intent to damage society through bombings and killing people might be considered an example of barbarians (within the gates), according to Hawes.

Historical reflections in this book show that we need to see others and understand their cultures, develop trust and employ *relational* approaches to resolve conflicts such as access to basic energy and food resources, learn from the values of others and navigate the *wicked issues* discussed in this and the previous volumes in this series. However, from the historical discourses on barbarians, summarised earlier, a fundamental existential threat of *barbarians at the gate* is clearly used by Putin to support his claims of a territorial threat from the North Atlantic Treaty Organization, in justification for his 'special operation' in Ukraine. With reference to the *Conceptual Framework for Action on the Social Determinants of Health* (see Figure I.1 in the Introduction to this book), the *structural* aspects of *culture and society* are influenced and can be manipulated by government. The crimes against humanity, identified by the United Nations High Commissioner for Refugees, justified by an existential threat cannot easily be explained by traditional approaches to social psychology in a tightly controlled society, in which freedom is suppressed and opposition to Putin met with long prison terms. Such deep-seated negative psychological factors mitigate against healthy relationships and are linked to conflict in the modern world of capitalism (Burrough and Helyar, 2009).

The way forward

The chapters in this book suggest a number of actions which might be considered in response to the ongoing war in Europe. These actions include:

- learning lessons from previous conflicts;
- supporting vulnerable people with less resilience relating to their social position;
- understanding the impact of traumatic effects on children and impact on their educational development;
- focusing on neonatal and post-natal care of children to live in a postwar world;
- developing targeted programmes for children in war zones and those displaced from their home countries;
- supporting fair and equitable resources;prioritisation to provide optimal support for conflict-affected populations;
- using the principles of *relationalism* in understanding and addressing conflict;
- adapting and developing existing rehabitation programmes,accommodation and employment/skill development facilities for displaced people.

Policy development frameworks, such as the *Conceptual Framework for Action on the Social Determinants of Health* model and the *Linking Relief,*

Figure C.2: Symbolic representation of 'Barbarians at the Gate'

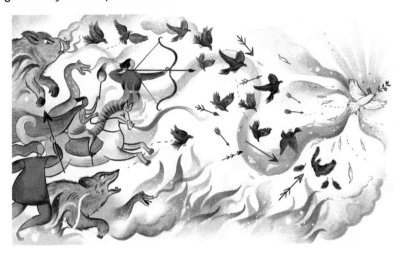

Note: This representation is inspired by the idea that the term 'barbarian' is derived from the Greek, meaning 'different from us'. The illustration therefore has a stylistic nod to Ancient Greek art and mythology. It also reflects the invasion of Ukraine by using images of crows, which are used in Ukrainian art as a significant symbol of 'the enemy' (Novobrantes, 2017). The dove, representing peace, provides a link with the quotation from *Le Morte d'Arthur* which was the inspiration for the final section of Karl Jenkins' *The Armed Man: A Mass for Peace* (see 'End comment').

Source: Illustration and caption provided by Clair Rossiter, copyright 2024

Rehabilitation and Development model, presented in Chapter 17 and the strategic model presented in Chapter 19 can help analysts and policy makers to identify levels of intervention and entry points for action with respect to *structural* and *intermediate* determinants. However, a consideration of the principles of *relationalism* (Introduction to Part III), promoting trusted relationships respecting the rights and values of others (not regarded as barbarians) should underpin responses of the various government and non-governmental agencies in responding to the direct and indirect consequences of war.

The four parts of this book provide an insight into the *structural* and *intermediate* determinants of the direct and indirect impact of the war in Europe, with a particular focus on vulnerable people who, defined within the *structural* and *social position* with the conceptual framework of social determinants of health (WHO, 2010), are most at risk from the *wicked issues* of viral epidemics, climate change and the socioeconomic impact of these global challenges.

In summarising the contents of this volume, which focuses on war in Europe, there is a need for a global approach to current and future *wicked issues*. A social justice perspective is needed. Currently the editor is working with international university collaborators, to promote a university-based network to work objectively with governmental and non-governmental agencies, in collaboration with the International Salvation Army, working in 136 countries. Application of a critical understanding of the *structural determinants*, which should include a grounded view of culture and societal values, and interlinked *intermediate determinants* will support the most effective collaborative interventions, particularly for the most vulnerable. *The Salvation Army International Collaborative University Network (SAICUN)*, working with government and non-government agencies is currently being developed to provide a critical review of *Global Determinants of Health in an Unstable World: Drivers of Climate Justice*. That edited book will be launched as the next volume in this series.

End comment

> Lancelot: Better is peace than always war.
> Guinevere: And better is peace than evermore war.
> (From *Le Morte d'Arthur*, Sir Thomas Malory (1485). Used as the basis of *Better is Peace* in the final section of *The Armed Man: A Mass for Peace* by Karl Jenkins, which ends the mass on a note of hope. This music was composed in recognition of the war in the Balkans, commissioned by the Royal Armouries; highly recommended listening to provide a background to Chapters 6, 15 and others in this book, providing a spiritual-emotional dimension to *structural* and *intermediate* dimensions of health and wellbeing)

References

Black, I. (2014) Obama: US will not be intimidated by Isis 'barbarism'. *The Guardian*, 3 September. Available at: https://www.theguardian.com/world/2014/sep/03/obama-isis-barbarism-steven-sotloff

Bonner, A. (ed) (2018) *Social Determinants of Health: An Interdisciplinary Approach to Social Inequality and Wellbeing*. Policy Press.

Bonner, A. (ed) (2022) *Local Authorities and Social Determinants of Health*. Policy Press.

Bonner, A. (ed) (2023) *COVID-19 and the Social Determinants of Health: Wicked Issues and Relationalism*. Policy Press.

Bowden, B. (2004) The idea of civilisation: its origins and social-political character. *Critical Review of International Social and Political Philosophy*, 7(1).

Burrough, B. and Helyar, J. (2009) *Barbarians at the Gate: The Fall of RJR Nabisco*. Arrow Book, first published in Great Britain by Johnathan Cape Ltd

Dench, E. (2022) Barbarian. *Oxford Classical Dictionary*. Available at: https://oxfordre.com/classics/display/10.1093/acrefore/9780199381135.001.0001/acrefore-9780199381135-e-1051#:~:text=28)%20suggests%20that%20barbaros%20originally,throughout%20and%20beyond%20classical%20antiquity

Garry, S. and Checci, E. (2020) Armed conflict and public health: into the 21st century. *Journal of Public Health*, 42(3): e287–e298.

Herclides, A. and Dialla, A. (2015) Eurocentrism, 'civilisation' and the 'barbarians'. Humanitarian intervention in the long nineteenth century. Manchester Scholarship Online, Oxford Academic. Available at: https://academic.oup.com/manchester-scholarship-online/book/16587/chapter/173644959

Jarus, O. (2022) Who were the Barbarians? *AWS*, September. Available at: https://www.livescience.com/45297-barbarians.html#

Lacey, J. (2022) How dangerous were the barbarians? In *Rome: Strategy of Empire*. Oxford Academic. Available at: https://academic.oup.com/book/43892/chapter-abstract/370130724?redirectedFrom=fulltext

Marmot, M. (2020) *Health Equity in England: The Marmot Review 10 Years On*. Institute of Health Equity. Available at: https://www.instituteofhealthequity.org/resources-reports/marmot-review-10-years-on/the-marmot-review-10-years-on-full-report.pdf

Novobranets, I. (2017) Oh, those crows Swooped down. https://holodomormuseum.org.ua/en/tema-pro-holodomor/oh-those-crows-swooped-down/#:~:text=The%20artist%20painted%20crows%20as,dress%20in%20traditional%20Ukrainian%20attire

O'Leary, C. and Chadha, R. (2023) Volunteering and small charities. In A. Bonner (ed), *COVID-19 and Social Determinants of Health: Wicked Issues and Relationalism*. Bristol: Policy Press, pp 258–267.

Racioppi, F., Rutter, H., Nitzan, D., Borojevis, A., Carr, Z., Grygaski, T.J., et al (2022) The impact of war on the environment and health: implications for readiness, and recovery in Ukraine. *The Lancet*, 17 September. Available at: https://www.thelancet.com/journals/lancet/article/PIIS0140-6736(22)01739-1/fulltext

Tully, M. (2005) Waiting for the barbarians. Available at: https://www.bbc.co.uk/programmes/m001ry2w

UN (2023a) *History of the United Nations*. Available at: https://www.un.org/en/about-us/history-of-the-un

UNHRC (2024) Ukraine Refugee Situation. Operational Data Portal. https://data.unhcr.org/en/situations/ukraine. Accessed on 1 09 2024.

Vlassopoulos, K. (2013) *Greeks and Barbarians*. CambridgeCore. Available at: https://www.cambridge.org/core/books/greeks-and-barbarians/CA8E4141E95FF846E3C4831FB8279DBF

WHO (2023) Key priorities for health system, recovery in Ukraine the focus of new paper. *WHO*, 7 February. Available at: https://www.who.int/eur ope/news/item/07-02-2023-key-priorities-for-health-system-recovery-in-ukraine-the-focus-of-new-paper

Wilson, A. (2019) The massacre that shook the empire. Review: TV presentation by Sathnam; the brutal truth of colonial India. *The Guardian*, 13 April. Available at: https://www.theguardian.com/tv-and-radio/2019/apr/13/amritsar-massacre-that-shook-the-empire-channel-4

APPENDIX A

Key dates in the history of the United Nations

---

24 October 1945: The UN Charter is signed by 50 countries in San Francisco

20 October 1947: The UN flag is adopted

29 November 1947: The UN committee agrees to partitioning Palestine into the State of Israel despite Arab anger

1947–1949: The Security Council orders a ceasefire between Indonesia, who declared unilateral independence, and its erstwhile colonial masters – the Dutch. UN sponsors Indonesian independence, which comes to fruition in 1949

10 December 1948: The UN General Assembly adopts the Universal Declaration of Human Rights

18 July 1949: India and Pakistan sign the UN-sponsored Karachi Agreement establishing a ceasefire line which the United Nations Military Observer Group in India and Pakistan (UNMOGIP) is to monitor

1950: The Security Council authorise the use of force under Chapter VII to defend South Korea

1956: A Security Council draft resolution calls on the Soviets to withdraw from Hungary. Moscow vetoes the resolution

19 October 1956: War between Egypt and Israel, supported by UK forces, breaks out over the former's decision to nationalise the Suez Canal. The Security Council orders Israel to withdraw from Egypt; the UK and France exercise their veto for the first time and the UN Emergency Force is formed and remains on the Egypt–Israel borders until 1967

1960: Seventeen newly independent states join the UN

1963: Cyprus gains independence from the UK. Civil war between Greeks and Turks in Cyprus breaks out. A UN peacekeeping force of 6,000 is sent to act as a buffer and remains until 1970

1964: Peacekeepers are sent to Cyprus

1965: The UN Children's Fund (UNICEF), which works towards securing children's rights, is awarded the Nobel Prize

1966: Mandatory sanctions imposed against Rhodesia (called Zimbabwe and Zambia)

1967: The Security Council calls for a ceasefire in the war between Israel and Arab states like Egypt, Jordan and Syria under Resolution 242. Though signed by all parties it fails to resolve the Israel-Palestinian conflict

1 July 1968: The Treaty of Non-proliferation of Nuclear Weapons (NPT) is signed. Evetnually, 189 countries sign the accord. India, Israel, North Korea and Pakistan have yet to sign

1969: The UN's International Labour Organisation (ILO) receives the Nobel Peace Prize

1971: China replaces Taiwan at the UN

1972: The first UN environment conference is held in Stockholm

1974: The UN recognised the Palestine Liberation Organisation (PLO)

1975: First UN conference on women

1977: Mandatory arms embargo against South Africa

1979: USSR vetoes Security Council resolution that demanded a Soviet withdrawal from Afghanistan

1980: Smallpox eradicated

1982: Convention on the Law of the Sea

1987: Treaty on protection of the ozone layer

1990: Convention on the Rights of the Child, World Summit on Children

---

August 1990: Security Council condemns Iraqi invasion of Kuwait

1992: The Security Council holds its first summit to look at reform and restructuring

1992: UN holds the first Earth Summit

1993: UN supervises elections in Cambodia

1993: The UN holds the World Conference on Human Rights

1994: Security Council authorises NATO airstrikes on Serb forces in Bosnia-Herzegovina

1995: UN convenes the first World Summit on Social Development

April 1995: UN authorised the oil-for-food programme to allow Iraq to sell oil in exchange for food, medicine, and other humanitarian requirements of its citizens

10 September 1996: The Comprehensive Nuclear Test-ban Treat is adopted by the UN General Assembly as a non-binding resolution

1 December 1997: The Kyoto Treaty is adopted to implement the UN Framework Convention for Climate Change

13 March 2002: The UN Security Council passes a resolution for the first time calling for a Palestinian state alongside Israel

8 November 2002: The UN Security Council unanimously adopts resolution 1441, drafted by the US and UK. Despite global criticism, the US later say that resolution authorised its invasion and occupation of Iraq

5 March 2003: France, Russia and Germany declare their opposition to a new US–UK draft resolution authorising war on Iraq

18 March 2003; Bush issues an ultimatum for Saddam and his sons to leave Iraq within 48 hours. Iraq rejects the ultimatum and the UN was obliged to pull its arms inspector out of the country

22 May 2003: The Security Council adopts resolution 1483, recognising the US and UK's occupation of Iraq and lifting economic sanctions. The resolution assigned the UN's role in a transition to democratic government

15 September 2005: Ariel Sharon, the Israeli prime minister, addressed the UN General Assembly and recognised Palestinian rights, but says that Israel has a right to a united Jerusalem, and will spare no effort to combat 'terrorism'

15 March 2006: General Assembly establishes the Human Rights Council

11 August 2006: The Security Council unanimously approves a proposal aimed at ending the conflict between Israel and Hezbollah

25 August 2006: The Security Council establishes the UN Integrated Mission in Timor-Leste (UNMITY) for an initial period of six months

31 July 2007: The UN establishes a peacekeeping mission in Darfur – UNAMID – in cooperation with the African Union

31 March 2008: A Security Council resolution removes the arms ban on the government of Democratic Republic of Congo

Source: Adapted from 'Timeline: the United Nations', *Al Jazeera*. Available at: https://www.aljaze era.com/news/2008/12/9/timeline-the-united-nations

Origin and development of The Salvation Army in Europe

Territory	Officers*	Staff	Members/volunteers
Denmark and Greenland Work commenced in Denmark in 1887 and Greenland in 2012.	64	78	901
Eastern Europe Work began in *Russia* in 1910 but withdrawn in 1912. Commenced in St Petersburg in 1913–1918. Proscribed in 1923. Recommenced in Russia in 1991, extended to *Ukraine* in 1993 and Moldova in 1994; Romania in 1999. Registration of the 'Moscow Branch' of The Salvation Army in 2009. Work began in Bulgaria in 2021.	94	53	2,500
Finland and Estonia Work began in Finland in 1889, Estonia in 1927–1940, recommenced in 1995.	110	317	800
France and Belgium Work began in France in 1881, Algeria in 1934–1970. Belgium in 1889. France–Belgium territory formed in 2009.	146	2,886	1,700
Germany, Lithuania and Poland Work began in Stuttgart in 1886, registered company in Berlin 1897, recognised as church and public corporation throughout Germany in 1967. Lithuania in 1998, Project Warsaw in 2008.	117	645	1,000
Italy and Greece Work began in Italy in 1887 however was not established until 1893. It received status as a philanthropic organisation in 1965 and religious body in 2009. Work commenced in Greece in 2007.	43	43	361
Netherlands, Czech Republic and Slovakia Work began in 1887, Netherland East Indies/Indonesia in 1894, Surinam in 1926 and Curacao in 1927. Czechoslovakia in 1919–1950. Slovakia in 2015.	289	7,865	4,500
Norway, Iceland and Faroes Work started in Oslo in 1888 and Iceland in 1895 spreading to The Faroes in 1924.	318	1,709	5,935

Territory	Officers*	Staff	Members/ volunteers
Russia See *Eastern Europe*. Separated from Eastern Europe in restructure in 2015.	28	(38)	450
Spain and Portugal Work began in Spain in 1971. Portugal in 1972, recognised by the Ministry of Justice in 1981.	37	105	500
Sweden and Latvia Work began in 1878, in Sweden;first women's home, 1890. Work with deaf and blind, 1895. Work began in Latvia in 1923, closed in 1939 due to outbreak of World War II, it was re-established in, 1991.	289	935	4,500
Switzerland, Austria and Hungary Geneva in 1882. Austria in 1927, recognised by Austrian Federal Ministry in 1952. Hungary, 1924–1950, re-established in 1990, legal status as a church in 2012.	347	2,040	3,600
United Kingdom and Ireland Christian Mission: London 1865, The Salvation Army, 1878.	2,175	3,783	29,000

Note: * Ordained Salvation Army ministers of religion.

Index

References to illustrative material such as maps, graphs and diagrams appear in *italic* type.